A DENTAL PRACTITIONER HANDBOOK
SERIES EDITED BY DONALD D. DERRICK, D.D.S., L.D.S. R.C.S.

AN OUTLINE OF ORAL SURGERY, PART II

H. C. KILLEY

F.D.S. R.C.S.(Eng.), F.D.S., H.D.D. R.C.S.(Edin.),
L.R.C.P.(Lond.), M.R.C.S.(Eng.)

*Professor of Oral Surgery, London University.
Head of Department of Oral Surgery, Eastman Dental Hospital.
Hon. Consultant, Eastman Dental Hospital and
Westminster Hospital Teaching Group*

G. R. SEWARD

M.D.S.(Lond.), M.B., B.S.(Lond.), F.D.S. R.C.S.(Eng.)

*Professor of Oral Surgery, London University.
Head of Department of Oral Surgery,
The London Hospital Medical College.
Hon. Consultant, The London Hospital Group*

and

L. W. KAY

M.D.S., F.D.S. R.C.S.(Eng.), L.R.C.P.(Lond.), M.R.C.S.(Eng.)

*Reader in Oral Surgery, London University.
Hon. Consultant, Eastman Dental Hospital*

Revised Reprint

BRISTOL: JOHN WRIGHT & SONS LTD.
1975

First edition, 1971

Revised reprint, 1975

Reprinted, 1979

ISBN 0 7236 0407 X

PRINTED IN GREAT BRITAIN BY
HENRY LING LTD., A SUBSIDIARY OF JOHN WRIGHT AND SONS LTD., BRISTOL,
AT THE DORSET PRESS, DORCHESTER

PREFACE

THIS *Outline of Oral Surgery* is written as a guide for postgraduate and senior undergraduate students and for practitioners with a special interest in oral surgery. It is not intended as a textbook for the established consultant in the speciality, for in a book of this size it is impossible to consider the subject in the necessary detail.

The field of oral surgery covers a wide range of topics and in a work of this nature it is impossible to discuss the entire speciality. Space has therefore been devoted to the more important aspects of oral surgery, but even so it has been necessary to divide the work into two volumes. Although these two books are complementary, each volume is more or less complete in itself. Part I is mainly devoted to the practical aspects of minor oral surgery and should be of value to all dental practitioners who perform surgery, while Part II deals with the needs of the dental surgeon working in a hospital.

At the request of the publisher, fractures of the mandible and middle third of the facial skeleton have not been discussed as these subjects have been dealt with elsewhere in the Dental Practitioner Handbook series, and illustrations have been cut to a minimum in order to reduce costs.

It is the authors' sincere hope that this *Outline of Oral Surgery* will be of help to students preparing for undergraduate final examinations and for higher examinations in dentistry.

H.C.K.

February, 1975
G.R.S.

L.W.K.

CONTENTS

ACKNOWLEDGEMENTS

THE authors' sincere thanks are due to Miss B. Richardson, of the Eastman Dental Hospital for much painstaking work in arranging and typing the manuscript of the first edition. We are also grateful to Mrs. B. Rayiru and Mrs. A. McMahon for typing and arranging the revised reprint. We should like to thank Miss P. Burgess, of the Photographic Department of the London Hospital, and Mr. J. Morgan, of the Photographic Department of the Eastman Dental Hospital, for their skilled photography. The illustrations *Figs.* 27, 28, and 29 are by Professor G. Seward and his co-authors are sincerely grateful. *Figs.* 14, 15, and 16 were originally published in *The Dental Practitioner and Dental Record* (**18**, 83–98, 1967), and the authors would like to thank John Wright and Sons Ltd., Bristol, for permission to reproduce them. *Figs.* 38, 39, 40, and 41 were published in *Oral Surgery, Oral Medicine and Oral Pathology* (**25**, 670–678, 1968, and **25**, 810–816, 1968), and we should like to thank the C. V. Mosby Co., St. Louis, for permission to include them. *Figs.* 9 and 10 were published in the *British Journal of Oral Surgery* (**3**, 36–47, 1965) and *Fig.* 32 was published in the same journal (**5**, 99–105, 1967), and the authors are indebted to E. & S. Livingstone Ltd., Edinburgh, for permission to use them.

Finally, we should like to express our sincere thanks to Mr. L. G. Owens, B.Sc., Publishing Director of John Wright of Bristol, for inviting us to write this work and for his great help and guidance in its preparation.

AN OUTLINE OF ORAL SURGERY, PART II

CHAPTER I

THE CASE HISTORY

THE art of taking an accurate case history is probably the most important single step in the diagnosis of a medical or surgical condition. Sometimes the disorder may be diagnosed from the history alone as many diseases have a characteristic story, but in every instance valuable diagnostic clues can be obtained and these leads may be followed up during the actual physical examination of the patient.

A case history may be divided into the following sections:—

1. The patient's name, age, occupation, address, and the address of his doctor and dental surgeon.
2. The nature of the complaint in the patient's own words.
3. The family history.
4. Personal or social history.
5. History of past diseases.
6. History of the present illness.

The order in which the information is obtained and recorded can vary due to personal preference, for example the history of the present illness may be placed after the complaint and before the family history, etc.

If the case to be examined falls within the province of the dental surgeon, it is unnecessary to consider each of the sections in the detail that a consultant physician would employ, but the same general scheme of history-taking should be followed and the detail may be adapted to the dental surgeon's requirements.

1. The importance of taking the patient's name, age, address, and doctor's address is too obvious to be commented upon. The patient's occupation is always of great interest and if it involves work with such substances as lead, mercury, arsenic, bismuth, etc., it may furnish a valuable clue to what might otherwise be an obscure oral condition. In this respect it is always worth while finding out exactly what people do at their place of employment. For instance, a worker in a lead paint factory may be engaged on clerical duties well away from any possible contamination.

2. The Complaint.—The nature and duration of the presenting symptoms should be considered briefly under this heading. Sometimes the patient will complain of several separate symptoms, in which case they should be listed, but with the major complaint first. Ask the patient: (*a*) 'What seems to be the main trouble?', (*b*) 'How long have you had this complaint?'

The nature of the complaint and its duration should be recorded in the patient's own words, but be careful to avoid using the patient's own diagnosis, i.e., neuralgia, sinus trouble, etc. Such diagnoses are usually incorrect and may lead the clinician astray. Re-frame the question and discover exactly what the patient does complain about, i.e., 'pain on the left side of the face which has been present for two months'. The complaint, therefore, represents the headings for the more detailed history of the present illness.

3. Family History.—The physician is interested in the health and medical history of all near relatives of the patient: the grandparents, parents, brothers, sisters, and any children. The wife or husband is, of course, not a blood relation, but their health may be relevant because of its impact on the spouse or perhaps because the illness may be infectious. If any member of the family is dead, the age at the time of death and the cause of the death are of importance. It is wise to inquire after all members of the family in turn. Often patients will assure you that there is no one ill in the family, and on further questioning it will be found that several members of the family have died from tuberculosis or some other disease.

Long or short lives, mental instability, epilepsy, migraine, high blood-pressure, diabetes, and some malignancies are sometimes found to occur in certain families, while in well-known hereditary diseases such as haemo-philia, and some congenital abnormalities, a study of the relatives is essential for the establishment of a diagnosis.

The state of the health of the patient's children or a history of mis-carriage or sterility may furnish valuable clues to such diseases as congenital syphilis. Much information in the family history is irrelevant, but some of the facts obtained may furnish conclusive evidence for a diagnosis.

The oral surgeon is interested in the family history in such conditions as haemophilia and congenital anomalies such as clefts of the lip or palate, congenital syphilis, emotional instability, etc.

Too much time should not be spent upon this part of the history, but only experience of case history taking will enable the clinician to decide whether it will prove a fruitful source of relevant information. Inquiry into the family history should never be omitted.

4. Personal History.—This part of the history enables the physician to build up a picture of the patient's background and much valuable informa-tion can be obtained by systematically covering the patient's entire life. The impact of the patient's disease and its treatment on his own life, his work, and the well-being of his family should be discovered.

a. School life: Did he play organized games? (Conditions such as congenital heart disease preclude normal activity at this age.) What was his age on leaving? What standard of education was reached?

b. Occupation: Here the physician wants to know the exact type of work in which the patient engages. Is he exposed to physical or mental strain? Is he exposed to weather or to noxious elements such as chemicals, dust, or fumes? Does he work with X-rays? Does he work long hours? Does he stick to one job or has he tried many? Does he like his work? These last two questions may give some clue as to the patient's mental state and give some idea whether the condition which is troubling him is of psychosomatic origin.

Every dental surgeon knows the difficult patient with the obscure pains or temporomandibular joint trouble. These symptoms may sometimes represent an escape mechanism.

c. Recreation: Does he take regular exercise? i.e., a man who plays football every weekend is probably a good risk for an out-patient general anaesthetic, etc.

d. Habituation to drugs: Few patients seen are drug addicts in the generally accepted sense of the expression, but many people habitually take sleeping tablets, tonics, or laxatives, or consume large quantities of alcohol. Many mysterious allergic rashes can be traced to such a source and excessive alcohol may lead to a vitamin-B deficiency, for alcoholics obtain their calorie requirements from the alcohol and do not feel the need for additional food.

e. Environment: The effect of a patient's home conditions on his general health cannot be over-emphasized and it is also of interest to know whether he lives in the town or the country.

f. Meals: Is he eating an adequate quantity of suitable food? Has he any food fads which might lead to a deficiency in the diet? Most patients will say that they have a normal diet. If there is a possibility of some deficiency disease being present, it is as well to ask the patient to describe the meals eaten during a typical day, and judge for yourself.

g. Holidays: Does he take regular holidays? Many symptoms can be ascribed to overwork and to too little time off.

h. Has he lived abroad? Could the condition be due to some tropical disease? Air travel increases the possibility of tropical disease being seen in countries where such conditions were previously unknown.

i. Worries: Has the patient either financial or domestic problems and what is his attitude to these worries? Does he think he is suffering from a serious disease such as cancer? It is always a good plan to ask the patient what he thinks is wrong with himself.

It may take both time and tact to elicit the relevant information. A proper rapport needs to be established before the patient will confide in the clinician. The key to an otherwise inexplicable problem may not be revealed until the patient has been seen several times.

5. Previous Diseases.—Inquire of the patient what *diseases, operations,* or *accidents* he has sustained and list them in chronological order. Always give the dates and do not write 'three years ago', etc.

Never accept the patient's diagnosis such as neuralgia, rheumatism, etc. Get him to describe the symptoms and judge for yourself.

Pay attention to time spent in hospital, what treatment was given, and whether the patient made a full recovery. Some diseases, such as rheumatic fever or chorea, are more likely to have left severe sequelae when the case has not been dealt with seriously, rather than when a history of strict bed-rest in hospital is obtained.

Patients often dismiss past illness in a light-hearted fashion. Put your questions as to illness in several ways. Have you ever been ill? Have you ever been under the doctor? Have you ever been in hospital? If you draw a blank on all these questions, ask incredulously, 'Have you *never* had anything the matter with you at all?' Occasionally the patient will then grudgingly admit that he had a bit of a touch of the rheumatic fever for a month or so, but never had anything *he* really calls an illness!

Direct questioning is often necessary to obtain a history of disease which the patient feels carries with it a social stigma, such as venereal disease or mental illness.

6. History of the Present Complaint.—This part of the story must be gone into in complete detail. It is best to start by asking, 'When were you last completely fit?', and then get the patient to tell the story in his own fashion. Never ask leading questions, for some patients are very suggestible and can readily be talked into a whole series of new symptoms. Ask what was the first thing that he noticed wrong. What other symptoms have occurred? What seems to be the main trouble now? What makes it better or worse? What treatment has he had and does it help? How much does this trouble incapacitate him (her)? What does the patient think he is suffering from?

Finally, ask about—Appetite, Weight, Bowel habits, Micturition, Sleep. And whether the patient has: Shortness of breath, Cough, Chest pain, Swollen ankles.

And whether any of these have been altered in any way since the onset of the illness.

If the patient is female, ask about menstruation. Menstrual history is recorded as 13 5/28 etc., that is,

$$\text{Age of onset in years} \ \frac{\text{Length of period in days}}{\text{Length of time between periods in days}}$$

The clinician must always consider whether the patient is a good witness and whether his statements can be relied upon. He will soon learn to assess such characters as the hysteric who sits back with a happy smile and describes his excruciating pains and unbearable sufferings.

Time spent in taking a case history is always well spent and the more skilled the physician or surgeon, the more time will he devote to this part of the examination. When the case history has been competently taken, the clinician is well on the way to a correct diagnosis before he even begins the actual physical examination of the patient.

When writing the patient's case notes or preparing a case history for publication, the facts should be recorded under the headings and in the order already listed. However, when interrogating a patient it is prudent to discuss the history of the present illness immediately after ascertaining the nature of the patient's complaint. The conversation then naturally leads on to the history of past diseases, personal history, and finally the family history. This is a matter of common sense, for a patient who is anxious to explain all about his illness is unlikely to see the relevance of explaining why his grandparents died. Taking the case history in this manner has the added advantage that when the family history is eventually discussed, the clinician will know whether it has any special relevance to the case under discussion.

CHAPTER II
CLINICAL EXAMINATION OF A PATIENT WITH A PAIN, A LUMP, OR AN ULCER

AFTER an accurate case history has been taken, the clinical examination is carried out. This consists of:—
1. A general physical examination of the patient.
2. A local examination of the lesion which carefully elicits all its clinical characteristics.

The majority of the patients who consult an oral surgeon complain of either a pain, a lump, or an ulcer. Each of these conditions have their own special characteristics which must be carefully elucidated by the clinician.

PAIN

Pain is a subjective symptom and unlike a lump or an ulcer which can be examined and assessed, in the case of a pain the clinician must rely on the description given by the patient. In the case of a pain, therefore, the history is of paramount importance. Careful consideration of the description of the pain frequently suggests the likely cause and the likely site of the cause. The clinician will direct his examination accordingly. With the account of a pain may go a story of associated phenomena—facial swelling, discharge, anaesthesia or muscular weakness, for example. The physical signs relevant to these complaints should also be sought at the examination.

There are ten questions which must be asked about any pain:—

1. Its Character.—Pains may be described as dull, sharp, throbbing, burning, etc. Patients with pain of psychosomatic origin often give bizarre descriptions of the pain, likening it to icy cold, red hot, or feathers running up and down their face, etc.

2. The Severity.—Owing to the varying degrees of pain threshold in different individuals, the intensity of a pain is difficult to ascertain accurately, for agony to one patient may be described as moderately severe by another. Relief afforded by a mild analgesic drug such as aspirin 300–900 mg. is a helpful indication of the degree of severity, for a pain which can be adequately controlled by a low potency analgesic preparation is not particularly severe. If more powerful analgesics such as pethidine 50–100 mg. are required to assuage the pain its severity must be correspondingly worse.

Interference with sleep is also a reliable guide to a pain's severity, for if the patient's sleep is not disturbed the pain cannot be too severe. Patients with pain of psychosomatic origin always exaggerate the pain and describe it as unendurable agony, but smile happily as they describe their symptoms. They usually complain of inability to eat or sleep, but invariably appear well rested and nourished. The patient's G.P. may well be helpful in providing background information about the patient. Great caution must be exercised before labelling a pain as psychosomatic in origin and even after such a diagnosis has been made, the patient should still be treated with great sympathy and understanding. The pain might be imaginary to the clinician but it is real enough to the patient.

3. Date of Onset.—The date of onset of a pain is of great importance and while most pains are of recent onset some may have been present for years. The likelihood of finding a previously unsuspected cause where the pain has been present for many years tends to be poor. Conversely the disease is clearly not of serious prognosis or progressive if the symptoms have remained unchanged over a long period of time.

4. Is the Pain Continuous or have there been Remissions?—Pain is seldom absolutely continuous, for even the most excruciating pains are relieved by occasional short remissions. Most patients with pain of psychosomatic origin describe it as continuous without any remissions.

5. Is it Increasing or Decreasing in Severity?—A pain which is increasing in severity will obviously require urgent investigation while a pain which is rapidly improving may allow a certain degree of procrastination on the part of the clinician. Of course, sometimes the pain persists at a uniform level.

6. Where is the Point of Maximum Intensity?—The most satisfactory method of ascertaining the point of maximum intensity of a pain is to get the patient to point to where it hurts most!

7. Area to which Pain spreads.—The pain usually spreads from the point of maximum intensity to involve the surrounding area to a greater or lesser extent. For instance, pain from an abscess on an upper canine may be most intense over the apex of the canine, but the entire side of the face may ache at the same time.

8. Area to which the Pain radiates.—The area to which a pain radiates is of considerable diagnostic significance. For example, the pain of coronary thrombosis is substernal, but the pain characteristically radiates down the left arm. In the mouth, pain from a carcinoma of the side of the tongue spreads to the ear on the same side and pains from infected lower 3rd molars often radiate in the same way. It must not be forgotten that pain in the mouth may be referred from one jaw to the other on the same side. In some cases the whole pain is ascribed by the patient to the site of radiation, so that the question of a referred pain should also be considered.

Hysterical subjects and other patients with pain of psychosomatic origin often describe pains radiating to areas to which it would be anatomically impossible. For instance, they may state that the pain radiates across the midline to involve the opposite side of the jaw.

9. What makes the Pain Worse?—Much useful information can be obtained by ascertaining what makes the pain worse or what aetiological factors are involved. For example, the excruciating pain of trigeminal neuralgia may be triggered off by a light touch on the face, while other pains are described as occurring when the patient is tired or worried. Pains which are produced when hot or cold drinks or foods are taken usually point to a purely dental origin. The pain of acute maxillary sinusitis is frequently exacerbated by biting, bending, lifting, straining, and by jarring movements.

10. Are there other Symptoms?—Local ones such as intra- and extra-oral swelling, discharge, bad taste, halitosis, discomfort on swallowing, and interference with mastication.

When the clinician has accurate information concerning the ten points enumerated in this examination, the pain can usually be accurately described and its possible aetiology ascertained.

Another way to prepare to examine a patient for the cause of a pain is to decide:—

1. **The Nerve Involved.**—In oral surgery it is usually the trigeminal, with the exception of pain over the angle of the mandible which may involve the great auricular, pain at the back of the tongue or in the throat which may be glossopharyngeal, or pain in the lower jaw associated with a tightness in the chest which may be cardiac in origin.

2. **Whether the Pain is Peripheral, Proximal, Intracranial, or Intracerebral in Origin or whether it conforms to None of these Patterns.**—If the cause is peripheral only one branch of the nerve will be involved.

If the cause is proximal, more than one branch will be involved; possibly more than one division, though this is uncommon.

If the cause is intracranial, more than one division may be involved and in advanced lesions there may be signs of a rise in intracranial pressure.

If the cause is intracerebral then there may be neurological deficits to be demonstrated on the other side of the body, due to involvement of the long tracts.

If the pain is due to trigeminal or glossopharyngeal neuralgia, Horton's syndrome, or is hysterical, it will not conform properly to any of the patterns.

3. **The Pathological Process to be looked for.**—Pain due to pulp disease or its sequelae is at some stage in its evolution intermittent and altered by hot and cold stimuli and the causative tooth becomes tender to bite on late in the course of the attack.

Pain due to gingivitis and periodontal abscesses tends to be constant and soreness or a tender tooth appears early on. A periodontal type of pain with a swollen cheek and limitation of opening suggests pericoronitis of a 3rd molar. Bilateral maxillary pain, pain and tenderness involving several maxillary teeth, and supra-orbital headache suggest sinusitis. If there is epiphora or a blood-stained discharge, carcinoma of the maxilla should be considered. Temporomandibular joint pain can radiate across either mandible or maxilla, but is often associated with a click in the joint or limitation of opening without swelling. Trigeminal neuralgia and Horton's syndrome have a characteristic pain pattern and negative findings on examination.

THE EXAMINATION OF A LUMP

Before carrying out a local physical examination of any lump or mass it is essential to ascertain:—

1. How long the swelling has been present.
2. Whether it is getting larger.
3. Whether there is any possible cause for the swelling, i.e., trauma, etc.

As far as the local examination of the lump is concerned, the most important facts to ascertain are as follows:—

1. **The Exact Anatomical Situation of the Mass.**—Lumps may arise from skin, subcutaneous tissues, muscle, tendon, nerve, bone, blood-vessels, or an organ, and if the examiner is unable to ascertain the exact structure

from which the mass arises then any attempt at differential diagnosis is likely to prove grossly inaccurate. For example, a swelling at the angle of the mandible may appear to originate from the hard tissues and the clinician will consider the possibility of a cyst, ameloblastoma, etc., when, in fact, the lump is arising from the soft tissues and is, indeed, a sarcoma of the masseter muscle.

Deciding the exact anatomical location of any mass or swelling is probably the most important single step taken in the physical examination and diagnosis of a lump.

2. **Are the Associated Lymph-nodes Enlarged?**—Whenever a lump or mass is examined, careful palpation of the associated lymph-nodes must be carried out. This important step must never be omitted. In fact, in the clinical investigation of an oral lesion, it is prudent to examine the cervical nodes first before inspecting the mouth, lest this vital stage in the local physical examination be overlooked once the clinician becomes engrossed by the findings in the oral cavity. The tender enlarged lymph-nodes associated with an inflammatory process are readily differentiated from the rock-hard nodes of a metastasizing malignancy.

3. **Is the Swelling Single or Multiple?**
4. **The Shape** and
5. **The Size** of any mass which is readily discernible.
6. **The Surface of the Mass.**—The surface of a mass may be smooth, lobulated, or irregular.
7. **The Edge.**—The edge of a lump may be clearly defined or diffuse, fading into the surrounding tissues as do most lumps or masses of inflammatory origin.
8. **The Consistency.**—The consistency of lumps or masses is defined surgically as *soft*, as in the case of the lipoma; *firm*, which is the consistency of a fibroma; *cartilage hard*, as in the pleomorphic adenoma; *bony hard*, as exemplified by the osteoma; *rock hard*, as seen in malignant lymphatic nodes; *rubbery hard*, which is the classic description of the consistency of the affected nodes in Hodgkin's disease. These descriptions of the consistency of lumps are surprisingly helpful and have been used by countless generations of surgeons.
9. **Is the Lump Tender or Warm on Palpation?**—Tenderness on gentle palpation is a valuable physical sign, for while it can be elicited with inflammatory lumps, neoplasms are commonly painless unless they just happen to be secondarily infected. The site of an acute inflammation is usually warmer than the adjoining areas.
10. **Is the Lump Attached to the Skin?**—During the physical examination of a lump an attempt should be made to move the skin over the lump to ascertain if the skin is tethered to it. The skin overlying an abscess may be fixed firmly to the inflammatory mass and a similar condition may occur with superficial malignancies. Of the benign lesions, the sebaceous cyst is characteristically tethered to the skin by the punctum of the sebaceous gland from which it arises.
11. **Care must be taken to ascertain whether the Lump arises from Deeper Structures.**—Can the overlying tissues move separately from it in any way. It is frequently helpful to get the patient to tense adjacent muscles to see whether the lesion is attached to them. In the differential

diagnosis of a swelling at the angle a soft mass partly within a muscle may be extruded during contraction and regress into the muscle again as it relaxes.

12. Is Fluctuation Present?—Fluctuation is a valuable physical sign indicating the presence of fluid within a lump. It is elicited by placing the tips of two fingers on the lump. When pressure is applied to the mass with one finger, a transmitted upward impulse is felt with the other finger-tip. A variation of this method, which can only be employed with large tumours, is to place two finger-tips of one hand on the mass and then press between these two fingers with the tip of a finger of the other hand. The transmitted impulse will be felt with the finger-tips of the opposite hand. It should be remembered that a false positive sensation may be felt if these tests are carried out on each side of the longitudinal axis of a muscle. A useful variation of this test can be carried out with fluid-containing cysts of the jaws even when they are covered with an appreciable thickness of bone. Firm intermittent pressure with the thumb over the suspected cystic area in the buccal sulcus will produce a transmitted pulsation which can be detected by the finger-tip of the other hand placed on the opposite side of the alveolar process in the palate or on the lingual side of the mandible.

13. Are there Signs of Inflammation Present?—The classic signs of heat, redness, swelling, and pain are indicative of either an inflammatory swelling or secondary infection in a non-inflammatory mass.

14. Transillumination.—The only readily transilluminable swelling of the head and neck is the cystic hygroma, but this test can sometimes be applied to nasolabial cysts.

15. Is there an Impulse on Coughing and Crying?

16. Does the Lump pulsate?—There are three types of pulsation which may occur in lumps:

a. The mass may be pulsatile, i.e., the entire mass pulsates. This is best exemplified by the aneurysm.

b. Transmitted pulsation occurs when the mass rests on a large artery. When such a mass is palpated, an impulse is felt which is transmitted from the artery. Salivary adenomas in the palate may sometimes transmit the pulsation of the greater palatine artery.

c. A mass lying deep in the tissues may displace an artery so that it lies superficially upon the mass. On palpation the mass will appear to pulsate though the clinician is, in fact, palpating an artery.

17. Any Mass may produce Pressure Effects on:—

a. Arteries: Pressure on arteries is evidenced by diminution of the pulse and in extreme cases by coldness of the dependent part and eventually by gangrene.

b. Veins: Pressure on veins may produce cyanosis and oedema on the distal side of the vessel.

c. Nerves: Pressure on nerves may produce paraesthesia, anaesthesia, or paralysis, etc.

d. Neighbouring organs: Pressure may be exerted by a mass on any neighbouring organ. In the head and neck two structures commonly affected in this way are the trachea and the oesophagus, with resultant respiratory embarrassment and dysphagia.

18. The Colour of the Lump.—This may be a helpful diagnostic sign.

Reddening may suggest an inflammatory aetiology, while a bluish swelling which blanches on pressure is most probably a haemangioma.

19. The General Condition of the Patient.—Massive swellings associated with cachexia of the patient are usually indicative of malignant neoplasms. Carcinoma of the head and neck does not commonly cause a severe deterioration in the patient's nutritional state until the terminal stages of the disease, unless the tumour involves the gastro-intestinal tract and mechanically interferes with ingestion and deglutition of food. Massive inflammatory swellings will produce a toxic effect on the patient. In these days, tuberculoma of the tongue or other oral tissues are rare in the extreme in this country, but are not in some others. Such lesions occur only in the advanced stages of the disease.

EXAMINATION OF AN ULCER

Before carrying out any local examination of an ulcer, ascertain whether there is any known exciting factor such as trauma, etc., and also establish the duration of the ulcer.

So far as the local physical examination of the ulcer is concerned, start the examination by palpating the dependent lymph-nodes associated with the ulcer. This essential step is best carried out at the onset of the examination in case it is inadvertently omitted.

With regard to the actual ulcer, ascertain:—

1. The Situation of the Ulcer.—Many ulcers occur in characteristic situations, for example the rodent ulcer at the side of the nose and beneath the eye, and the carcinoma of the tongue at the side of the tongue, while the gummatous ulcer often occurs at the junction of the hard and soft palates. Some indication of the nature of an ulcer may be obtained from its situation alone.

2. Is the Ulcer Single or Multiple?

3. Note the Size of the Ulcer.

4. Examine the Shape of the Ulcer.—Ulcers may be round, oval, crescentic, serpiginous, irregular, punched-out, etc.

5. Note the Base of the Ulcer.—The base of an ulcer may be indurated, soft, or fixed to deeper structures. Marked induration or fixation to deeper structures may be indicative of malignancy.

6. The Floor of the Ulcer may be covered by:—

a. Granulations. These may be red, pale, or flabby and may or may not bleed.

b. The floor may be smooth.

c. It may be covered with slough, membrane, scab, etc.

d. The floor may be adherent to soft parts or bone.

e. The floor may be fungating as seen in some clinical varieties of malignant disease.

7. The Edge of the Ulcer may be:—

a. Undermined (as seen in tubercular ulcers).

b. Punched-out (as found in gummatous ulcers).

c. Rolled (as characteristically occurs in rodent ulcers).

d. Rolled, raised, and everted (as characterized by malignant ulcers).

8. The condition of the parts surrounding the ulcers must be examined.

They may be inflamed, healthy, oedematous, pigmented and, in some instances, the adjoining area may have impaired sensation.

Most long-standing areas of ulceration are surrounded by zones of pigmentation and this condition is well exemplified by the varicose ulcer over the internal malleolus. When the region surrounding an ulcer is anaesthetic, as on the sole of the foot with a tabetic ulcer, the area of anaesthesia is, of course, largely responsible for the ulceration, for the normal response to pain is absent and existing irritation is therefore ignored by the patient. Similar ulcers may be seen in the palate after alcohol injection of the trigeminal ganglion.

9. If there is a discharge from the ulcer, its colour, and smell should be noted and a bacteriological smear taken for culture.

10. Is the Ulcer Painful?—Inflammatory and traumatic ulcers are usually painful while tuberculous ulcers in the mouth are often extremely painful, but in the early stages most malignant ulcers are painless. However, when the malignant ulcer becomes established and increases in size it may cause extreme discomfort.

11. The General Condition of the Patient must always be considered.— Patients become very cachetic when a malignant ulceration involves the gastro-intestinal tract. Tubercular ulceration of the mouth may be associated with pulmonary tuberculosis, while severe ulceration in the oral cavity may occur in diabetes, leukaemia, uraemia, agranulocytosis, scurvy, syphilis, etc.

One final point: Be cautious about handling ulcers you do not understand with ungloved fingers. Always wash your hands well after examining an ulcerated mouth.

CHAPTER III

SOME ADDITIONAL EXAMINATIONS CARRIED OUT WHEN INVESTIGATING A LESION

ALL patients admitted to a ward routinely have their temperature, pulse, and respiration rates recorded. They are weighed and their blood-pressure is measured, and routine blood investigations include their haemoglobin, differential white cell-count, sedimentation rate, and Wassermann reaction.

THE TEMPERATURE

A patient's normal temperature is 98·4° F. or 37° C. when taken in the mouth. Axillary temperatures are about ½° lower and rectal temperatures about 1° higher than the mouth reading. Rectal temperatures are usually taken in infants, for it is unsafe to place a thermometer in the mouth of most young children, as they usually chew the glass. There may be slight variations from the normal bodily temperature due to meals, hot baths, etc., and the evening temperature is usually 1° F. higher than the morning temperature. The temperature may fall as low as 95° F. in severe shock and pyrexia occurs in all fevers.

THE PULSE

The pulse should be felt in both wrists, for there may be variations between the sides. The normal adult pulse-rate is usually 72 per minute, but it is more rapid in children, being about 140 at birth and gradually becoming slower with age until it reaches the adult rate at about 15 years of age. In old age the pulse becomes slower and may be 55–65 per minute. Bradycardia is also seen in some athletes. Tachycardia occurs following exercise and also in fevers, thyrotoxicosis, and emotional upsets.

The rhythm of the pulse tends to increase with inspiration and decrease with expiration and when this alteration is marked the term 'sinus arrhythmia' is used. This condition is comparatively common in young adults. Common irregularities are extra systoles which are of no clinical significance and which disappear with exercise. A more sinister irregularity is atrial fibrillation which is described as an 'irregular irregularity'. This is an irregularity which generally occurs with serious heart disease and is commonly associated with mitral stenosis, thyrotoxicosis, and ischaemic heart disease.

BLOOD-PRESSURE

The blood-pressure is measured with a sphygmomanometer. The average blood-pressure in a group of healthy adults tends to increase with age and is 120/80 at about the age of 20 years, rising to about 160/90 at the age of 60 years. There are, however, wide variations in the blood-pressures within such a group of adults, but for life insurance examinations and similar medical examinations, 150/90 is usually taken as the upper limit of normal. Moderate elevations of the systolic pressure are of less clinical significance than rises in the diastolic pressure. Gross elevation of the blood-pressure is always a matter of concern and necessitates a full clinical examination. About 80 per cent of cases of hyperpiesis are due to essential (idiopathic) hypertension and 19 per cent to renal disorders. Rare diseases such as Cushing's syndrome, phaeochromocytoma, or coarctation of the aorta account for the remainder of the causes. Malignant hypertension carries an especially grim prognosis.

Fall in blood-pressure is found in collapse, shock, and following severe haemorrhage. Hypotension in the elderly is seen following cerebral or cardiac catastrophes, and in this age-group is an especially valuable sign in the diagnosis of the so-called 'silent coronary'.

RESPIRATORY RATE

The normal respiratory rate is 16–20 per minute and like the pulse-rate it is faster in children and slower in old age. An increase in the rate of respiration occurs following exercise and in fever, thyrotoxicosis, etc., while the rate decreases during sleep and under the influence of narcotic drugs. Cheyne-Stokes respiration consists of an apnoea followed by respirations which increase in magnitude to a maximum and then diminish until apnoea occurs again. This type of respiration is found in grave illness such as cerebral haemorrhage, meningitis, uraemia, etc.

WEIGHT

A patient may be above or below the normal weight, but more important are rapid alterations in the weight. Loss of weight is a presenting symptom in diabetes, pulmonary tuberculosis, thyrotoxicosis, etc., and is also seen in its extreme form in anorexia nervosa and malignant disease which affects the gastro-intestinal tract. An increase in weight is most commonly caused by over-eating which is often due to an emotional factor, but it is also seen in pregnancy and in all conditions where fluid retention occurs in the body.

Particularly sad is the sudden increase in weight which occurs in patients with extreme cachexia due to malignant disease which has become widely disseminated throughout the body. This increase is, of course, due to ascites and is frequently a terminal event.

HAEMATOLOGICAL INVESTIGATIONS

Haemoglobin.—The average haemoglobin content of normal blood is 14·8 g. per 100 ml. (Haldane 14·6 g. per 100 ml.), but variations in men from 13·56 to 18 g. per 100 ml. and in women from 11·56 to 16·4 g. per 100 ml. are seen. The figure of 14·8 g. per 100 ml. is usually taken as an arbitrary 100 per cent in most laboratories, but as there is some controversy on this point, the haemoglobin should always be expressed in grams per 100 ml.

The Red-cell Count.—The red-cell count tends to be inaccurate unless the counting is done by an experienced and careful worker, but the information is only required in some obscure anaemias. Iron deficiency can be more readily diagnosed by the Mean Corpuscular Haemoglobin Concentration (MCHC). The normal red-cell count is subject to wide variations. Normal for men is 5·4 million ±0·8 and in women 4·8 million ±0·6. As the red-cell count, except in very experienced hands, is an inaccurate measurement, the indices derived from it, i.e., colour index, mean corpuscular haemoglobin, and mean cell volume, are correspondingly inaccurate.

The opinion of a haematologist on the appearance of the red cells is much more valuable than a red-cell count. The mean cell diameter is 7·5 μ ± 0·3 μ and is the same for men, women, and children, though at birth it is 8·6 μ and falls to 7·4 μ at six months.

Haematocrit Value (Packed cell volume).—This is the volume occupied by red cells in 100 ml. of centrifuged blood and is normally about 45 ml. per cent.

Mean Corpuscular Haemoglobin Concentration (MCHC).—This value is obtained by dividing the haemoglobin in grams per 100 ml. by the packed cell volume in ml. per 100 ml. and then multiplying by 100. The normal is 32–38 g. per cent and values below this figure invariably indicate the need for iron therapy. The MCHC is the most reliable evidence for the recognition of iron-deficiency anaemia.

Mean Corpuscular Volume (MCV).—The mean corpuscular volume is the average volume of a single red cell in cubic microns and is obtained by dividing the packed cell volume in ml. per 1000 ml. of blood by the red cells in millions per c.mm. The normal is 78–94 c.μ. The MCV is therefore an indication of the size of the red cell in three dimensions.

Colour Index.—The colour index is obtained by dividing the haemoglobin percentage by the red-cell count expressed as a percentage of the normal figure of 5 million and therefore indicates the mean haemoglobin content of a single red cell. The normal figure is 1.

Red Cell Appearance and Abnormalities.—

Reticulocytes.—Reticulocytes normally form 1·5 per cent of the total red-cell count but up to 6 per cent is normal in children. They are found when increased marrow activity occurs, particularly in pernicious anaemia when treatment is started. They are also present after acute or chronic bleeding.

Nucleated Red Cells.—Nucleated red cells are not normally seen but occur in any very severe anaemia and in leukaemia, multiple myeloma, carcinomatosis, pernicious anaemia, and in newborn infants.

Punctate Basophilia.—Punctate basophilia is not normally present, but occurs in lead poisoning.

Sickle Cells.—Sickle cells occur in sickle-cell anaemia and are usually seen during suboxygenation.

Polychromasia.—Variable staining of the red blood-cells occurs during conditions of increased marrow activity.

Anisocytosis.—A condition where the red blood-corpuscles are unequal in size.

Poikilocytosis.—An alteration in the shape of the red cells.

Anisochromia.—Which denotes irregular staining.

These last three are all seen in severe anaemia.

White Cells.—The normal total white-cell count is 4000–11,000 c.mm. There is a leucopenia in haemopoietic disorders such as aplastic anaemia, aleukaemic leukaemias, pernicious and iron-deficiency anaemias. It also occurs in bacterial infections, such as typhoid, brucellosis and in any overwhelming pyogenic infection, as well as in many virus diseases such as influenza, measles, rubella, etc. The white-cell count can also be depressed as a result of drugs and toxic chemicals such as benzene, nitrogen mustard, thiouracil, chloramphenicol, amidopyrine, phenylbutazone, etc.

The Polymorphonuclear Leucocyte Count is normally 35–75 per cent of the total count and is raised in all acute infections and following trauma, blood-loss, and after cardiac infarction. It is also raised in rheumatic fever, rheumatoid arthritis, gout, and polyarteritis nodosa. The polymorph count is greatly raised in myelogenous leukaemia, but the cells are, of course, abnormal. The polymorphonuclear leucocyte count is lowered in acute leukaemia and as a result of drug therapy with thiouracil, amidopyrine, gold, and arsenic and occasionally with sulphonamides. The condition is known as 'neutropenia', and an extreme reduction is called 'agranulocytosis'.

The Lymphocyte Count is normally 15–60 per cent of the total and is raised in pertussis, lymphocytic leukaemias, and in glandular fever where there are abnormal forms. The lymphocyte count is lowered in whole body radiation exposure. The lymphocytes are increased and the polymorphs decreased in children as compared with adults as a normal state of affairs.

Monocytes usually account for 2–9 per cent of the total count and the count is raised in all protozoal infections and in monocytic leukaemia. It is also raised in infective mononucleosis or glandular fever.

Basophils normally constitute 0–2 per cent of the total white count and are rarely increased to any considerable extent.

Eosinophils account for 1–6 per cent of the total count and are raised in all parasitic diseases and intestinal worm infestations as well as in some allergic diseases such as asthma and urticaria.

Bleeding Time.—The normal bleeding time by Duke's method is 2–7 minutes. It is raised in idiopathic and symptomatic thrombocytopenia and in secondary non-thrombocytopenic purpuras and Von Willebrand's disease. The bleeding time is normal in haemophilia, Christmas disease, hereditary telangiectasia, anaphylactoid purpuras, and is usually normal in prothrombin deficiency.

Clotting Time.—The clotting or coagulation time is usually measured by the Dale and Laidlaw method and the normal is 1 minute 40 seconds. The clotting time is increased in haemophilia and Christmas disease, but it may be normal during their quiescent periods. It is also raised in conditions of fibrinogen deficiency and in patients being treated with anticoagulant therapy such as heparin, etc. The clotting time is normal in all purpuras.

Red Cell Sedimentation Rate.—The Westergren method is usually used and the normal for men is 3–5 mm. in 1 hour and women 4–7 mm. in 1 hour. It has recently been recommended that the upper limit of normal should be: men 15 mm./hour, women 25 mm./hour (below 50 years) and men 20 mm./hour, women 30 mm./hour (above 50 years).

The sedimentation rate is raised in any condition of raised plasma fibrinogen or of increased or abnormal globulins. This test is especially useful for assessing the progress in rheumatic fever, pulmonary tuberculosis, and rheumatoid arthritis. However, a normal E.S.R. cannot exclude serious disease and if the test is normal, it may engender a false sense of security in the clinician. On the other hand, a high sedimentation reading may occasionally prevent an erroneous diagnosis of psychosomatic illness being made. The sedimentation rate is especially high in multiple myelomatosis, carcinomatosis, and polyarteritis nodosa.

EXAMINATION OF THE URINE

The normal daily urinary output in a healthy adult is about 1500 ml. but it may vary between 400 and 3000 ml. depending upon fluid intake and loss by sweat, etc. It is important to maintain an adequate fluid intake and urinary output in all hospitalized patients and to ensure satisfactory levels a fluid balance chart is kept. This record is especially important in cases of facial fracture, when pain on deglutition may discourage the patient from drinking and in the unconscious or semi-conscious patient who is being fed via a transnasal gastric tube or by intravenous fluids. It should be remembered that following a severe accident or operation there is an impairment of water excretion which lasts for 24–36 hours and is characterized by a low output of urine which has a high specific gravity. A high fluid intake is required for patients on sulphonamide therapy to prevent crystalluria and again a fluid balance chart must be kept.

Specific Gravity.—The specific gravity of urine is measured with a hygrometer and varies between 1024 and 1032.

Proteinuria.—Protein in the urine may be due to an infection of the urinary tract (cystitis, pyelitis, etc.) or to excess protein leaking from the blood to the urine across the glomerular membrane. Albumin has the smallest molecule and leaks most easily, but all fractions of the plasma proteins appear in the urine if the glomerular leak is severe.

Proteinuria is found in every variety of renal disease, but the quantity present is not related to the severity of the disease. It should be remembered that a trace of protein may be seen as a contaminant in routine urine specimens especially in women, and whenever possible a catheter specimen should be sent for examination.

Bence-Jones Proteose.—Bence-Jones proteose is the name given to a protein precipitate which occurs at 55° C. and disappears at 85° C. when a urine specimen is heated in a water bath. The condition occurs in multiple myelomatosis.

Cells in Urine.—If 10 ml. of urine are centrifuged and the deposit examined under a ⅙th objective occasional cells may be seen. This test should be carried out in cases of suspected subacute bacterial endocarditis when excess red cells may be seen as a result of minute emboli in the uriniferous tubules, and in patients under protracted sulphonamide therapy when crystalluria will also produce multiple red cells in the urine.

Blood in Urine.—The urine of all accident cases, especially the first specimen passed after the injury, should be examined for blood which may indicate damage to some part of the urinary tract. Patients with facial fractures caused by accidents while riding two-wheeled vehicles are especially liable to damage to the urethra from the saddle. If in a patient with a fractured pelvis a drop of blood appears at the urethral meatus and a ruptured urethra is suspected, the patient should not be encouraged to pass urine until a surgical opinion has been obtained. If the urethra is torn across, extravasation of urine could follow an attempt to pass it.

Glycosuria.—The presence of glucose in the urine in large amounts or on repeated tests gives rise to a suspicion of diabetes mellitus, especially if acetone is also present. It should be remembered that glucose may be present in the urine following subarachnoid haemorrhage and is also found in early specimens of urine from patients who have sustained a severe fracture of the middle third of the facial skeleton

WASSERMANN REACTION, KAHN TEST, V.D.R.L., AND PRICE'S PRECIPITATION REACTION

Of the standard tests for syphilis, the Wassermann reaction is a complement-fixation method, the Kahn and V.D.R.L. (Venereal Disease Reference Laboratory) tests are flocculation reactions, and Price's precipitation reaction is a precipitation with antigen test.

These tests form a useful screening measure for syphilis. The V.D.R.L. slide test is claimed to be more specific for syphilis than the W.R. and Kahn methods. The tests are expressed as positive, negative, or doubtful and they become positive about four weeks after the primary infection or one week after the chancre appears. Tests for syphilis before this time are carried out by dark ground illumination examination of a smear of the chancre when the *Treponema pallidum* are seen. True positive reactions occur in bejel, pinta, leprosy, sleeping sickness, and yaws, as well as in syphilis. False positive reactions occur in about 1/3000 normal people as well as in 20 per cent of cases of *Leptospiro-ictera haemorrhagica* (rat bite fever) and relapsing fever. False positive reactions are seen in bacterial infections such as leprosy (50 per cent of cases), advanced tuberculosis, scarlet fever and pneumococcal pneumonia, protozoal infections such as acute malaria (100 per cent of cases), and virus infections such as virus pneumonia, glandular fever, infective hepatitis, vaccinia, mumps (20 per cent of cases), measles, lymphogranuloma venereum (2–5 per cent of cases), as well as in certain miscellaneous conditions such as the collagen diseases.

False negative reactions occur in about 10 per cent of patients with tertiary syphilis, particularly in tabes dorsalis. False negative results seldom occur in active cardiovascular disease.

RADIOLOGY

Radiology plays an important role in the differential diagnosis of lesions of the jaw. Most pathological conditions of the mandible or maxillae can be satisfactorily demonstrated by routine radiography, but occasionally special radiographical techniques are required to elucidate some particular facet of the case under investigation.

Routine Radiography.—
The Lower Jaw.—The routine radiographs required for a lesion of the mandible are:—

1. Left and right oblique lateral jaw views of the appropriate regions.
2. The postero-anterior jaws view.
3. The true lateral.
4. Intra-oral periapical views.
5. An occlusal view.
6. Modified reverse Towne's (to show condylar necks).
7. Temporomandibular joint views with the mandible in the open and closed positions.

The Upper Jaw.
1. Occipito-mental views. The standard view is taken with the radiographic base line at 45°, but other tilts such as 15° are sometimes used. Also the tube may be tilted caudally 30° for the 30° O.M.

2. Postero-anterior jaws view, penetrated for the maxilla.
3. Intra-oral periapical views.
4. True, lateral, or oblique occlusals.

One or more of these radiographs will usually demonstrate any bony lesion of the upper and lower jaw in a satisfactory fashion, but occasionally they must be supplemented by radiographs which make use of additional radiographical techniques. Some of these special X-ray examinations are:—

1. Tomography.—Tomographs are used to demonstrate lesions at varying depths in the body. Using a technique whereby both the film and the X-ray source move at the time of exposure, only the layer of the body which is stationary relative to both is shown on the film and all other parts are blurred. Radiographs can be taken to depict layers at 0·5 cm. and 1 cm. intervals through the thickness of the part under investigation and the depth of a cavity in, for example, the lung can then be estimated. The routine postero-anterior radiograph of the chest would, of course, only show the area of the lesion. In the jaws the tomogram is principally used to demonstrate intra-capsular fractures of the condyle which cannot be seen with any clarity on the P.A., oblique lateral, and modified reverse Towne's views. Tomograms are sometimes used to demonstrate the exact size and shape of lesions such as an osteoma in the maxillary sinus or to search for destruction of the bony wall as evidence of the presence of a carcinoma.

2. Soft Tissue Radiographs.—These are very helpful in showing the exact relationship of the soft tissues to the underlying bone. They are employed for assessing the degree of deformity in skeletal anomalies such as prognathism and they are also used for orthodontic investigations.

3. Pantomography.—Pantomography is useful for demonstrating the upper and lower teeth on a single X-ray film. Rotational tomography uses similar principles to planar tomography except that curved layers are recorded. One centre (concentric) or two or three centres (eccentric) of rotation or a continuously varying centre of rotation which follows a semi-elliptical path may be used to demonstrate the whole of the upper and lower dental arches on one film. These machines can also be used to produce tomographic views of the nasal sinuses and temporomandibular joint.

4. Bite Wing Films.—In the bite wing film attention is directed principally to the crowns of the teeth. The technique is mainly used for demonstrating carious lesions, but is also valuable for assessing early periodontal bone loss.

5. Stereoscopic Radiographs.—To produce a stereoscopic effect, two radiographs are taken of the same area but at a slightly different angle to each other, the difference between the positions of the X-ray tube representing the distance between the eyes. These films are placed on two viewing boxes which are fixed facing each other at either end of a six-foot viewing table. In the centre of the table, exactly between the viewing screens, are two plane mirrors with their mirrored surfaces facing the viewing screen at each end of the table. These central mirrors are hinged together at their anterior edges and the clinician stands facing this anterior edge. By manipulating a simple screw device which pushes the distal edge of the mirrors apart, the mirrors can be angled so that the films in the viewing box come into focus stereoscopically. This form of investigation enables the exact relationship of the fragments in fractures of the middle third of the facial skeleton to be studied. For small films a prismatic stereoscope, which is like a pair of binoculars, can be used.

6. Cineradiography.—Cineradiography has been used to study the movements of the tongue and palate in speech and deglutition. It is especially useful for observing variations of the normal in such conditions as the cleft palate.

7. The Use of Radio-opaque Materials.—The principle of using radio-opaque materials in conjunction with routine or special radiographs can be applied in many ways:—

a. Radio-opaque Probes.—Soft silver probes can be inserted down sinuses in the jaw prior to taking radiographs in order to demonstrate the path, depth, and extent of the sinus. The same principle can be used by inserting one or more needles into the tissue in order to localize a foreign body such as a broken needle in the soft tissues.

b. Localization of Roots using a Removable Appliance.—In order to localize roots in the upper or lower jaw some authorities use a wax plate containing metal markers which can be placed over the alveolus prior to taking radiographs. The position of the roots can then be ascertained in relation to the metal markers and the plate is removed prior to surgery.

c. Sialography.—Neohydriol solution can be injected into the ducts of glands in order to demonstrate the glandular structure. By this method such conditions as duct stricture or dilatation, glandular dilatation (sialectasis), and intra-glandular space-occupying lesions can be demonstrated. (*See* The Major Salivary Glands, p. 216.)

d. Barium Swallow.—In this technique postero-anterior and lateral radiographs are taken as a patient swallows a solution containing barium. This technique demonstrates deviations, strictures, space-occupying lesions, and foreign bodies in the oesophagus. It is an invaluable technique for demonstrating a radiolucent foreign body such as a broken acrylic denture impacted in the oesophagus.

e. Following the marsupialization of a large cyst the cavity can be packed with cotton-wool soaked in lipiodol. Used in conjunction with routine radiographs of the jaw, this will demonstrate the exact area involved by the cyst and follow-up radiographs will show any regression of the lesion. The injection of radio-opaque material into maxillary cysts prior to operation is not particularly helpful in delineating the extent of the cyst, for it obscures the adjacent bony structures and the lipiodol could, of course, be injected in error into the maxillary sinus.

f. Angiography.—The injection of a radio-opaque material into blood-vessels is useful in the head and neck for demonstrating aneurysms. The material used is Hypaque which is completely inert. At one time radio-active materials such as diadrast and thoratrast were used, but they carried a risk of causing a sarcoma of spleen and should not be employed.

Arteriovenous shunts occasionally occur in the mandible, especially at the angle and they may resemble a residual cyst, for they appear as a radiolucent area in the jaws.

g. The Exploration of Sinuses and Fistulae.—Water-soluble radio-opaque media can be injected into external sinuses and fistulae on the face and neck and a postero-anterior and lateral radiograph will clearly demonstrate the path and extent of the track. This technique is invaluable for demonstrating thyroglossal and branchial fistulae.

ADDITIONAL BLOOD AND SEROLOGICAL TESTS

Glucose.—The normal fasting glucose or blood-sugar is 70–120 mg. per 100 ml. and the blood glucose is raised in diabetes mellitus, Cushing's syndrome, haemochromatosis, and subarachnoid haemorrhage. It is also raised in various other conditions such as acute pancreatitis, Wernicke's encephalopathy, etc., which are of little dental interest. There is, however, often a raised glucose level following severe head injury and raised levels are often seen in fractures of the middle third of the facial skeleton immediately after injury. In such cases the blood-sugar level returns to normal within a few days.

In all cases where glycosuria is present, a full glucose tolerance test should be carried out for one random test is of little value.

Glucose Tolerance Test.—The glucose tolerance test is represented as a 2-hour curve showing the response to 50 g. of glucose by mouth. A fasting blood-sugar together with a urine examination for sugar is made and then the patient is given 50 g. of glucose by mouth. Further glucose and urine examinations are carried out at 1 hour and 2 hours and the results plotted as a curve.

The normal fasting level is 70–120 mg. per 100 ml. which rises by 30–60 mg., but not above 170 mg., the normal renal threshold. At 2 hours the normal reading will be about 120 mg. A level of less than 170 mg. at 1 hour excludes frank diabetes.

Paul-Bunnell Test.—The Paul-Bunnell test is a serum agglutinin test and when agglutination at serum dilutions of 1/128 occurs it is diagnostic of glandular fever (infective mononucleosis). Positive results can also be obtained with trypanosomiasis.

Blood-urea.—The normal blood-urea is 15–40 mg. urea per 100 ml. and it is raised (azotaemia) in primary renal disease and other conditions with impaired renal function. Hence, an increased blood-level is to be expected in acute and chronic glomerulonephritis, chronic bilateral pyelonephritis, and renal tubular necrosis. The blood concentration is also elevated in lower urinary tract obstruction due to prostatic obstruction, increased tissue protein metabolism associated with a negative nitrogen balance (e.g., in fevers, thyrotoxicosis, wasting diseases, diabetic coma, or after a major operation) and in extra-renal uraemia due to impaired renal circulation and dehydration.

Blood Uric Acid.—The normal blood uric acid is 1·5–3·9 mg. per 100 ml. and a high level is suggestive but not diagnostic of gout.

It is also raised in any condition where there is excessive breakdown of cell nuclei such as carcinomatosis, polycythaemia, chronic myeloid leukaemia, and often in pernicious anaemia.

Alkaline Phosphatase.—The normal alkaline phosphatase in adults is 4·5–12 units per 100 ml. by the King-Armstrong method and 1·5–4 units per 100 ml. by the Bodansky method. Higher values, up to 25 King-Armstrong units, are normal for children. The alkaline phosphatase is raised in Paget's disease, hyperparathyroidism (when there are bone changes), carcinomatosis metastasizing to bone, rickets, osteomalacia, renal rickets, fibrous dysplasia, and in patients with healing fractures. The highest readings are seen in Paget's disease, especially during the active phase of the disease.

Acid Phosphatase.—The normal acid phosphatase is 1–3 King-Armstrong units per 100 ml. or 0·5–1·5 Bodansky units. It is raised in metastasizing carcinoma of the prostate as well as in osteogenesis imperfecta and marble bone disease. It is also raised in any condition where there is a very high serum alkaline phosphatase.

Serum Calcium.—The normal blood or serum calcium is 9·6–10·9 mg. per 100 ml. and it is raised in hyperparathyroidism, vitamin D intoxication, sudden immobilization as after fractures, idiopathic hypercalcaemia of infants, and after excessive milk or alkali therapy. It is also raised in some malignant diseases involving bone such as multiple myeloma, skeletal metastases, etc. The serum calcium is lowered after total parathyroidectomy.

Inorganic Phosphates.—The normal value of the serum inorganic phosphates is 2–4 mg. per 100 ml., but these are slightly raised in infancy.

The inorganic phosphates are raised in renal failure from any cause and values over 8 mg. per 100 ml. indicate severe renal failure. They are also raised in vitamin D overdosage, in acromegaly, and in cases of diminished parathyroid function.

The inorganic phosphate level is lowered in hyperparathyroidism, Fanconi syndrome, and in conditions caused by a vitamin-D deficiency, i.e., rickets and osteomalacia.

BIOPSY

The term 'biopsy' is most frequently used to indicate the removal of tissue and its histological examination. It is the least equivocal of all the diagnostic procedures performed in the laboratory and it should be carried out whenever a suspicious lesion is encountered.

Excision and Biopsy.—Where the clinician is reasonably certain on clinical grounds that a lesion is benign it should be excised and sent for histological examination.

Incisional Biopsy.—If the lesion under examination is extensive, if its nature is uncertain or if it is suspected that it might be malignant, then an incisional biopsy is the method of choice. This consists of removing one or more portions of representative tissue from the lesion. The material should be taken from the edge of the lesion so as to include some normal tissue. In taking a margin of normal tissue unnecessary risks of spreading the lesion should be avoided. However, care must be taken to ensure that an adequate amount of the abnormal tissue is included. Where the lesion is very small an adequate sample may include all the visible part. Obviously no attempt should be made to remove a curative margin on the assumption that it is malignant as this may cause unnecessary mutilation. Care must be taken, however, to record accurately the pre-biopsy appearance and a decision on treatment must be made while the site is still clearly visible in the patient. Three modifications of the incisional biopsy are the punch biopsy, the needle biopsy, and curettage.

Punch biopsy is performed with a surgical instrument which punches or bites out a portion of tissue. It has no advantage over the incisional biopsy and can result in the material being bruised or otherwise damaged.

Needle or drill biopsy has been employed for obtaining material from deep-seated lesions, but histological diagnosis of such material is difficult and it has a very limited place in oral surgery.

Curettage biopsy suffers from the same disadvantage for again the material obtained tends to be damaged and unsuitable for histological examination. For the same reason any manipulation and grasping of the specimen during excisional or incisional biopsy must be minimal so as to preserve the tissue structure intact.

Dangers of Biopsy.—The spreading of tumour cells along lymphatic and vascular channels by biopsy is a possibility and gross manipulation of a tumour may possibly increase the number of cells released. However, the risk of spreading cells from a malignant tumour during a biopsy is secondary to establishing a diagnosis so that correct treatment can be instituted. Other dangers of biopsy are haemorrhage, infection, and failure of the tissue to heal.

Haemorrhagic tumours should be biopsied with extreme caution and intra-oral biopsies of tumours such as an adamantinoma may result in an infected area in the mouth which is slow to heal. This might preclude the insertion of an immediate bone-graft following resection of the portion of mandible containing the tumour. Nevertheless the most direct approach to the mass is appropriate to avoid opening unnecessarily the tissue planes of the face or neck.

Aspiration Biopsy.—Aspiration biopsy is a most valuable investigation and should be carried out on all cystic and fluctuant lesions. It is a simple examination and causes the patient minimal inconvenience. Local analgesic is injected over the lesion after which a wide-bore needle attached to a 10-ml. syringe is inserted into the lesion. Inability to aspirate usually indicates that the lesion is solid. Aspiration of air in the molar region of the upper jaw indicates that the needle is in the maxillary sinus and is a valuable method of differentiating the sinus from a suspected cyst. Aspiration of air from a cystic lesion in the lower jaw usually indicates a solitary bone cyst (traumatic, haemorrhagic, etc.). Aspiration of pus indicates an abscess or an infected cyst and aspiration of chronic abscesses around the jaws often confirms the diagnosis of actinomycosis. Keratin, which has the clinical appearance of pus without its unpleasant smell, denotes the presence of a keratocyst (primordial) while periodontal and dentigerous cysts contain straw-coloured fluid containing cholesterol crystals. Aspiration of blood denotes a haemorrhagic tumour or a blood-vessel. The inspissated material contained in a dermoid cyst is aspirated with extreme difficulty. Aspiration of cyst contents may prove to be an important aid to the diagnosis of the odontogenic keratocyst. If the aspirate is subjected to electrophoresis a soluble protein level below 4 g. per 100 ml. is very suggestive of keratocyst, whereas a level above 5 g. per 100 ml. favours apical, dentigerous, or other non-keratinizing cysts. An even simpler aid to diagnosis is to examine a stained film of the cyst fluid to demonstrate keratinized squames.

Oral Cytology.—Cytological examination for tumour cells was first described by Papanicolaou (1946) as a diagnostic procedure in the detection of uterine malignancy. Scrapings are taken of the suspected lesion, after which the cells obtained are smeared on to a clean slide, stained and examined. The report is based on the morphological features and staining quality of the cells.

The technique can be applied to oral lesions, but should be employed as an adjunct to, and not a substitute for, biopsy as it is not so uniformly reliable as the excisional or incisional biopsy.

Postal Regulations.—If biopsy specimens are sent by post the postal regulations must be complied with.

REFERENCE

PAPANICOLAOU, G. N. (1946), 'Diagnostic Value of Exfoliated Cells from Cancer Tissue', *J. Am. med. Ass.*, **131**, 372.

CHAPTER IV

THE DIFFERENTIAL DIAGNOSIS OF SWELLINGS OF THE NECK

SWELLINGS of the neck may be conveniently divided into three main groups: (1) Lymphatic swellings, (2) Cystic swellings, (3) Other swellings.

LYMPHATIC SWELLINGS OF THE NECK

The cervical lymph-nodes are arranged in two main groups:—

1. **A Circular Group** around the base of the skull which includes the submental, submandibular, pre- and post-auricular, parotid, retropharyngeal, and occipital lymph-nodes. Above this level there is the isolated facial gland on the cheek.

2. **The Vertical Chain of Nodes** running down the neck. These consist of a relatively unimportant *superficial chain* which includes the anterior jugular, prelaryngeal, pretracheal, and paratracheal, and a deep chain which is arranged in four main groups according to the level at which they lie and their relation to the internal jugular vein. They are:—

a. The upper anterior deep cervical lymph-nodes in the upper part of the anterior triangle in front of the jugular vein.

b. The upper posterior deep cervical nodes in the upper part of the posterior triangle.

c. The lower anterior group in the lower part of the anterior triangle.

d. The lower posterior group which lie in the posterior triangle along the posterior belly of the omohyoid.

In examining enlarged lymph-nodes of the neck, attention must be given to:—

1. **Pain.**—Pain is usually only severe in acute pyogenic lymphadenitis.

2. **The Age of the Patient.**—For example, the predominant cause of enlarged cervical nodes in childhood is chronic upper respiratory tract infection and tuberculosis, while in old age secondary carcinoma is a more likely diagnosis.

3. **The Duration.**—The duration of the enlarged gland characterizes the swelling as acute, subacute, or chronic. For example, an acute swelling of short duration is almost certainly pyogenic in origin. A subacute swelling may, for example, be tubercular or syphilitic, while chronic swellings may possibly be tubercular or neoplastic.

4. **The Number of Nodes Involved.**—The number of nodes involved may give some indication of the aetiology. Numerous nodes are involved in infective mononucleosis, leukaemia, etc., while solitary nodes may be due to lymphosarcoma and secondary carcinoma. Whenever more than one cervical node is enlarged, an examination must be carried out for lymphadenopathy elsewhere in the body, for the condition may be generalized.

5. **The Site of the Nodes.**—The site of the enlarged nodes is especially helpful where lymph-node enlargement is of pyogenic aetiology, especially when the source of the infection is in the mouth.

6. The Consistency of the Enlarged Glands.—The consistency of the enlarged gland may be of diagnostic significance. The enlarged gland in Hodgkin's disease feels rubbery, the secondary carcinoma feels rocky-hard, enlargements due to pyogenic infection are tender and relatively soft while the glands of tuberculosis may be fluctuant or matted together.

The primary cause of a cervical lymphadenopathy must be sought in the area drained by the gland or glands in question. However, if there is a generalized lymphadenopathy involving axillary, inguinal glands, etc., there is more likely to be a generalized systemic cause for the lymphatic enlargements.

When the occipital or post-auricular glands are enlarged, the scalp is examined. The submental glands drain the lower lip, the lower incisor area, and the tip of the tongue and part of the floor of the mouth, the submandibular glands drain much of the face, the mouth, and anterior two-thirds of the tongue excluding the tip. The upper anterior cervical glands are usually involved from the fauces and pharynx. In the case of a pyogenic infection, the instigating focus of infection may have healed and search should be made for a scar or other evidence of recent infection. Difficulty may be experienced in secondary involvement of the cervical glands with carcinoma, for the primary lesion may be extremely small and may be merely a crack in the lip or a minute ulcer in the vallecula or the piriform fossa. The primary lesion may also be hidden in the nasopharynx, subglottic region, or the paranasal sinuses. Malignant lesions in the nasopharynx are notoriously difficult to find. The skin should be examined for rashes which are seen only fleetingly in such diseases as rubella and tularaemia, but are more obvious in secondary syphilis. Other investigations include the temperature, which may be raised in infective mononucleosis, tularaemia, etc., while a blood examination establishes a diagnosis of leukaemia and infective mononucleosis. However, many lymphadenopathies require special investigations in order to elucidate their aetiology, and the Wassermann reaction for syphilis, the Paul-Bunnell test for infective mononucleosis, and the examination for viral antibodies are obvious examples of this group.

7. The Histology and Bacteriology of the Nodes.—Should a diagnosis not be possible after the above measures, then a few drops of sterile saline may be injected into one of the nodes and aspirated. The aspirate can be used to produce a smear, or it can be cultured or used for guinea-pig inoculation. In this way various causative bacteria may be isolated including the tubercle bacillus.

Excision of a node for biopsy should be performed where histological examination is necessary. In such a case it may be helpful to send half of the specimen unfixed for bacteriological examination.

Examination of an Enlarged Lymph-node should include:—

Aspiration ⎰ Smear
          ⎱ Culture   ⎰ Pyogenic organism
            Guinea-pig inoculation ⎱ Tubercle

Excision of a node or biopsy: half for histological examination and half for bacteriological examination.

Classification

Lymphatic swellings of the neck may be pyogenic, viral, tubercular, syphilitic, or malignant in origin.

1. Pyogenic Origin.—Pyogenic lymphadenopathy may arise from the lips, incisor region, and chin when the submental glands are involved. Infection from the face, mouth, and front of tongue usually involves the submandibular glands while the upper anterior cervical group of glands are involved from a focus in the fauces and pharynx. A not uncommon cause of extensive cervical lymphatic enlargement is a septic focus in the scalp, and the hair of the head of a child should always be searched for head lice when painless glands of recent origin are found involving the occipital chain of glands or the superficial cervical glands on either side of the neck. The infective source may be a septic cut or scratch and it is prudent to remember that pediculosis capitis is by no means uncommon and gives rise to extensive septic involvement of the scalp through scratching. Grossly enlarged lymphatic glands may break down and suppurate.

2. Viral Origin.—

German Measles (rubella).—This mild disease practically always produces enlargement of the cervical nodes which persists long after the rash, which may be transient, has disappeared. Although a harmless disease which is never fatal, it may give rise to congenital deformities in the developing foetus if the mother is affected during the first four months of pregnancy. The history of a mild febrile illness with a macular type of eruption lasting 1–3 days may help to make the diagnosis in an otherwise inexplicable lymphadenopathy. Identification of the rubella virus during the first three days of the illness is now feasible by means of a haemagglutination-inhibition procedure.

Infective Mononucleosis (glandular fever).—This common disease usually affects young adults. There is low protracted pyrexia and general malaise often associated with a sore throat. Many cases present with severely affected gums which may be erroneously diagnosed as ulcero-membranous gingivitis. A generalized lymphadenopathy develops which can sometimes be prolonged and recurrent. The diagnosis is confirmed by the blood picture, for there is a raised lymphocyte count and atypical mononuclear cells are plentiful in the film. Additional confirmation of the diagnosis is made with the Paul-Bunnell test which is positive in about 90 per cent of cases.

Cat Scratch Fever.—This febrile disease is transmitted to man by a scratch or bite from an apparently healthy cat. It may also enter the body through scratches made by thorns, wood splinters, or fishbones. The causal agent is a virus of the lymphogranuloma-psittacosis group. An ulcer occurs at the site of inoculation and a low-grade fever develops together with a regional adenitis which may be extremely protracted. Occasionally the glands break down and suppurate—often with sinus formation. Recovery is gradual. The only diagnostic test is the positive skin reaction obtained by intradermal injection of heated pus obtained from another case or from the patient himself. Frei antigen gives a negative reaction.

Tularaemia.—This highly infectious disease is normally enzootic in rodents. The clinical disease in man is characterized by a focal ulcer at the site of infection with marked lymphadenopathy, and severe constitutional symptoms. The condition is caused by the *Pasteurella tularensis* and diagnosis is made by recovery of the organism from the primary lesion or lymph-nodes.

Glanders.—This disease is due to an infection with *Pfeifferella mallei* (*Malleomyces mallei*) and occurs in horses and similar animals, but rarely may be transmitted to man. There is severe ulceration at the site of infection and enlargement of the cervical lymph-glands which may suppurate. The constitutional symptoms are severe. Diagnosis is by isolation of the causative organism.

Toxoplasmosis.—Toxoplasmosis in adults due to *Toxoplasma gondii* (a protozoan) often presents as a lymphadenopathy of the cervical lymph-nodes. The glands are smooth and mobile and may be mistaken for those in Hodgkin's disease. There is malaise but no fever. Diagnosis can be difficult and culture has only been successful in living cells. A complement-fixation test and a dye test using the patient's serum can be carried out by certain public health laboratories. The intraperitoneal inoculation of white mice with infected biopsy or autopsy tissue will cause infection in which *T. gondii* can be recovered.

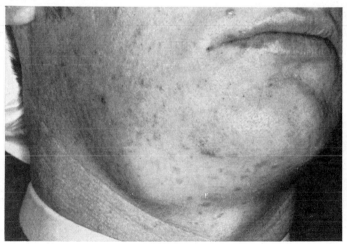

Fig. 1.—Tuberculous abscess.

3. Tubercular.—
Tuberculosis.—Tuberculous cervical lymphadenitis usually arises from an initial infection in the tonsillar crypt and spreads to the cervical lymph-nodes. These may become chronically enlarged and heal by fibrosis and calcification, but they may break down and caseate (*Fig.* 1). Initially the glands may be discrete, but when they become large they may become matted together and form an indurated mass.

Occasionally when they undergo caseous necrosis the pus tracks through the fascial planes to form a superficial cold abscess at some distance from the involved node. This is known as a 'collar-stud abscess'. Tuberculous cervical adenitis is seen in patients who have no immunity to tubercular infection and is often diagnosed in patients from Southern Ireland and from Norway. In such individuals the Mantoux test is often negative. Diagnosis is made either by biopsy of an affected lymph-node or by aspiration biopsy of a broken down lymph-gland when the characteristic acid-fast organisms of the tubercle bacillus are seen. The diagnosis may be confirmed in doubtful cases by animal inoculation. Occasionally the primary focus is on the gingivae and the submandibular nodes are affected. The primary oral lesion is granular, flat, and pale red and resembles a capillary haemangioma in appearance. Pressure with a glass slide may reveal 'apple jelly' nodules.

In some countries tuberculous lymphadenitis is becoming less frequent, and being replaced by unclassified or anonymous mycobacterial infections which also cause cervical lymphadenitis. The distinction is not merely academic. In addition to the eventual culture of the mycobacterium responsible, differentiation from classic tuberculosis can often be made by showing lack of contact with known cases of tuberculosis, lack of evidence of tuberculous foci elsewhere in the body, especially in chest radiographs, and the greater skin sensitivity to PPD (Purified Protein Derivative)-B (from unclassified mycobacteria) than to PPD-S (from *Mycobacterium tuberculosis*).

4. Syphilitic.—

Syphilitic Lymphadenopathy.—Enlargement of the cervical lymph-glands is seen in primary syphilis when the chancre is in the mouth or on the lips. There is a generalized enlargement of the submental, submandibular, pre-, and post-auricular, and the occipital glands, a condition known as a syphilitic collar. The glands are usually non-tender and discrete. Confirmation of the diagnosis of syphilis at this stage is made by darkground illumination of a smear taken from the suspected chancre in which the *Treponema pallidum* can be identified. It should be remembered that at this stage the Wassermann reaction will not be positive.

In the secondary stage of syphilis there is a generalized lymphadenopathy and again the individual glands are discrete, non-tender, and freely mobile. At this stage there may be an accompanying skin rash with mucous patches in the mouth or condylomata and the Wassermann and Kahn reactions are positive.

5. Malignant.—

Leukaemia.—Leukaemia is a disease characterized by proliferation of abnormal leucopoietic tissue throughout the body. It is divided according to the type of leucocyte affected into myeloid, lymphocytic, and monocytic varieties, but they all present a similar clinical picture in the acute phase. They occur at any age but are most common in young patients and at the start about a third of the patients are aleukaemic. The onset is sudden with fever, sore throat, bleeding mouth and the patient is gravely ill. In approximately one-third of patients, lymph-node enlargement is the first sign of acute leukaemia, generalized in the lymphocytic form but it may be inconspicuous in the myelocytic type. There may be ecchymosis, petechiae, and an enlarged spleen. The blood picture may show a raised white-cell count or it may be aleukaemic, but the most important feature is that the white cells are abnormal forms. This may lead to difficulty in distinguishing which of the white cells are predominantly affected during the acute stage.

There is a severe reduction in the red-cell and platelet count and the patient is markedly anaemic. The disease is fatal within a matter of days, weeks, or months.

Chronic Myeloid Leukaemia.—Chronic myeloid leukaemia occurs in early adult life and middle age. It usually presents as a progressive tiredness due to the anaemia together with a dragging feeling in the abdomen due to the enlarged spleen.

The total white count with abnormal forms is in the region of 500,000–1 million associated with a reduced red-cell count and haemoglobin.

Chronic Lymphatic Leukaemia.—Chronic lymphatic leukaemia occurs in late middle age and has a reasonable prognosis. The lymph-nodes in the neck are markedly enlarged. The blood picture is similar to that seen in myelogenous leukaemia, but the cells affected are small lymphocytes.

Hodgkin's Disease (*lymphadenoma*).—Hodgkin's disease is a progressive and fatal disease of lymphoid tissue characterized by lymph-node swellings which are first localized and later generalized, accompanied by splenomegaly and progressive cachexia.

The disease starts in a superficial group of lymph-glands, but eventually all the lymph-nodes in the body may become affected. In a majority of cases the first symptom is an enlargement of a cervical lymph-node. The glands are painless, rubbery, and firm. Diagnosis is made by biopsy of an affected gland when Virchow and Dorothy Reed cells are seen. Eosinophilia is seen in about 10 per cent of cases, but is of little diagnostic significance.

Lymphosarcoma.—Lymphosarcoma may affect any lymphatic tissue, but is more common in the neck. The glands affected may be single or multiple and histologically the tumour is seen to be composed of lymphoblasts. Diagnosis is by biopsy.

Secondary Carcinoma.—An enlarged cervical lymph-node in an adult patient over 40 years old is likely to have a sinister significance, and is frequently a sign of malignant neoplasia. Indeed, it has been widely taught for many years that all painless swellings of the neck are malignant unless proved otherwise. It is also important to realize that in middle-aged individuals, non-specific lymphadenitis is not uncommonly related to a nearby malignant tumour which has not actually invaded the node.

Secondary carcinoma in the neck, as elsewhere in the body, takes the form of a rocky hard swelling of one or more lymph-nodes. The swelling is painless and in time becomes fixed to the surrounding tissues. Eventually it penetrates the overlying skin and may fungate. Enlargement of a cervical lymph-node in relation to a known primary lesion is not necessarily due to a secondary neoplasm, for it may be a pyogenic lymphadenitis.

Malignant enlargement of cervical lymph-nodes may precede the diagnosis of the primary lesion which may be in the nasopharynx or some similar location where it cannot be readily detected. According to Aird (1957), in one-third of all nasopharynx tumours neck swelling is the first symptom.

Malignant Melanoma.—Malignant melanoma is a rare tumour of the head and neck, but if the patient lives long enough, metastases will occur in the lymph-glands of the neck. These secondary deposits may be blackish in colour.

In childhood various neoplastic conditions produce enlargement of the lymph-nodes. Leukaemia is probably the commonest and after that lymphosarcoma, especially in the first decade of life. Hodgkin's disease and other lymphomas account for a small proportion of cervical masses.

Drugs.—Lymphadenopathy may be a rare complication of anti-convulsant therapy with the hydantoins and primidone, and the condition clinically and morphologically resembles a reticulosis. The exact mechanism by which the disease occurs is unknown, but the nature of the condition has been considered to be a hypersensitivity reaction.

Immunological Factor.—A symptom-complex can occur in young children characterized by generalized lymphadenopathy (involving the cervical nodes) and hepatosplenomegaly. This simulates a malignant lymphoma, and, although of unknown aetiology, it is suggested that this condition may be a primary immunological disorder.

CYSTIC SWELLINGS OF THE NECK

1. The Sublingual Dermoid Cyst.—Sublingual dermoid cysts may be central or lateral, a classification originally described by Barker (1883). These cysts always originate above the mylohyoid but occasionally they may penetrate it (Seward, 1965). Usually such cysts give the appearance of a 'double chin', but occasionally there is considerable sublingual swelling. This intra-oral swelling is exacerbated if the cyst becomes infected. Under these circumstances the swelling of the floor of the mouth gives the appearance of a Ludwig's angina with the tongue pressed up against the roof of the mouth.

2. The Thyroglossal Cyst.—The thyroglossal cyst may present in any part of the thyroglossal tract in its course from the foramen caecum to the isthmus of the thyroid. The most common situations in order of frequency are: (*a*) Beneath the hyoid; (*b*) In the region of the thyroid cartilage; (*c*) Above the hyoid bone.

It is a midline swelling except in the region of the thyroid gland where the thyroglossal tract is pushed to one side, usually the left. According to Aird, 25 per cent are either to the left or right of the midline. As with all thyroid swellings, the thyroglossal cyst moves on swallowing but in addition the cyst also moves upwards when the patient protrudes the tongue. Very rarely the thyroglossal cyst can present in the mouth and interfere with speech. Thyroglossal cysts have a tendency to recurrent attacks of inflammation and may be mistaken for abscesses and incised. In this way a thyroglossal fistula may be formed. The thyroglossal cyst is often not noticed by the patient until middle or old age, but about 10 per cent are present in infancy (Aird, 1957).

3. Branchial Cyst.—The branchial cyst is said to arise from the second branchial cleft. The cyst is often seen for the first time between the ages of 20 and 25 years, but the swelling may present much later in life. Its position is characteristic in the upper part of the neck beneath the upper third of the sternomastoid muscle, protruding beneath its anterior border (*Fig.* 2). It is a smooth, globular, tense swelling and if the cyst becomes very large the patient may complain of discomfort, dysphagia, and even huskiness of the voice.

Many of these cysts are diagnosed as tubercular glands and clinically the differential diagnosis may be difficult. On aspiration of the branchial cyst, however, fluid containing cholesterol crystals is obtained. Occasion ally a branchial cyst becomes infected and this increases its similarity to an abscess.

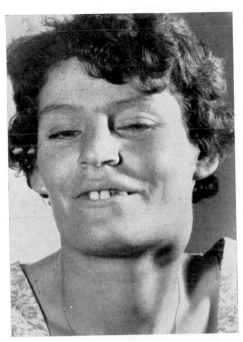

Fig. 2.—Branchial cyst.

4. Cystic Hygroma.—Cystic hygromas are formed by sequestration of the lymphatic endothelium of the jugular sac, the sequestrated endothelium retaining independently its power of irregular growth. The cystic hygroma may be present at birth or become manifest during infancy or childhood. It forms a soft translucent tumour usually situated in the lower third of the neck, but they can also occur in the axilla. When extremely large they may even interfere with labour.

It is the only tumour of the head and neck which is brilliantly translucent. The tumour may continue to grow during infancy, in which case it may interfere with respiration by compressing the trachea, and require urgent decompression by aspiration. At other times it may become infected and spontaneous regression may follow the successful treatment of this complication. Uncontrolled secondary infection, on the other hand, may be fatal. Pathological examination of the tumour shows an aggregation of cysts like masses of soap bubbles. These cysts are lined by endothelium and contain lymph and tend to infiltrate the underlying muscle layers.

OTHER SWELLINGS OF THE NECK
(i.e., Non-Lymphatic and Non-Cystic)

1. **Sternomastoid Tumour.**—The sternomastoid tumour is a hard spindle-shaped tumour which occurs in the lower third of the sternocleidomastoid muscle and makes its appearance ten days to two weeks after birth. It is usually unilateral, but rarely bilateral tumours are present. The mass can be moved laterally but cannot be moved vertically up and down the muscle. After remaining quiescent for some weeks it decreases in size and tends to disappear before the sixth month. However, the patient may be left with a permanent torticollis (wry-neck). The sternomastoid tumour may be due to haematoma formation following birth trauma, or the lesion may be vascular in origin. Ischaemia of the muscle may be responsible and by some it is considered to be a pure fibroma. The permanent wry-neck becomes manifest at the age of about 4 years. If this is untreated, secondary cranial and facial asymmetry develops. Histologically the sternomastoid tumour is found to be a mass of fibrous tissue.

2. **Cervical Rib.**—Cervical ribs usually arise from the seventh cervical vertebra and in about half the cases they are bilateral. They may vary in size and extend from a complete rib to a fibrous band in the scalenus medius muscle. In some cases the rib ends in a large bony mass and in others the rib is connected to the scalene tubercle of the first rib by a fibrous band. A complete or incomplete cervical rib may be felt as a bony swelling in the neck and it may, of course, be unilateral or bilateral. Symptoms from cervical rib may be nervous or vascular. The sensory phenomena include pain, paraesthesia, and anaesthesia of the little and ring fingers, the ulnar border of the hand, and the forearm. There may be motor weakness which affects the small muscles of the hand and some-times the flexors of the wrist and fingers. Some 5–6 per cent of patients suffering from neurological manifestations of cervical rib have vascular anomalies of the upper extremity. In the shoulder these may take the form of excessive pulsation and thrill of the subclavian artery above the clavicle, while distally there may be a weakness or obliteration of the radial pulse. The hand may exhibit pallor, cyanosis, paraesthesia, Raynaud's pheno-mena, acrocyanosis, or even gangrene of the finger-tips.

3. **Lipoma.**—Lipomas can occur anywhere in the neck and form soft lobulated tumours of varying size. They are most commonly seen bilaterally at the back of the neck beneath the occiput.

4. **Carotid Body Tumour (Non-chromaffin Paraganglioma).**—The carotid body tumour is a rare swelling which generally first becomes apparent in middle life. It is usually unilateral but may occur bilaterally. When this occurs the second swelling arises some time after the first. The tumour arises from the bifurcation of the carotid artery and is therefore localized to this area. After remaining localized for many years the tumour may metastasize. From its shape, lobulation, and colour, it has become known as a 'potato' tumour. The swelling is usually painless and symptomless, but compression effects are sometimes observed while some patients complain of attacks of faintness—the carotid sinus syndrome.

5. **Branchial (Branchiogenic) Carcinoma.**—'Branchial carcinoma' is the term used for a tumour lying deep to the upper part of the sternomastoid

in a patient who apparently has no primary lesion. It is probable that all the so-called 'branchial carcinomas' are, in fact, metastases from a minute primary concealed in the nasopharynx, paranasal sinuses, pyriform fossa, etc., which can easily be overlooked. The more careful and exhaustive the examination made for inconspicuous primaries, the less frequently the diagnosis of branchial carcinoma is made.

6. Aneurysm.—Aneurysms of the neck are usually related to the common carotid artery and they produce a pulsatile swelling of the neck which may compress the trachea, oesophagus, larynx, or recurrent laryngeal nerve. A prominent carotid in an elderly subject should not be mistaken for an aneurysm.

7. Neurofibromas.—Multiple neurofibromas may be seen on the neck in Von Recklinghausen's neurofibromatosis and similar lesions will, of course, be seen elsewhere on the body.

8. Carcinomatous Deposits in Left Supraclavicular Lymph-nodes.—A rock-hard swelling of the left supraclavicular lymph-node indicates a carcinomatous metastasis from a gastric carcinoma. This physical sign is named after Troisier.

9. Enlargements of the Thyroid Gland.—Any enlargement of the thyroid gland is known as 'goitre'.

Classification of Enlargements of the Thyroid

1. Non-toxic
   - Physiological
     - Puberty
     - Pregnancy
     - Menopause
   - Colloid
   - Nodular
     - Multiple
     - Solitary (adenoma)

2. Toxic
   - Primary
   - Secondary to an existing non-toxic goitre

3. Inflammatory
   - Acute pyogenic
   - Chronic
     - Tubercular
     - Syphilitic
     - Actinomycotic

4. Riedel's thyroiditis (Riedel's struma)

5. Hashimoto's disease (struma lymphomatosa)

6. Carcinomatous
   - Follicular
   - Papilliferous
   - Anaplastic

1. Non-toxic Goitres.—

a. Physiological Goitre.—The physiological goitre is almost exclusively confined to females and presents as a swelling in the neck in the thyroid region which requires no specific treatment as it usually subsides in the course of time. However, some of these parenchymatous goitres fail to subside completely and constitute a potential colloid goitre.

b. Colloid Goitre.—Colloid goitres are seen between the ages of 15 and 30 years and are usually physiological goitres which have failed to subside.

c. *Nodular Goitre.*—Nodular goitre is seen after the age of 30 years and the entire gland is studded with rounded swellings of varying size. Patients with colloid goitre tend to develop nodular goitres with age. Pressure on the trachea may occur especially if haemorrhage into one of the cysts occurs.

2. Toxic Goitre.—Toxic goitre may be primary or secondary and while symptoms often occur between 20 and 40 years, they may develop either earlier or later. The condition is more common in females and is usually characterized by exophthalmos and enlargement of the thyroid gland. Symptoms and physical signs occur in several bodily systems.

a. *Cardiovascular Signs and Symptoms.*—
  i. Tachycardia.
  ii. Extrasystoles.
  iii. Raised pulse pressure.
  iv. Atrial fibrillation.
  v. Enlargement of the heart.
  vi. Systolic murmur.
  vii. Heart failure.

b. *Central Nervous System.*—
  i. Irritability.
  ii. Fatigue.
  iii. Nervousness.
  iv. Manic depressive insanity.

c. *Gastro-intestinal Tract.*—
  i. Voracious appetite.
  ii. Diarrhoea.
  iii. Vomiting.

d. *Metabolic.*—
  i. Loss of weight.
  ii. Alimentary glycosuria.
  iii. Raised E.S.R.
  iv. Accelerated tendon reflexes.

e. *Genital.*—
Amenorrhoea.

f. *Integumentary.*—
  i. Lips are red due to vasodilatation.
  ii. Skin delicate, glossy, and moist.

g. *Eye Signs.*—
  i. Exophthalmos.
  ii. Lid lag sign (von Graefe's sign).
  iii. Absence of wrinkling of forehead when head is bent down and patient looks up (Joffroy's sign).
  iv. Difficulty in convergence (Moebius's sign).

Examination of a Patient with an Enlarged Thyroid.—
1. Feel the gland which may be diffuse or localized, smooth or nodular.
2. Watch and feel the gland on swallowing.
3. Is the trachea displaced? Palpate and radiograph.
4. Is there a retrosternal extension? Percuss and radiograph.
5. Listen to breathing for stridor.

6. Examine the eyes. Remember that in secondary thyrotoxicosis positive eye signs are usually absent.
7. Feel pulse and measure blood-pressure. Look for tachycardia, atrial fibrillation, and raised pulse pressure.
8. Watch the outstretched hand for tremor.
9. Examine the condition of skin, nails, hair, and demeanour of the patient.
10. Ascertain whether there is paralysis of recurrent laryngeal nerve. Listen to voice and perform laryngoscopy.

3. Inflammatory.—The thyroid gland may be the seat of acute pyogenic infection or chronic infections of tubercular, syphilitic, or actinomycotic origin.

4. Riedel's Thyroiditis.—Riedel's struma or thyroiditis presents as a small stony, hard thyroid which often causes pressure symptoms. It cannot be differentiated from a scirrhous carcinoma on physical examination alone, and must be confirmed by operation and biopsy.

5. Hashimoto's Disease.—Hashimoto's disease or struma lymphomatosa usually affects middle-aged women and is becoming more common. The entire gland is enlarged and feels like india-rubber and is seldom tender on palpation. Confirmatory diagnosis from carcinoma of the thyroid gland is made by operation and histological examination.

6. Carcinoma of the Thyroid Gland.—Carcinoma of the thyroid gland shows wide histological variations, but three main types are seen:—

1. *Papilliferous:* This often occurs in young persons, frequently in a solitary node and may remain quiescent for long periods eventually metastasizing to the cervical lymph-nodes.

2. *Follicular:* This variety of carcinoma occurs in the middle-aged and is more malignant than the papilliferous variety and rapidly metastasizes to the bone and lungs via the blood-stream.

3. *Anaplastic:* This variety occurs in the elderly and often in a previously normal gland.

In some instances the primary carcinoma of the thyroid may remain small and be overlooked clinically. Eventually metastasis to a bone takes place. Metastases of a carcinoma may also exhibit sufficient secretory activity for the patient to present as a case of mild thyrotoxicosis.

REFERENCES

AIRD, I. (1957), *A Companion in Surgical Studies*, 2nd ed. Edinburgh: Livingstone.
BARKER, A. E. (1883), 'Sebaceous or Dermoid Cyst of the Tongue; Removal by Submental Incision; Cure', *Trans. clin. Soc. Lond.*, **16**, 215.
SEWARD, G. R. (1965), 'Dermoid Cysts of the Floor of the Mouth', *Br. J. oral Surg.*, **3**, 36.

Chapter V

SKIN INCISIONS IN ORAL SURGERY

SOME oral surgery operative wounds are opened through intra-oral incisions and these have been dealt with in Part I. To perform other procedures, the surgical field is approached through a skin incision. One of the major disadvantages of incisions in the skin of the face and neck as opposed to incisions in the mucous membrane of the mouth is that the healed scars are exposed to view. They are not even normally covered by clothing. Therefore, every care must be taken to see that the resulting scars are inconspicuous.

This objective can be achieved in a number of ways: firstly the incision can be placed in a relatively hidden area, such as within the hairline, or in the shadow of the lower border of the mandible. Secondly, the incision can follow Langer's lines. Incisions placed parallel to these lines of tension in the collagen fibres of the dermis do not gape and when they are sutured a thin scar is formed. Should incisions be placed at right angles to Langer's lines the wound edges are pulled apart and a broad, stretched scar is the result after the sutures have been removed. Thirdly, incisions should not be placed in a direction such that muscles which are inserted into, or attached to, the skin can pull on the edges of the wound and widen the scar. The best place for an incision is therefore in a skin crease, that is where there is a local excess of skin and where muscular activity tends to approximate the skin edges. Incisions so placed will, of course, be hidden in the skin crease, or one placed parallel to a skin crease will be mistaken for a further skin crease once the scar has completely matured. Lastly, the wound should be closed with care and sutured skilfully.

The skin creases, as a result of the manner of their formation, represent areas where muscular pull is absent. The direction of skin creases and lines at right angles to the direction of muscle pull do not necessarily follow Langer's lines, but the general direction is similar and conformity to one, or the other, will not seriously affect the quality of the final scar.

Certain factors out of the control of the surgeon mitigate against the formation of a cosmetically acceptable scar. It must, of course, be recognized that all soft tissue wounds heal by scar formation. The question is one of degree. Some persons have a propensity for the formation of hypertrophic or keloid scars. Such persons are more common in certain racial groups. As most older children and adults have suffered accidental cuts, or surgical incisions, such a likelihood can be ascertained by questioning the patient and by a physical examination. The distinction between a hypertrophic and a keloid scar is, to some extent, a matter of degree. Hypertrophic scars are unusually thick, prominent scars confined to the line of the incision. They remain a dusky red colour for longer than normal scars. Keloid scars are even more thickened and lumpy and the process spreads into the tissue adjacent to the margin of the wound.

Occasionally they reach enormous proportions. Mildly hypertrophic scars will flatten in time. The condition may be improved by the intradermal injection of triamcinolone and a jet injection device is ideal for this purpose. Keloid scars can be treated by excision, followed by a small dose of X-irradiations to the new wound as it heals.

Incisions in growing children tend to heal with a broad scar. A possible explanation is the increase in volume of the tissues beneath as a result of somatic growth so that the newly formed scar is stretched. Broad or hypertrophic scars also result when all the first three principles outlined above are transgressed because of the need to make the most direct approach to the operation site. Emergency tracheostomy when a vertical incision is made in the front of the neck is an example of such an occasion.

Before the surgeon puts knife to tissue he should plan the incision. In some situations it may be sufficient to visualize the site and extent of the cut. On the face it is advisable to map the incision out with pen and Bonney's blue. For incisions in the neck it is satisfactory to scratch the line of the cut with the back of the point, provided that the scratch is not carried too deep. Lengthy incisions should be cross-hatched at about three places with Bonney's blue on the face, or with scratches on the neck. Such marks help in the correct approximation of the wound edges at the end of the procedure.

The skin is incised at right angles to the surface except within the eyebrow where the cut should be angled along the line of the eyebrow hairs. Skin and subcutaneous tissue should be penetrated in one sweep if possible, down to the subjacent layer. The tissues should be separated on both sides of the wound over the surface of each succeeding layer and each is opened in turn. In this way, proper layer-by-layer closure is facilitated. Where the subcutaneous fat is thick a subcutaneous suture will be required and the wound edges should be undercut to a depth of about 2 mm., about 4 mm. deep from the surface. This will permit proper eversion of the wound edges without unnecessarily deep stitches and minor corrections can be made in the lie of the wound margins with the skin sutures. Such undercutting should be done as the wound is established, so that proper haemostasis has been ensured by the time that closure is undertaken. It is particularly important to undercut the opposite edge of a wound where one edge is raised as a skin flap. Unless both margins are equally mobile a nice closure is difficult. Undercutting is also necessary where there is oedema of the skin, as, for example, when osteomyelitis or certain fractures are operated upon. Otherwise the stiff skin is difficult to suture.

The skin edges of neck and facial wounds should not be grasped with dissecting forceps, tissue forceps, or towel clips or they will be crushed and damaged. Where a wound is to be open for some while it must be protected from organisms brought to the surface of the adjacent skin as the patient sweats. Plastic sprays, adhesive drapes, and skin towels should be applied to overcome this problem, particularly where bone surgery is involved. Where skin towels are applied, they should be sewn on with loosely tied horizontal mattress sutures and not clamped on with towel clips. Should a skin flap be everted as the tissues are retracted, a moist pack should be applied to the underside of the subcutaneous fat to prevent drying in the heat of the operating room.

The deep layers should be closed neatly with 3·0 or 4·0 plain catgut. Often a continuous suture is satisfactory, but the stitch should not be drawn up tight like a purse string and the knots should be buried on the deep surface of the layer. Skin hooks and 5·0 or 6·0 nylon on atraumatic curved cutting needles should be used to close the skin. Some surgeons prefer braided silk as it is softer and knots more easily. The stitches should enter not more than 2 mm. from the wound edge and pass to a depth of about 4 mm., embracing a greater width of subcutaneous tissue. Each edge should be dealt with separately so that accurate passage of the needle through the tissues is ensured. The suture should pass to the same depth through each wound margin to avoid overlapping or stepping of the skin and it must lie at right angles to the wound. When it is closed the wound surfaces should be approximated so that no dead spaces are left and the cut edges at the surface should be slightly raised in order to produce a final scar that is flat and level with the rest of the surface. A spray-on plastic dressing is sufficient since a dry wound stands the best chance of remaining uninfected, unless, of course, a pressure dressing is applied.

Neck Incisions.—Incisions in the neck are made to follow the skin creases. In general, therefore, they are horizontal or sloping somewhat downwards from behind forward. The major exception is the incision for a block dissection of neck which has a vertical component.

Incisions in the submandibular region are placed in, or parallel to, the skin creases. When the mandible is to be exposed they should be about 1 cm. below the lower border so that the final scar is in the shadow of the jaw. Regard should not be paid to the position of the mandibular branch of the facial nerve. The latter lies deep to the platysma. More posteriorly, it is deep to the deep fascia as well, so that if it is necessary to include the nerve in the upper flap the incision in the platysma can be adjusted to the appropriate level. It is in any case best to identify the nerve, regardless of the way the incision is made, so that it may be preserved.

In the submental region the skin creases run transversely, so it is difficult to join an incision posteriorly to one below the chin. Neither does a submental scar always heal to give a good aesthetic result. The midline of the mandible is best reached by a degloving incision made in the lower buccal sulcus, or by retraction forwards of a submandibular incision.

Peri-orbital Incisions.—Incisions are made in this region to expose the zygomatico-frontal region, the floor of the orbit and infra-orbital margin and the medial wall of the orbit. The zygomatico-frontal region can be exposed by an incision in the lateral end of the eyebrow carried backwards in the line of a crow's foot crease. An alternative is a V-shaped cut made just internal to the lateral margin of the orbit, in the lax tissue lateral to the upper and lower eyelids.

Medially an incision can be made medial to the supra-orbital notch and within the eyebrow. If necessary, such an incision can be extended across the root of the nose so as to expose the nasal bones.

Inferiorly the incision is usually made in a curve following the line of the infra-orbital margin. It should not encroach on the lateral third of the orbit or the lymphatic drainage from the lower lid is affected. For resections of the maxilla the incision runs through the upper lip, lateral to the philtrum, around the ala of the nose, and then up to the margin of the lower lid lateral to the lacrimal canaliculus. It is carried laterally through the lower conjunctival fornix and may be extended further laterally in a crow's foot crease (Crockett, 1963). Incisions involving the free margin of the lip should be broken by lateral cuts and sutured in a Z. Special care should be given to approximating the muscle layer. Both measures are necessary to prevent notching of the lip as the scar contracts. Stepping of eyelid incisions is also necessary to prevent a coloboma of the lid as the wound heals (Kazanjian and Converse, 1959). ... That is, the conjunctival incision is made a short distance to one side of the skin incision so that a step is created through the muscle layer.

Opposite the lower lateral rim of the orbit a radial incision is made. Such cuts not only follow the skin creases, but also do not interfere with the lymphatic drainage of the lower lid.

Pre-auricular Incisions.—Pre-auricular incisions are required to approach the zygomatic arch, temporomandibular joint, and parotid salivary gland. Such incisions should start within the hairline, slope backwards to the pinna, and follow the anterior attachment of the auricle on to the free margin of the tragus. From there they may be extended down and then back beneath the cover of the lobe of the ear. If further extension is required, it may be made backwards into the hairline again or downwards and forwards into a submandibular crease.

REFERENCES

CROCKETT, D. J. (1963), 'Surgical Approach to the Back of the Maxilla', *Br. J. Surg.*, **50**, 819.
KAZANJIAN, V. H., and CONVERSE, J. M. (1959), *The Surgical Treatment of Facial Injuries*, 2nd ed. pp. 72. Baltimore: Williams & Wilkins.

CHAPTER VI

THE MANAGEMENT OF HAEMORRHAGE IN ORAL SURGERY

HAEMORRHAGE is encountered to a greater or lesser degree in all surgical operations and its management depends upon whether the patient is haematologically normal or suffers from some upset in the clotting mechanism. Anomalies of bleeding occur as a result of a diathesis or from some form of disease or drug therapy which adversely affects haemostasis.

THE MANAGEMENT OF HAEMORRHAGE IN THE NORMAL PATIENT

Haemorrhage during the Operation.—The overwhelming majority of patients seen by the oral surgeon have a normal haemostatic mechanism and are not suffering from diseases or taking drugs whose effects might produce the problem of prolonged haemorrhage. Even so, excessive loss of blood during the operative procedure can only be avoided by meticulous attention to haemostasis. The management of haemorrhage during the operation can be considered under the following headings:—

1. Planning of the incision to avoid large blood-vessels.
2. The securing of bleeding vessels with haemostats.
3. Haemostasis through the application of pressure with swabs.
4. The use of haemostatic agents.
5. Hypotensive anaesthesia and vasoconstriction.

1. *Incision Planning.*—In the performance of any operation it is mandatory to plan the various incisions so that unduly large blood-vessels are not severed. Intra-oral and extra-oral incisions have already been discussed (*see* p. 17, Part I; p. 36, Part II), but it should be remembered that even in the normal patient haemorrhage may be profuse if the area to be incised is inflamed as a result of local infection. Once the wound has been opened further dissection should be conducted in such a manner that sizeable blood-vessels are identified and dealt with in a systematic fashion. This presupposes that the surgeon is adequately acquainted with the normal anatomy of the part.

2. *The Securing of Bleeding Vessels with Haemostats.*—The most effective haemostats for use in oral surgery are the curved or straight Halsted's mosquito artery forceps and no incision should ever be made through the skin unless an adequate number of haemostats is available for immediate use. Intra-orally the use of haemostats is somewhat limited, but occasionally a moderate-sized aberrant vessel is encountered in the cheek and has to be ligated, or one of the greater palatine arteries requires clamping. It is, of course, impractical to clamp the inferior dental artery within the bone and the use of haemostats on the lingual aspect of the mandible in the lower 3rd molar area is also unwise, since the lingual nerve may be included in the seized tissue which could lead to a protracted anaesthesia of the anterior two-thirds of the tongue. When operating on the face and neck, arteries and veins should, of course, be carefully

identified and, if they have to be divided, haemostats should be applied above and below the point at which they are to be incised before dividing the vessel. The tips of the curved haemostats should be applied so that the curve of the instrument causes the tips of the blades to face upwards and out of the wound so that each severed end of the vessel can be properly exposed by the assistant in order to facilitate the tying off of the vessel with catgut. Size 3·0 (metric size 2·5) catgut is satisfactory for most purposes in oral surgery. Many small vessels do not require tying and if the end of the haemostat is twisted a couple of times before removing it the haemorrhage will usually cease. Small vessels can also be sealed by briefly touching the haemostat with a diathermy set for coagulation before removing it from the vessel.

3. *Haemostasis through the Application of Pressure with Swabs.*—If bleeding points cannot be secured with haemostats, haemorrhage should be controlled by pressure from swabs and this is undoubtedly the most effective method for almost all intra-oral wounds. A dry gauze swab is packed into the wound over the bleeding area and digital pressure is maintained over the swab for a minimum of two and a half minutes. The normal coagulation time is just over two minutes and it is useless to expect to control haemorrhage from a wound by pressure with a swab for a shorter period than this. Pressure is a simple but most effective method of controlling haemorrhage, and the authors have witnessed bleeding from the maxillary artery successfully arrested in this manner. If there is a large raw area which is oozing blood, some operators prefer to use a hot, wet swab to control the haemorrhage. The swab is soaked in hot normal saline solution (temperature 48·8° C., 120° F.), and then it is well wrung out before applying it to the wound. This method is no more effective than the use of ordinary dry swabs and is dangerous when used in the mouth as the delicate tissues of the floor of the mouth may be scalded, especially if there is any excess fluid in the swab. Occasionally the haemorrhage shows a tendency to persist even after pressure with a dry swab for an adequate period of time. This can occur when an artery such as the inferior dental within its canal is incompletely severed and, therefore, the ends are unable to contract. In such circumstances a pack can be left in the wound. To reduce any risk of infection, half-inch (1·25 cm.) ribbon gauze soaked in Whitehead's varnish (benzoin 10 parts, storax 7·5 parts, balsam of Tolu 5 parts, iodoform 10 parts, and solvent ether to 100 parts) should be packed into the wound. The pack should be sewn into position to prevent its subsequent displacement and this precaution is especially important if the patient is being operated upon under general anaesthesia. Such packs will always control a persistent haemorrhage, but they should be removed within 48 hours if they have been packed into a bleeding tooth socket or they may give rise to a dry socket (alveolar osteitis).

4. *The Use of Haemostatic Agents.*—Every dental surgeon is familiar with the multiplicity of topical haemostatic agents which have at some time or other been advocated for the control of dental haemorrhage. Some of these materials, such as turpentine or tannic acid applied on gauze packs or cotton-wool, can be frankly dangerous and the authors have seen second-degree burns at the angle of the mouth and on the lips where the material has leaked over the face. The various commercial

preparations are often of dubious efficacy and obviously more costly than the dry gauze swabs which are infinitely more efficient. Thrombin and Russell viper venom will certainly precipitate clot formation when applied on a pledget of cotton-wool, but again both are expensive. One of the best of the commercially absorbable haemostatic agents is oxidized regenerated cellulose (Surgicel). Unlike most of the other preparations, it works very efficiently and as it is absorbable it can be safely buried in the tissues. Several absorbable gauzes and sponges act merely as a mechanical trap for fibrin and are otherwise inert. Surgicel partially dissolves to form acid products which coagulate plasma proteins together with haemoglobin so as to form a black, sticky clot. The pH of the mass remains acid and may theoretically interfere with normal clotting locally. However, this is not a practical disadvantage since the Surgicel clot is not formed by the normal physiological mechanism. Nevertheless, because of the low pH thrombin solutions should not be used with the gauze because the activity of the thrombin will be rapidly destroyed.

A purely mechanically acting haemostatic agent is Bone Wax (Horsley's) which consists of beeswax (yellow) 7 parts by weight, olive oil 2 parts, phenol 1 part. This substance is packed into bleeding bone ends to control the haemorrhage. Some operators still use this substance, but it should not be used with any frequency as appreciable quantities can result in the formation of wax granulomas.

5. *Hypotensive Anaesthesia and Vasoconstriction.*—Hypotensive anaesthesia can be employed when working under general anaesthesia in order to reduce operative haemorrhage to a minimum. In this technique the patient's blood-pressure is lowered by the anaesthetist through the use of hypotensive agents such as Arfonad and bleeding is greatly reduced. There are disadvantages to this procedure, for during the operation sizeable vessels may be cut without any obvious bleeding and, if overlooked, they are not then tied off with catgut. However, when the operation is over and the patient's blood-pressure is allowed to return to normal, such damaged vessels bleed profusely and the patient may have to be returned to theatre for haemostasis to be effected. There is also a risk of encouraging thromboses, especially in elderly patients with hyperpiesis, when the blood-pressure is lowered to such an extent, and the method itself is not without risk. Hypotensive anaesthesia should therefore be reserved for operations where excessive haemorrhage due to oozing can be anticipated or where visibility is of the utmost importance and a dry field cannot be obtained by other methods. In such cases it is of considerable value.

The use of vasoconstrictors: Vasoconstrictors are incorporated in local analgesic solutions in order to prolong their analgesic effects and they are employed when working under general anaesthesia in order to reduce capillary haemorrhage. The usual vasoconstrictor employed in local analgesic solutions such as Xylocaine (lignocaine) is 1/80,000 adrenaline, but in Citanest (prilocaine) the strength is 1/300,000 and this has been found sufficient in combination with this drug. Adrenaline is alleged, however, to produce undesirable cardiac arrhythmias, especially when a halogenated anaesthetic agent is employed. Further, when used as a vasoconstrictor to facilitate visibility during an operation, it has the disadvantage of producing local tissue cyanosis and acidity. Therefore, as the effect of the adrenaline passes off, a reactive hyperaemia occurs which potentially can result in postoperative haemorrhage and haematoma formation. However, according to Shanks (1963) Octapressin (felypressin) does not produce such undesirable sequelae during halothane anaesthesia and, used in a concentration of 0·03 I.U. per ml. with prilocaine 3 per cent, a satisfactory degree of vasoconstriction is obtained without the same risk of postoperative haemorrhage. Felypressin solutions without prilocaine are not generally available and have not, so far, been widely used as a surgical vasoconstrictor. Not more than 8–10 ml. of the 0·03 I.U. per ml. solution should be injected into an adult at one time.

Postoperative Haemorrhage.—Postoperative haemorrhage may be due to: (1) Failure to control haemorrhage at the conclusion of the operation; (2) A factor restarting haemorrhage in the early postoperative period; (3) Infection at the wound site leading to secondary haemorrhage.

1. *Failure to effect Haemostasis.*—Failure to effect adequate haemostasis at the conclusion of an operation comes under the heading of negligence and it causes great inconvenience to the patient, the nursing staff, and the operator. It is obviously more simple to deal with haemorrhage at the time of operation than have to contend with haemorrhage in the ward or in the out-patient department. No wound should ever be sutured until adequate haemostasis has been effected, for even though the haemorrhage may not be sufficiently severe to necessitate re-opening the wound in order to control it, the patient will inevitably bleed into the tissue planes of the neck and this results in an unsightly ecchymosis, or there may be haematoma formation of considerable dimensions. In the extreme case this could even result in fatal pressure on the trachea.

2. *Factors restarting Haemorrhage.*—Haemorrhage may start again during the first few hours after the operation. During this time haemostasis in the smaller vessels is largely due to contraction of the vessel and platelet thrombus and the mechanism monitoring the former is altering. Blood-clots, too, have not yet matured and contracted. Mechanical injury of the wound, application of heat to the wound inducing local hyperaemia, reactive hyperaemia resulting as the effect of adrenaline wears off, violent exercise with general peripheral vasodilatation and a rise in blood-pressure, or the consumption of a number of alcoholic drinks, perhaps for their analgesic or euphoric effect, again with general peripheral vasodilation, all may trigger off such a haemorrhage. A fit of coughing, as for example in response to a small trickle of blood or saliva, may produce venous congestion and restart substantial haemorrhage from the wound. The classic reactionary haemorrhage, of course, is that which supervenes with the rise in blood-pressure during the initial recovery from a severe operation.

3. *Infection at the Wound Site.*—Secondary haemorrhage is usually due to a partial division of a blood-vessel in combination with sepsis and according to Aird (1957) sepsis alone rarely causes secondary haemorrhage. Provided the operation is carried out with careful attention to asepsis and haemostasis and postoperative infection is prevented, secondary haemorrhage on the classic tenth day should largely be of purely historical interest.

One operation of interest to oral surgeons carries a particular risk of such a haemorrhage. This is the radical neck dissection. The carotid vessels are stripped clean of tissue on their superficial aspect. If the tri-radiate part of the suture line lies over these vessels and wound dehiscence occurs, there is a considerable risk of ulceration and rupture of a carotid.

Bleeding from a Tooth Socket.—Bleeding from an extraction socket is the most common postoperative haemorrhage encountered by the dental surgeon. As with other wounds bleeding may be a continuation of the primary haemorrhage, reactionary haemorrhage occurring after the passage of a few hours, or secondary haemorrhage occurring 7–10 days after the extraction.

The most common cause of persistent primary haemorrhage is *pre-existing local inflammation* at the site of the wound. The sockets of teeth extracted for advanced periodontal disease are notorious for the way they bleed and the routine suturing of such sockets has much to commend it. *Hypertension* either as the patient's normal state, or as a result of the emotional stress associated with the extraction, is another cause. *Small puncture wounds* in the sulcus opposite an upper canine, or a lower second molar, due to a slip with an instrument, can damage the upper labial artery or the facial artery, respectively, and can be a cause of profuse, persistent haemorrhage which may be thought mistakenly to be coming from the socket.

All of the factors mentioned under Section 2 above may result in reactionary haemorrhage from a tooth socket. Secondary haemorrhage is fortunately a rare complication of tooth extraction. It is most likely to be seen where a patient develops a Vincent's acute ulcerative gingivitis during the days following the extraction. Because the haemorrhage under such circumstances is not severe, but may recur persistently, a defect in the haemostatic mechanism may be suspected rather than the true cause. The exhibition of antibiotics together with appropriate haemostatic manoeuvres will control the bleeding.

Treatment depends upon identifying the source of the bleeding. First, the patient's mouth should be washed out with cold water and adherent clot removed with a gauze swab, so that the bleeding socket can be accurately visualized and identified. The operator then places the thumb and forefinger on either side of the socket and applies pressure to the gingivae covering the buccal, lingual, or palatal alveolar process. If this pressure controls the haemorrhage, it implies that the source of the bleeding is in the gum and a suture across the socket will effect haemostasis by compressing the mucoperiosteum against the underlying bone. If such pressure fails to control the blood-flow it is obvious that the source of the haemorrhage originates within the bony cavity and some form of socket pack is required, i.e., Whitehead's varnish on ribbon gauze or one of the absorbable haemostatic agents such as gelatin sponge or Surgicel. Suturing across the socket will not control this type of haemorrhage, for the bleeding will continue in the depths of the socket, and as it is unable to escape from the socket owing to the suture it will extravasate into the tissue planes of the neck.

Haematoma Formation.—Postoperative haematoma formation is due to a combination of inadequate postoperative haemostasis or lack of drainage where this is appropriate. All potential dead spaces should be drained and pressure dressings applied to their flaps to discourage capillary ooze and the consequent accumulation of blood. In intra-oral surgery lack of drainage may be due to over-tight suturing of the wound. It may result in a considerable facial swelling which is tender on palpation. The condition is usually present on the first postoperative day and should be treated by removal of one or more sutures and evacuation of the haematoma possibly by aspiration with a sterile wide bore needle. In the mouth it is usually sufficient to institute an intensive régime of hot saline mouthbaths. These effusions of blood often become infected and if the patient has a pyrexia, suitable antibiotic therapy should be instituted. An infected haematoma inevitably leads to breakdown of the suture line and protracted healing of the wound.

THE HAEMORRHAGIC DISEASES

The haemorrhagic diseases can be divided into three main groups: (1) Diseases where there is a defect in coagulation; (2) Diseases where there is a thrombocytopenia; (3) Diseases where there is an abnormality in the capillaries.

1. *Diseases where there is a Defect in Coagulation*

A defect in coagulation occurs in (*a*) haemophilia and its related diseases and (*b*) in conditions where there is hypoprothrombinaemia.

Coagulation.—The mechanism of the coagulation of blood is still imperfectly understood and the views expressed in this text are those of MacFarlane (1965). According to Professor MacFarlane the natural haemostatic mechanism is an interlocking mechanism of three processes: fibrin formation, platelet aggregation, and vascular contraction. Immediately after vascular injury the platelets adhere to the damaged tissue' and to each other to build up a haemostatic plug which in the case of very small vessels is sufficient to stop bleeding, but in larger vessels must be reinforced by fibrin in order to withstand the blood-pressure. Vascular contraction is important as it reduces the diameter of the vessel and so helps to consolidate the haemostatic plug. The mechanism of vascular contraction is imperfectly understood but it may occur as a result of the direct effect of trauma on the muscle of the vessel wall or to nervous impulses, but it is also due to vaso-active substances, e.g. 5 hydroxy-tryptamine, 5HT, released by the platelets and to substances formed in the blood as a result of clotting. Platelet aggregation is probably due to adenosine diphosphate; a powerful platelet agglutinin which is known to be released in areas of damage and also by the platelets themselves when they are exposed to foreign surfaces or the action of thrombin.

Fibrinogen is a glycoprotein composed of three pairs of polypeptide chains, α, β and χ. Thrombin is a proteolytic enzyme which removes first of all 19 amino-acids from one end of both α chains and then more slowly 14 amino-acids from one end of both β chains. The remainder of the molecule forms the fibrin monomer which polymerizes end to end to form a soluble polymer, fibrin Ia. Insoluble fibrin Ib is precipitated by Factor XIIIa which results from the action of thrombin on Factor XIII. Thrombin is generated from prothrombin by the action of thrombo-plastin now called prothrombinase. Prothrombin is therefore a pro-enzyme. Prothrombinase is generated by the combination of Factor Xa (which results from the activation of Factor X) with the phospholipid platelet Factor 3 (PF3) and Factor V in the presence of calcium ions.

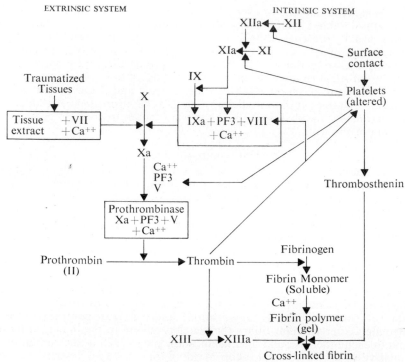

The Coagulation Pathway
(after Boulton, 1973)

Two systems may activate Factor X to Xa: the so called extrinsic system, and the intrinsic system which is formed in normal blood which has been left to stand. In the body both systems probably function together.

In the extrinsic system a phospho-lipo-protein is released from traumatized tissue and combines with Factor VII in the presence of calcium ions. This molecular complex then activates Factor X as described above. In the intrinsic system Factor IXa produces another macro-molecule with PF3 and Factor VIII in the presence of calcium ions. Factor IX is activated to Factor IXa by Factor XI which itself is activated, either by platelets which have been altered by contact with exposed collagen, or by Factor XIIa which arises as a result of the contact of Factor XII with a foreign surface, all this in the form of a 'cascade' reaction (MacFarlane, 1965):

$$
\begin{array}{rcl}
XII & — & XIIa \\
XI & — & XIa \\
IX & — & IXa \\
VIII & — & VIIIa \\
X & — & Xa \\
II & — & thrombin \\
I & — & fibrin
\end{array}
$$

Once thrombin is formed it too induces the release of PF3 so that the two processes of clotting and platelet aggregation are interlocked (*see diagram on* p. 52).

Each of these clotting factors may be deficient as a result of hereditary defects or disease or the action of drugs. The most important are haemophilia due to a deficiency of Factor VIII, Christmas disease which is due to deficiency of Factor IX, and deficiencies of Factors V and VII. A review of the blood clotting mechanism and haemostasis in general is to be found in a paper by Boulton (1973).

a. Haemophilia

Haemophilia has an incidence of 1 or 2 per 100,000 of the population and it is caused by a deficiency of antihaemophilic globulin (AHG or · Factor VIII) in the plasma. It is inherited as a sex-linked recessive character appearing only in males and is transmitted to them by clinically normal female carriers. All sons of haemophiliacs are free from the haemophiliac gene and all daughters are carriers. When a female marries a normal man half the sons are haemophiliacs and half the daughters are carriers. If a haemophiliac carrier marries a haemophiliac it is possible for their daughter to be a haemophiliac. A case of female haemophilia has been reported by Gilchrist (1961).

The defective gene on the X chromosome causes a deficiency of Factor VIII which can be complete or partial. If the level is 25–50 per cent of normal the patient has no trouble unless he suffers from major trauma. Minor injuries do not bleed abnormally owing to the fact that haemostatic function is quantitative and what is enough for minor injuries is insufficient for major trauma. At levels of 10–25 per cent more serious bleeding occurs after minor injuries and below 10 per cent bleeding into muscles and joints occurs. The blood coagulation time is normal with Factor VIII levels above 1–2 per cent, but the severe haemophiliac usually has 0 per cent Factor VIII. Of the severe haemophiliacs most cases appear to have a plasma factor which cross-reacts with human Factor VIII, but a few do not. This implies that there are two populations of haemophiliacs: the larger one having a non-functioning Factor VIII analogue and a smaller one which does not even produce the abnormal Factor VIII. These latter patients are particularly liable to develop Factor VIII antibodies as a result of transfusions.

Symptoms of Haemophilia.—The principal symptoms are persistent bleeding after cuts and abrasions and especially after tooth extraction. There is also bleeding into the large joints especially the knee-joint. . .

The Investigation and Management of a Haemophiliac requiring Oral Surgery.—

The History.—The medical history of an adult haemophiliac will leave no doubt in the mind of the clinician concerning the diagnosis, for it will consist of numerous accounts of severe bleeding episodes following trivial trauma, most of which will have resulted in the patient being hospitalized.

Clinical Examination.—Clinical examination of the patient usually reveals evidence of haemarthrosis in the form of limitation of movement of large joints such as the knee, and in more recent episodes there may be evidence of swollen painful joints and possibly swollen areas elsewhere in the body. The bleeding is deep in the tissues and ecchymosis is not a prominent feature. The patient may also give a history of episodes of haematuria and haematemesis.

Selection of Time for Operation.—A study of the medical history will show that the bleeding episodes tend to be grouped together and are separated by periods when the patient appears to have been relatively free of the disease. An intelligent adult haemophiliac can usually be relied upon to inform the clinician when he is in a 'good phase' and if surgery is contemplated, it is prudent to select such a time.

Diagnosis.—The investigation of a suspected case of haemophilia requires the services of a skilled haematologist, and once the missing factor in the coagulating mechanism has been identified the patient can be rendered fit for surgery by injecting the missing factor intravenously. The clotting time in haemophilia is not prolonged until the level of AHG falls below 1 per cent and a relatively normal reading could prove most deceptive to the surgeon. The only safe test for haemophilia is to estimate the AHG level in the patient and this requires the services of a specially equipped laboratory.

Treatment.—The treatment of haemophilia is essentially a problem for the haematologist, first, by diagnosing the exact nature of the disorder, and then, by replacing the missing factor in the blood, it may be possible to render the patient relatively normal so far as the surgery is concerned. The blood level of Factor VIII can be raised by the injection of various substances, but the effect is short-lived. The preparations which contain Factor VIII are:—

1. Fresh whole blood.
2. Fresh or frozen plasma.
3. Cryoprecipitate prepared from human plasma.
4. Freeze-dried animal AHG (antihaemophilic globulin).
5. Freeze-dried human AHG (antihaemophilic globulin).

Fresh whole blood and plasma have low concentrations of Factor VIII and as one can only give a certain volume without overloading the circulation, only a limited blood level can be attained. Even when fresh blood containing its full complement of Factor VIII is used, it cannot be transfused into the patient quickly enough to achieve a level of Factor VIII which will bring about haemostasis. The policy, therefore, should be to give blood transfusions only to replace blood-loss and not to use as a source of Factor VIII. The best Factor VIII level which can be attained with whole blood is 5–7 per cent and with frozen or fresh plasma 15–20 per cent. By using human AHG a level of 50–60 per cent can be obtained and a level of 60–100 per cent can be attained by using animal AHG. There is a shortage of human AHG and the supplies are inadequate for the demand, but animal AHG which is derived from ox or pig blood is readily available. Unfortunately, this material is a foreign protein and is antigenic, and if treatment with this agent is unduly protracted the patient will develop resistance and there will also be a loss of therapeutic effect and probably an allergy will develop. Animal AHG should, therefore, be reserved for emergencies, for a second course of the drug would probably result in anaphylaxis.

Cryoprecipitate and fresh frozen plasma are the preparations usually used to cover exodontia. Of the two preparations, cryoprecipitate is the more concentrated (anything from 5 to 15 times more concentrated) so that higher blood levels of AHG are more easily obtained and there is less risk of overloading the circulation, particularly in a child. Further, cryoprecipitate can be given intravenously with a syringe, while fresh frozen plasma requires an intravenous infusion. Cryoprecipitate is prepared by freezing fresh plasma and re-thawing in a controlled manner at +4°C. so that AHG and fibrinogen are precipitated. Plastic bags containing 5–20 ml. of plasma are in use and concentrations are between 15 and 45 New Oxford units per ml. Each pack will, on average, increase the level of Factor VIII in the blood of a 70-kg. man by $3\frac{1}{2}$ per cent so that about 8–10 packs may be needed preoperatively. While much AHG is lost in the preparation the technique is comparatively simple compared with the preparation of dried human AHG. The excess of fibrinogen does not normally matter.

The half-life of injected Factor VIII in the body is about 12 hours and 24 hours after an injection it will be down to a quarter of its immediate postinjection level. According to MacFarlane (1965) a level of 20 per cent Factor VIII falling to 5 per cent is adequate for minor injuries and single tooth extractions (i.e., use of plasma). More serious traumas such as multiple extractions require 40 per cent falling to 10 per cent which can be achieved with human AHG. Major trauma or surgery will probably require a 100 per cent Factor VIII level, and therefore animal AHG will have to be used. It should be stressed, however, that most patients become resistant to treatment with the particular animal AHG within 7–10 days of starting treatment and their Factor VIII response after transfusion of the dose gradually diminishes.

Management of the Haemophiliac undergoing Oral Surgery.—The management of the haemophiliac is essentially a haematological problem which consists of an exact diagnosis of the condition followed by the replacement of the missing factor. There are, however, certain additional steps which should be taken by the oral surgeon. The most likely operation to be performed is, of course, the extraction of a tooth or teeth, for no one would advocate more major surgery unless it was absolutely vital. Every effort should be made to conserve teeth and no more extractions should be carried out than are absolutely essential.

Anaesthesia.—In some ways local analgesia is preferable to general anaesthesia, for bleeding could occur at the back of the throat and the region of the glottis as a result of passing an endotracheal tube. In some cases a nasal inhalation anaesthetic after full premedication is satisfactory, in others a nasopharyngeal tube is used, or an orotracheal tube is passed in the relaxed patient under direct vision. Mandibular block injections are absolutely contra-indicated in view of the danger of persistent haemorrhage into the parapharyngeal tissues. Death following a mandibular block injection for conservative treatment has been reported (Parnell, 1964). Local infiltration causes bleeding at each point where the needle is inserted and the only absolutely safe site for injection is down the periodontal membrane. This is painful and infection could be introduced by the needle, but it gives good analgesia and the area is to be disrupted by the forceps beaks anyway.

A haemorrhage plate should be constructed prior to operation, not to control the haemorrhage, which it is incapable of doing, but to protect the blood-clot from the trauma of food and the patient's tongue during the postoperative period. The tooth to be removed should be extracted as atraumatically as possible, after which the sides of the socket are gently squeezed together. The socket should not be sutured, for not only would the needle wounds bleed but blood which could not escape into the mouth would merely be directed down the fascial planes of the neck. If the patient does bleed postoperatively it is preferable for the blood to flow into the mouth where it can be seen and be treated. A small pledget of cotton-wool soaked in Russell viper venom should be placed over the socket or Surgicel can be used for the purpose, after which gentle pressure is maintained until coagulation occurs.

It should be remembered that unless the patient has a 0 per cent concentration of AHG, coagulation will eventually occur and if, for example, the coagulation time is half an hour, gentle pressure for just over half an hour will eventually succeed in staunching the flow. Normally the missing factor will, of course, have been replaced by the intravenous route shortly before operation and so coagulation can be confidently expected in a comparatively short time. The patient is returned to the ward and subjected to the following régime:—

1. The patient should be nursed in the sitting position.

2. The patient should be on absolute bed-rest.

3. To prevent breakdown of the clot by muscular movement, the mandible should be immobilized by applying a barrel bandage.

4. A lukewarm liquid diet should be ordered.

5. The patient should not have hot drinks or any form of alcohol.

6. The patient is best in a room on his own so that the bleeding is not started by excessive talking.

7. Visitors should be kept away for the same reason.

8. In order to endure this régime, the patient should be sedated with phenobarbitone 30 mg. b.d.

Additional booster doses of Factor VIII (e.g., cryoprecipitate) should be administered daily and the patient must be hospitalized until five days have elapsed without bleeding. It need hardly be added that such analgesics as aspirin are absolutely contra-indicated in view of the danger of severe haematemesis and even in small doses aspirin is known to impair platelet function, and this added haemostatic defect in the haemophiliac can make him prone to bleed. As an alternative to aspirin as an analgesic, paracetamol or dihydrocodeine may prove effective.

EACA.—In recent years epsilon aminocaproic acid (EACA), an antifibrinolytic substance, has been used to increase the stability of the clots formed after extractions in haemophiliacs. EACA has been used in combination with various local measures but without AHG replacement, and also in combination with AHG replacement. The drug is not free from possible unpleasant side-effects, but no treatment in haemophiliacs is without risk (Cooksey and others, 1966; Reid and others, 1964). Tranexamic acid reduces plasminogen activity by competitive inhibition and it also reduces the activity of preformed plasmin. Pell (1973) suggests that as it is a safer drug than EACA it should be used in preference to the latter in the treatment of haemophiliac bleeding.

If the patient has Christmas disease or an absence of Factor V or VII, the necessary modifications are made to this treatment.

Christmas Disease.—Christmas disease has the same inheritance and clinical features as haemophilia, but the Christmas factor (Factor IX) is much more stable than antihaemophilic globulin and stored blood can be used in its treatment. As in the case of haemophilia some patients appear to have an inactive material which cross-reacts antigenically with the normal factor, that is Factor IX. A few cases do not have this abnormal material. Some cases have a factor which appears to inhibit both normal Factor IX and normal Factor VII *in vitro*. These cases have been designated Haemophilia B.M. Cryoprecipitate does *not* contain Factor IX and is not appropriate in the treatment of Christmas disease. Fresh frozen plasma or, if they are available, Factor IX concentrates are used. As the half-life of Factor IX is $2\frac{1}{2}$ days, smaller amounts of infusion material are required.

Factor V Deficiency is inherited in some families as a dominant trait, but is extremely rare. It can be treated with fresh blood.

Factor VII Deficiency is seen in patients under anticoagulant therapy and occasionally in advanced liver disease. Treatment is with stored blood.

Other Deficiencies.—From time to time patients with a deficiency of other factors—for example, Factor X (Quast and others, 1971) and Factor XI (Williams, 1972) are reported. Such cases are rare and specialist advice by a haematologist is necessary to unravel their diagnostic problems.

b. Conditions in which there is a Hypoprothrombinaemia

Prothrombin is produced in the liver and vitamin K (napthaquinone) is required for its synthesis. Factors VII, X, and IX also require the presence of vitamin K for their production in the liver. There are two sources of vitamin K—an exogenous source in the diet and an endogenous source from the intestines where it is synthesized by certain bacteria. Vitamin K is not properly absorbed in the absence of bile-salts. Clinical prothrombin deficiency is therefore seen in:—

1. Newborn babies in whose intestines the vitamin-K-forming organisms have not yet become established, i.e., haemorrhagic disease of the newborn. This condition can be largely prevented by giving intramuscular vitamin K either to the mother before birth or to the baby as soon as it is born.

2. Patients with obstructive jaundice who should also be given vitamin K analogues if any surgical operation is contemplated, otherwise serious haemorrhage can occur.

3. Patients in whom the vitamin-K-forming organisms have been greatly reduced as a result of protracted therapy with broad-spectrum antibiotics, or who are 'washed-out' through severe dysenteries. In these patients vitamin K production may be inadequate and so again haemorrhage may occur. The conditions also can be corrected by administering water-soluble vitamin K analogues.

4. Patients with severe liver damage as a result of hepatitis, multiple metastases, etc., in whom again there is a failure to produce prothrombin,

but this condition is not wholly dependent on the lack of vitamin K and may be improved, but cannot be corrected by its administration.

5. Conditions of extreme malnutrition.

6. Patients receiving an oral anticoagulant.

7. Patients suffering from fatty diarrhoea, e.g., coeliac disease and sprue.

8. Patients who have a rare form of congenital hypoprothrombinaemia. Such patients are on maintenance doses of vitamin K for life.

The main importance to the oral surgeon of all these conditions is that he should be aware of the possibility of severe haemorrhage following even minor surgery when working upon any of these categories of patients. Water-soluble vitamin K analogues given i.m. for three days preoperatively may be helpful in such cases—except, of course, for patients on phenindione, etc., where vitamin K_1 (phytomenadione) given intravenously is usually advocated for the emergency reversal of the anticoagulant effect. Frequently all that is needed is to stop treatment with the anticoagulant, but if urgent reversal of the anticoagulant is required fresh frozen plasma should be given. This measure is safer and rather more constant in its effect than the administration of vitamin K. Whatever treatment is used the effect should be monitored by prothrombin time tests.

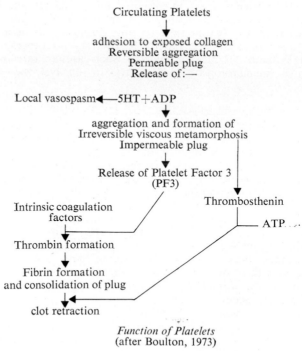

Function of Platelets
(after Boulton, 1973)

2. Diseases where there is a Thrombocytopenia

Essential Thrombocytopenia (Idiopathic Thrombocytopenic Purpura).— This is a rare disease of young adults characterized by episodes of skin purpura, epistaxis, and alimentary and uterine haemorrhage. The platelet count is low (below 40,000 per c.mm.) and the bleeding time is prolonged but the coagulation time is normal. The Hess test is strongly positive. As a result of recurrent haemorrhages the patient may have an iron-deficiency type of anaemia. In some patients the spleen is palpable.

Treatment is by splenectomy, but this carries a high mortality if carried out during the acute phases of the disease. Adrenocortical steroids may also be used in treatment and these must be considered if surgery is contemplated.

Bleeding in thrombocytopenia is excessive after even minor trauma so that tiny wounds such as needle punctures can bleed for prolonged periods, or give rise to a spreading haematoma (Seward, 1962). Widespread bruising and petechial haemorrhages are also characteristic of a platelet deficiency or abnormality rather than a clotting defect. Boulton (1973) lists the following drugs which may cause thrombocytopenia:—

1. Those associated with pancytopaenia:

Cytotoxic drugs	Tolbutamide
Gold	Chlorpropamide
Chlorthiazides	Organic arsenicals.

2. Those causing selective thrombocytopenia:

Quinidine	Phenobarbitone
Quinine	Butobarbitone
Digitoxin	Cephalothin sodium

Salicylates.

There are also a number of diseases in which the platelets are normal in number but abnormal in function. For example, part of the cause of bleeding in Von Willebrand's disease is due to defective platelet adhesion, and in Glanzmann's disease, or thrombasthenia, there is a defective platelet aggregation in the presence of ADP and defective clot retractions (Wood, 1973). Skilled haematological testing is required to sort out these abnormalities.

In thrombocythaemia the number of platelets is increased. If their function is normal a hyperthrombotic state exists. If they are abnormal the patient bleeds abnormally. In macroglobulinaemia the platelets tend to become coated with protein and their function is impaired.

3. *Diseases in which there is an Abnormality of the Capillaries*

Purpura may be seen in any of the acute fevers, especially meningococcal infections, and can also occur as a result of drug sensitivity with agents such as heavy metals, sodium salicylate, isoniazid, thiouracil, chlorpromazine, etc. Senile purpura occurs in elderly people and purpura also occurs as a result of avitaminosis (scurvy).

Anaphylactoid Purpura

The Schönlein-Henoch syndrome is characterized by purpura and allergic manifestations such as urticaria, joint pains, joint swelling, and angioneurotic oedema which also affects the gut causing intestinal colic. Henoch's purpura is associated with abdominal colic and Schönlein's purpura with joint pains, but both conditions may occur in the same patient. Severe haemorrhage may occur when operating on patients suffering from these conditions.

The Ehlers-Danlos Syndrome

The Ehlers-Danlos syndrome (E.D.S.) was originally described by Van Meekeren in 1682. Ehlers (1901) described the hyperelastic skin, skin haemorrhages, and loose jointedness, while Danlos (1908) reported the cutaneous pseudotumours and peculiar scarring. The syndrome is inherited as an autosomal dominant trait and the condition is said to be more common in males. The basic defect in E.D.S. is unknown. Wechsler and Fisher (1964) carried out histochemical and electron microscopy investigations without elucidating the basic defect, but most authors consider it to be a collagen defect. Jansen (1955) considered that the cross linkages between the collagen fibres were defective.

Clinical Features.—

Fragility of the skin: The skin has a velvety feel and is hyperelastic and brittle. Minor trauma results in gaping wounds of the skin which are difficult to suture because the sutures tear out.

Scarring: When the lacerations heal they form thin papyraceous scars which, instead of contracting, tend to spread.

Hyperextensibility of the skin: In pronounced cases the skin can be pulled into large folds, but when it is released it snaps back into its normal position.

Hypermobility of the joints: Joints may be extremely mobile (double-jointed). Thexton (1965) reported a case who had to have bilateral condylectomy following repeated dislocations of the mandible. This characteristic of joint hypermobility is shared with Marfan's syndrome, osteogenesis imperfecta, and some cases of cleidocranial dysostosis.

Pseudotumours: Resolving haematomas and excessive scarring form 'pseudotumours' over prominences such as the elbows and knees.

Subcutaneous spherules: These small, hard, mobile nodules occur in the subcutaneous tissues. They are said to be fat lobules which have a fibrous tissue capsule and later they become calcified and are rendered radio-opaque.

Excessive bruising: After minimal trauma there is extensive ecchymosis and haematoma formation.

Protracted bleeding after extractions: Protracted post-extraction haemorrhage has been reported by Tobias (1934), Johnson and Falls (1949), and Jacobs (1957), but in the 9 cases described by Barabas and Barabas (1967) only one suffered from post-extraction bleeding. Five of their 9 cases were subjected to a haematological examination which included bleeding time, whole-blood clotting time, one-stage prothrombin time (Quick's method), serum prothrombin consumption index, thromboplastin generation test, antihaemophiliac globulin assay, clot retraction, and the Hess test for capillary fragility. The Hess test was positive but all other tests were negative, including the case in which post-extraction haemorrhage had occurred.

Von Willebrand's Disease

Von Willebrand's disease has also been known as 'pseudohaemophilia' and was first described in 1926. It is transmitted as an autosomal dominant and occurs as frequently in men as in women. It is a haemorrhagic disorder characterized by a protracted bleeding time thought to be due to capillaries which do not contract normally and there is an associated deficiency of antihaemophilic Factor VIII. The abnormal capillaries may be seen with a dissecting microscope in the nail bed. Platelet adhesion is also reduced. Infusions of plasma or cryoprecipitate not only correct the Factor VIII deficiency but also correct the platelet abnormality. Following such an infusion the patient's own Factor VIII synthesis temporarily increases. Curiously the infusion of haemophiliac plasma will also stimulate Factor VIII synthesis. Patients suffering from Von Willebrand's disease are subject to exacerbations and remissions of their condition. Viral infections particularly may incite an exacerbation and surgery should be avoided during these illnesses. Haemorrhages follow trivial trauma and menorrhagia, haematoma formation, epistaxis, and gingival bleeding may occur. The bleeding tendency may improve in middle or old age. Treatment is effected by the administration of fresh blood or plasma.

Hereditary Haemorrhagic Telangiectasia
(Osler-Weber-Rendu Disease)

Hereditary haemorrhagic telangiectasia (H.H.T.) is not a true intrinsic bleeding state and in patients suffering from the disorder all the currently recognized haematological investigations are within normal limits. The disease involves the cutaneous, visceral, and mucosal surfaces and the disease is characterized by its familial occurrence and is transmitted as an autosomal dominant, both sexes being affected equally. The disease was first described by Sutton in 1864, who reported epistaxis as a disease or a prime symptom of a diseased state. In 1865 Babington described a disorder characterized by epistaxis which he had traced through five generations and in 1896 Rendu referred to the disease as 'pseudohaemophilia', a familial condition with epistaxis. However, Osler (1901) first provided a full clinical description of the disease, while Weber in 1907 made a clear-cut distinction between H.H.T. and the haemophilias. Hence, the eponym 'Osler-Weber-Rendu Disease'.

Clinical Features.—The diagnosis is made on the basis of the clinical triad of the characteristic telangiectatic lesions, a hereditary incidence, and a haemorrhagic diathesis. The angiomatous skin or mucous membrane lesions may be punctiform, spider-like, and nodular, and may all bleed when traumatized. There is a wide distribution of the telangiectases including the lips, tongue, nose, and more rarely the brain, spinal cord, gastro-intestinal tract, lungs, eye, bladder, and uterus. The defect has usually been attributed to a purely mechanical defect in the vessels. These fragile vessels are liable to rupture when subjected to minimal trauma. Ullman (1890), however, regarded the telangiectases as a new capillary formation of vessels. The haemorrhagic episodes are usually of short duration, but may occur so frequently that the patient becomes anaemic. However, some patients have a protracted bout of bleeding. The disease usually presents as recurrent epistaxes in youth with the cutaneous manifestations appearing in the second and third decades. The disease tends to become progressively more severe with age and many of the symptoms of the elderly sufferer are attributable to chronic anaemia. The disease is of particular interest to oral surgeons for the lips, tongue, cheeks, and floor of the mouth are the areas most commonly affected. The lesions present as tiny bright red or violaceous raised haemangiomas about 2 mm. in diameter which blanch on pressure. Even the minor trauma sustained during conservative dental treatment can lead to haemorrhage from one or more lesions through their surfaces being abraded. Protracted haemorrhage is unusual, but Killey and Kay (1970) reported a case in which a palatal lesion bled profusely on two separate occasions, and in 1908 Phillips reported a fatality following the use of a toothbrush on the gingival tissues.

Treatment of a telangiectatic area which tends to bleed persistently is effected by cautery excision, but this method is, of course, impractical when it comes to dealing with all the lesions present in the mouth. Nasal intubation for endotracheal anaesthesia is, of course, contra-indicated owing to the risk of a severe epistaxis.

Acute Fibrinolytic States in Surgery

One cause of acute failure of haemostasis during surgical operations is pathological fibrinolytic activity.

The fibrinolytic enzyme system or plasminogen–plasmin system is believed to have a physiological role complementary to that of the coagulation system in maintaining an intact, patent, vascular system. It is believed that the two systems are in a state of dynamic equilibrium, the coagulation system sealing with a fibrin plug any solution in continuity of the system and the fibrinolytic enzyme then removes such fibrin deposits after endothelial repair has been effected. The main components of the fibrinolytic enzyme system are plasminogen, plasmin, activators, and inhibitors. Plasminogen is normally an inert plasma globulin which is converted by activators to plasmin, a proteolytic enzyme which can digest many proteins including fibrinogen, fibrin, antihaemophilic globulin (AHG), and Factor V. The activators of plasminogen include a plasma activator, tissue activators present in high concentrations in lungs, prostate, thyroid, and uterus, and certain bacteria which can also produce plasminogen activators. Urinary activators may play a part in producing the ooze of blood which may take place from the gland bed after a prostatectomy. Surgeons have been aware for many years that fear increases haemorrhage and that sedation can be an aid to haemostasis. While the elevation of blood-pressure which accompanies fear may be one mechanism by which this occurs, fibrinolysis may also play a part because fear can cause the liberation of plasminogen activators.

Normal plasma probably contains inhibiting mechanisms to control the small amounts of plasminogen in the tissues. If large amounts of plasminogen activator are suddenly released into the circulation, plasminogen is suddenly converted into plasmin. This overwhelms the antiplasmin mechanism and the presence of free plasmin in the circulation results in digestion of fibrinogen, Factor VIII, and Factor V and a grave coagulation defect occurs. The products of fibrinolysis are also capable of interfering with the polymerization of fibrin and the formation of a clot. This condition may occur in thoracic surgery, especially when the heart-lung machine is employed, but it can also occur as a result of transfusing a patient with blood which is contaminated with bacteria. Certain bacteria (cryophilic) can actually breed in the chilled state in which blood used in transfusions is stored. A transfusion with such blood would result in a surgical disaster. EACA has been used in the treatment of this condition, combined, of course, with massive replacement transfusion.

Plasmin therefore removes fibrin after endothelial repair of a break in a vessel and probably in the tissues as well as a normal event. Fibrinolysins produced by bacteria also act in a similar fashion, but to facilitate the spread of the organisms through the tissues. Plasmin activators may be used to promote the removal of unwanted clot, as in venous thrombosis and pulmonary embolism, and fibrinolysins have been tried as a means of cleaning wounds and as a way of reducing postoperative swelling.

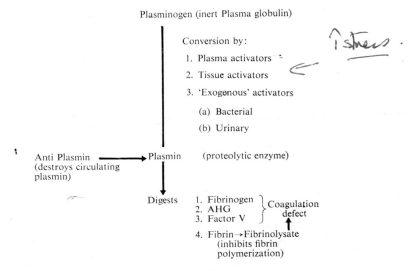

Plasminogen (inert Plasma globulin)

Conversion by:
1. Plasma activators
2. Tissue activators
3. 'Exogenous' activators
  (a) Bacterial
  (b) Urinary

Anti Plasmin ——————▶ Plasmin   (proteolytic enzyme)
(destroys circulating
plasmin)

Digests   1. Fibrinogen ⎫ Coagulation
             2. AHG   ⎬ defect
             3. Factor V   ⎭
             4. Fibrin→Fibrinolysate
               (inhibits fibrin
               polymerization)

LEUKAEMIA

Leukaemia is generally regarded as a neoplastic process, but its exact aetiology is unknown. The part which viruses play in human disease is uncertain. It is a disease characterized by abnormal proliferation of leukopoictic tissue throughout the body and it is classified according to the type of leucocyte which is affected into lymphatic, myeloid, and macrocytic varieties.

Acute Leukaemia.—The clinical picture in acute leukaemia is similar in all varieties. It can occur at any age, but it is more common in children. During the early stages of acute leukaemia there is usually a leucopenia and this is associated with low red-cell and platelet counts. Recurrent infective lesions and purpuric manifestations occur at this stage. The onset is usually sudden with fever, sore throat, and bleeding from the mouth and nose. The patient is pale and has a generalized lymphadenopathy and is obviously severely ill. There is usually tenderness on palpation over the sternum and the diagnosis is confirmed by examination of the bone-marrow, when abnormal varieties of white cells are seen. Protracted post-extraction haemorrhage can be a presenting symptom and the authors have seen several cases which have been diagnosed in this fashion. Postoperative bleeding can be anticipated in all types of chronic leukaemia and especially in the terminal stages of leukaemia when the patient becomes aleukaemic and there are severe haemorrhages and infections.

Anticoagulants and Surgery.—Anticoagulants are used in the treatment of a variety of thrombo-embolic conditions such as myocardial infarction and pulmonary and venous thrombosis, and the oral surgeon is increasingly confronted with the problem of having to carry out surgery on such patients. Minor surgery can be safely effected provided the patient is having a correct normal or slightly reduced maintenance dose of an anticoagulant drug, but many patients presenting for surgery have not been adequately supervised and have a higher than necessary or desirable level of the anticoagulant. In such patients severe postoperative bleeding can be anticipated.

Prior to oral surgery, the patient's anticoagulant level must be correctly regulated and this is confirmed by measuring the prothrombin level. This is done by:—

1. Owren's thrombotest method, when the value should be 7–15 per cent of normal.

2. Quick's test, where the level should be 15–30 per cent of normal.

3. Prothrombin and proconvertin method, when it should be 10–25 per cent of normal.

Provided that the patient's therapeutic level is within range of normal, forceps extractions can be undertaken without undue risk of postoperative haemorrhage. The reflection of flaps and multiple extractions necessitate a reduction in anticoagulant dosage. It is dangerous in some patients to stop the anticoagulant therapy prior to operation, for sudden withdrawal of the drug may lead to a tendency to an overswing towards thrombosis which may have serious and even fatal consequences. This phenomenon, which is especially liable to occur when anticoagulants of the dicoumarol group are suddenly discontinued, has been termed 'anticoagulant rebound' or 'rebound thrombosis' and may possibly be due to excessive concentration of Factor VIII.

REFERENCES

AIRD, I. (1957), *A Companion to Surgical Studies*, 2nd ed. Edinburgh: Livingstone.
BABINGTON, B. G. (1865), 'Hereditary Epistaxis', *Lancet*, **2**, 362.
BARABAS, G. M., and BARABAS, A. P. (1967), 'The Ehlers-Danlos Syndrome', *Br. dent. J.*, **123**, 473.
BOULTON, F. E. (1973), 'A Review of Haemostasis', Suppl. to *Lond. Hosp. Gaz.*, **76**, No. 1.
COOKSEY, M. W., PERRY, C. B., and RAPER, A. B. (1966), 'Epsilon-aminocaproic Acid Therapy for Dental Extractions in Haemophiliacs', *Br. med. J.*, **2**, 1633.
DANLOS, H. (1908), 'Un cas de cutis laxa avec tumerus par contusion chronique des condes et des genoux', *Bull. Soc. fr. Derm. Syph.*, **19**, 70.
EHLERS, E. (1901), 'Cutis laxa, neigung zu hemorrhagien in der haut, lockerung mehrerer artikulationen', *Derm. Z.*, **8**, 173.
GILCHRIST, L. (1961), 'A Case of Female Haemophilia', *Proc. R. Soc. Med.*, **54**, 813.
JACOBS, P. L. (1957), 'Ehlers-Danlos Syndrome', *Archs Derm.*, **76**, 460.
JANSEN, L. H. (1955), 'Le mode de transmission de la maladie d'Ehlers-Danlos', *J. Génét. hum.*, **4**, 204.
JOHNSON, S. A. M., and FALLS, H. F. (1949), 'Ehlers-Danlos Syndrome: A Clinical and Genetic Study', *Archs Derm.*, **60**, 82.

KILLEY, H. C., and KAY, L. W. (1970), 'Hereditary Haemorrhagic Telangiectasia', *Br. J. oral Surg.*, **7**, 161.

MACFARLANE, R. G. (1965), 'The Haemostatic Defect in Haemophilia and its Temporary Correction', *Proc. R. Soc. Med.*, **58**, 251.

OSLER, W. (1901), 'Family Form of Recurring Epistaxis', *Bull. Johns Hopkins Hosp.*, **20**, 63.

PARNELL, A. G. (1964), 'Danger to Haemophiliacs of Local Anaesthesia', *Br. dent. J.*, **116**, 183.

PELL, G. (1973), 'Tranexamic Acid—its Use in controlling Dental Postoperative Bleeding in Patients with Defective Clotting Mechanisms', *Br. J. oral Surg.*, **11**, 155–164.

PHILLIPS, S. (1908), 'Case of Multiple Telangiectasia (shown for Dr. Sidney Phillips by Sir F. Semon)', *Proc. R. Soc. Med.*, **1**, 44.

QUAST, U. R., SIBINGA, T. A., and WIJNJA, L. (1971), 'Stuart-Prower Factor Deficiency in Oral Surgery', *Br. J. oral Surg.*, **9**, 146.

REID, W. O., LUCAS, O. N., FRANCISCO, J., and others (1964), 'The Use of EACA in the Management of Dental Extractions in the Haemophiliac', *Am. J. med. Sci.*, **248**, 184.

RENDU, M. (1896), 'Epistaxis répétées chez un sujet porteur de petits angiomes cutanes et muqueux', *Bull. Mém. Soc. méd. Hôp. Paris*, **13**, 731.

SEWARD, M. H. (1962), 'An Unusual Presentation of Acute Leukaemia', *Dent. Practit.*, **13**, 143.

SHANKS, C. A. (1963), 'Intravenous Octapressin during Halothane Anaesthesia', *Br. J. Anaesth.*, **35**, 640.

SUTTON, H. G. (1864), 'Epistaxis as an Indication of Impaired Nutrition and of De-generation of the Vascular System', *Med. Mirror*, **1**, 769.

THEXTON, A. (1965), 'A Case of Ehlers-Danlos Syndrome presenting with Recurrent Dislocation of the Temporomandibular Joint', *Br. J. oral Surg.*, **2**, 190.

TOBIAS, N. (1934), 'Ehlers-Danlos Syndrome', *Archs Derm.*, **30**, 540.

ULLMAN, K. (1890), *Arch. Derm., Syph.*, **35**, 195.

WEBER, F. P. (1907), 'Multiple Hereditary Developmental Angiomata of the Skin and Mucous Membranes', *Lancet*, **2**, 160.

WECHSLER, H. L., and FISHER, E. R. (1964), 'Ehlers-Danlos Syndrome', *Archs Path.*, **77**, 613.

WILLIAMS, J. L. (1972), 'Plasma Thromboplastin Antecedent Deficiency', *Br. J. oral Surg.*, **10**, 126.

WOOD, N. (1973), 'Management of Extractions in a Case of Glanzmann's Disease', *Ibid.*, **11**, 152.

CHAPTER VII

SOME NON-MALIGNANT LESIONS IN AND AROUND THE JAWS

PAPILLOMA

THE papilloma is one of the more common benign neoplasms of the oral cavity and occurs with equal frequency on the cheek, soft palate, fauces, posterior wall of the pharynx, and tongue. They may be pedunculated or sessile and consist of keratinized epithelium on a connective tissue base. They are particularly common in children and young adults and in this age-group may be caused by the same virus that produces the multiple warts on the hands. They are usually single, occasionally multiple, pale pink to white in colour, irregular and often exhibit finger-like processes or have a knobbly or cauliflower-like surface. They are usually only a few millimetres in diameter, but may occasionally reach about 1 cm. in size. The surface over them is usually unbroken.

Treatment.—Treatment is by surgical extirpation and excision is effected through an incision round the base of the tumour. The incision need only be sufficiently deep to allow complete removal of the base of the attachment. Any haemorrhage from the base of the tumour can be controlled by a mattress suture or by electrocautery, after which the wound is allowed to granulate. However, if an elliptical incision is used the edges of the wound can be undermined to allow primary closure.

FIBROMA AND FIBROUS OVERGROWTHS

Fibrous overgrowths of the oral mucosa are comparatively common, but the majority of these are hyperplastic in origin and the true fibroma is a relatively rare tumour in the mouth. Barker and Lucas (1967) reviewed 171 fibrous lesions of the oral mucosa and in this series they excluded lesions due to denture irritation. There were 62 lesions from the cheek, 39 from the lip, 45 from the palate, and 25 from the tongue. Histological examination showed that 169 of the lesions were hyperplasias and only two of the lesions possessed a distinct capsule confining a mass of collagen fibres which differed both in character and size from those of the surrounding tissue. According to Barker and Lucas only these two lesions conformed to the generally accepted textbook definition of a fibroma.

The true fibroma is a firm, pink, sessile or pedunculated slow-growing tumour which cannot be differentiated on other than histological grounds from the more common fibrous overgrowths seen in the mouth. Fibrous hyperplasias in the mouth may be single or multiple and occasionally attain a considerable size. These benign tumours can be sessile or pedunculated and the pedunculated variety often occur in the palate where they may cover its entire surface, constituting a severe impediment to denture construction. The sessile variety are often found on the gingiva and may contribute to loss of teeth from caries as they tend to act as a food trap. Large fibrous overgrowths may become traumatized and ulcerated when they come into contact with teeth of the opposing jaw (*Figs.* 3, 4) and occasionally they become partially ossified, a fact which may be demonstrated by radiographs. The 'fibro-epithelial polyp' is a popular term for hyperplastic lesions of the palate, cheek, lips or tongue. The condition resembles a fibroma, but it is simply non-neoplastic reparative scar tissue (*Fig.* 5).

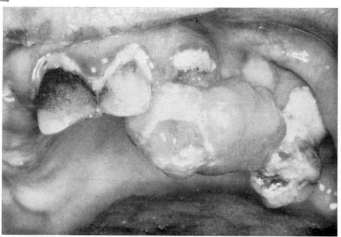

Fig. 3.—Fibrous epulis which has been traumatized by the opposing teeth in the lower jaw. The oral hygiene is poor.

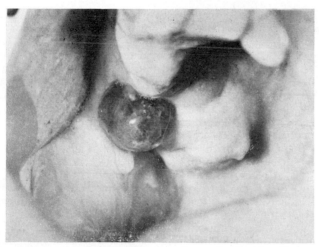

Fig. 4.—A prolapsed antral polyp; not to be confused with a fibrous or giant-cell epulis. The lesion is soft and a blunt probe can be introduced into an antro-oral fistula by the side of the peduncle.

Treatment.—Excision of a fibroma or a local fibromatous overgrowth is a simple matter, especially if the lesion is pedunculated. An incision is made round the base of the mass at mucosal depth and the lesion is dissected off the underlying tissues. A stitch passed through the mass to act as a handle facilitates the dissection. If a small raw area results it can be left to granulate, but the wound edges of a larger area should be undermined to allow primary closure. In the palate haemorrhage may be brisk, but can be controlled with a mattress suture.

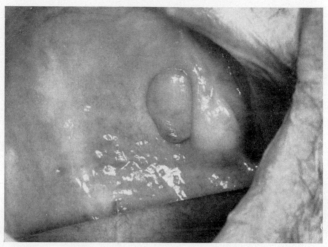

Fig. 5.—Fibro-epithelial polyp in the palate.

FIBROMATOSIS GINGIVAE

Fibromatosis gingivae (hereditary gingival fibromatosis) is a rare condition in which a diffuse mass of fibrous tissue is present within the gingivae of the upper and lower jaw. The mode of transmission of the disorder is usually a dominant trait, but occasionally it is the result of a new mutation. Although the hyperplasia is usually the only abnormal finding, there may be other associated defects particularly hypertrichosis, the onset of which may be at birth or puberty and is unrelated to the time of appearance of the gingival lesion. The second most frequent association is mental retardation. Clinically the condition is characterized by a firm painless nodular overgrowth of the palatal or gingival tissues of one or both arches. The tissue is pink in colour and very firm. The condition usually begins with the eruption of the permanent dentition, occasionally with the eruption of the deciduous dentition, and rarely is present at birth. According to Rushton (1957) a few cases have arisen in adult life. The lesional hypertrophic tissue may cover the whole or part of the dentition and even prevent the eruption of teeth into the mouth, although they erupt through the alveolar crest in the normal way. Histologically there is an increase in submucosal fibrous tissue. This syndrome is not only a diagnostic possibility when patients with gingival hyperplasia present with concomitant idiopathic hirsutes or mental retardation, but also when individuals show even more infrequent features of the disorder such as epilepsy, large ears, nasal abnormalities, and defective limb appendages.

Treatment.—Treatment is by a gingivectomy-type surgical removal of the excess tissue in order to expose the teeth and correct what is often a marked cosmetic deformity. The tissue seldom recurs if the excision has been radical.

GINGIVAL HYPERPLASIA FOLLOWING DRUG THERAPY

Fibrous hyperplasia of the gingiva may occur as a result of therapy with Epanutin or Dilantin Sodium (diphenylhydantoin), which is used as an anticonvulsant in the treatment of epilepsy. This side-effect only occurs in a minority of patients under treatment and it only affects areas where teeth are present. The gingival enlargement is lumpy with a smooth surface which is pink, firm, and shows no tendency to bleed. The enlargement may become so gross that the occlusal surface of the teeth is enveloped. At this stage ulceration from opposing teeth may occur and there is usually secondary infection.

Treatment.—Treatment is by surgical removal of the excess tissue in a gingivectomy type operation. If the patient continues the drug therapy recurrence is almost inevitable unless meticulous attention is paid to oral hygiene, but following removal of the teeth the condition will not recur.

DENTURE HYPERPLASIA

Denture hyperplasia or denture granuloma occurs as a response of the underlying tissues to a mobile, ill-fitting denture (*Fig.* 6). It may be

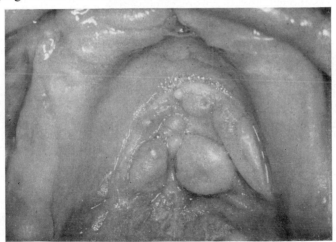

Fig. 6.—Denture hyperplasia from an ill-fitting upper denture.

localized or generalized and in some instances both the upper and lower ridges merely consist of several successive masses of fibrous tissue. Often the denture granuloma presents two flaps of tissue with a deep groove between, in which the flange of the denture fits. One flap of tissue lies against the fitting surface of the denture and may fill the gap left as the original ridge shrinks. The other flap overlaps the flange on the outer aspect. The course of events leading to the formation of a denture granuloma is probably as follows. There is repeated ulceration of the tissues where the flange presses into the sulcus. As a result of the irritation, there is a proliferation of granulation tissue particularly from each edge of the ulcer, so starting the two flap arrangement. Sometimes the underlying bone is affected by the denture trauma and becomes resorbed so that the ridge is soft and spongy. This happens especially in the upper incisor area when the full upper denture is opposed by the six standing lower incisor teeth. Occasionally a localized denture granuloma may be due to the denture cutting into the underlying tissues as a result of a cyst or other neoplasm growing within the bone. The possibility of a carcinoma of the maxillary antrum must always be considered when a denture granuloma occurs in the buccal sulcus in the upper molar area in a patient who has hitherto worn the upper denture without irritation of the underlying tissue.

Treatment.—Treatment of denture hyperplasia in the first instance should consist of leaving the denture out and this often results in quite a remarkable regression of the gingival hyperplasia. If the dentures are old or ill-fitting new dentures must be constructed. Residual masses of denture granuloma should be excised. The incision should be made at mucosal depth after which the mass is held up with toothed forceps or a series of transfixing sutures and dissected off the underlying tissues with McIndoe's scissors. If possible, primary closure of the wound should be carried out after undermining the edges of the wound with blunt-ended scissors. If the raw area is too extensive for primary closure it should be covered with a split skin-graft.

BILATERAL FIBROUS ENLARGEMENT OF THE TUBEROSITY

This condition has been described as symmetric gingival keloids (Rahb, 1936); diffuse fibroma of gums (Buchner, 1937); symmetrical hyperplasia of gingiva (Axhausen, 1940); (Linderman, 1941); fibroma of palate tuberosity (Straith, 1942); fibroma of tuberosity of maxilla (Cook, 1950), and fibroma symmetrica gingivalis (Fogh-Andersen, 1943).

The condition consists of bilateral hard fibromatous masses in the tuberosity region of the palate. While mild cases are not rare, sizeable examples are relatively uncommon. In a review of the literature, Fogh-Andersen (1943) found 40 cases, 27 occurring in men and 13 in women. The tumours are often present early in life, many being diagnosed in childhood. They may enlarge slowly, giving rise to impairment of tongue movements. With large lesions this can lead to speech difficulties and the impaction of food on the upper surfaces of the masses where it cannot be reached by the tongue. These are two reasons why the patients themselves seek medical advice. The only other symptoms described are gagging or retching (Beers Morrison, 1953) and pain on mastication due to the lesions impinging on the lower teeth and becoming ulcerated (Hiebert and Brooks, 1950). More often, it is the dental surgeon who advises their removal as a preliminary to the construction of dentures.

Fogh-Andersen describes a case where mother and daughter were affected, but a hereditary predisposition is not proved. He also describes a case where there was an associated mandibular protrusion. Most recorded cases mention associated dental sepsis in the region either from roots or abnormally placed teeth. It has been suggested that dental sepsis may play a part in causing enlargement of the tumour, but it can also be argued that the growing lesion may produce food traps around the teeth and result in extensive caries. The masses may also be responsible for abnormal positioning of the teeth if they happen to be present when the teeth are erupting.

The fibromatous masses are smooth, firm, pale pink in colour, and are usually sessile. They may become ulcerated on their undersurface by impinging on the lower teeth. In some cases the masses are so large they almost meet in the midline. Not infrequently the retromolar pad and the lingual gingivae in the lower molar region are also enlarged in the more marked cases. Such a finding suggests a possible relationship to fibromatosis gingivae, but if this is so it is curious that it is the palatal and lingual tissues which are involved.

Hiebert and Brooks (1950) suggest that they may become necrotic due to poor blood-supply and state that sarcoma may supervene. They also mention that the mass may become so enlarged that deglutition and even respiration are impaired.

Treatment.—Treatment is by surgical excision. As the fibromatous tissue is firmly adherent to the mucosa covering the area there is no plane of cleavage between the two and it is difficult to strip the mucosa from its surface.

Some authorities advocate excision of the masses subperiosteally, followed by fulguration of the cortex of the bone. They make no attempt to salvage the mucous covering. It would seem logical to raise a flap on the surface of the mass and use it to cover the raw defect, but this is difficult to achieve except in the edentulous patient as the underlying fibrous tissue is bound down to the surface epithelium and there is no tissue plane for dissection. If this operation is attempted, care must be taken to avoid damaging the greater palatine vessels or the flap will undergo necrosis. Excellent results can, however, be achieved by merely slicing the mass with a scalpel to restore the normal contours of the palate. This leaves an extensive raw area which can be left to granulate and epithelialize or can be grafted. The epithelium can be shaved off the surface of the part to be trimmed before the operation proper is started. This is stored in a swab moistened with saline until paring of the tuberosity has been completed and haemostasis obtained by firm pressure. A previously-constructed acrylic plate is lined with gutta-percha in the operation area and the pieces of graft assembled in a strip of tulle gras of appropriate size and shape. The graft is then applied to the raw area as a patch graft and held in place by the plate for 10–14 days.

NEUROFIBROMATOSIS

'Neurofibromatosis' is a term applied to a number of pathological conditions in which tumours of neurofibromatous material may occur singly or in various combinations. An inheritance factor may be detected in some instances and Freeman and Standish (1965) state that 41 per cent of cases show an inherited transmission. These tumours are slow-growing, cause pressure resorption of bone, do not have a capsule, and are radio-resistant. In either the solitary or generalized forms of the disease sarcomatous degeneration may occur and the incidence is about 8–15 per cent. Malignant change tends to follow chronic trauma or incomplete surgical excision.

Nerve-sheath tumours are not particularly common, but Heard (1962) collected 264 cases. There are numerous classifications of the condition and Aird's (1957) is both simple and comprehensive: (1) Generalized neurofibromatosis of Von Recklinghausen; (2) Plexiform neurofibromatosis; (3) Cutaneous neurofibromatosis; (4) Elephantiasis neuromatosa; (5) Solitary neurofibroma; (6) Neurofibrosarcoma.

1. Von Recklinghausen's Neurofibromatosis.—Generalized neurofibromatosis is a widespread thickening of nerves and tumour formation within them which may or may not be accompanied by plexiform and cutaneous forms of the disease or by elephantiasis. The essential feature of the disease is a proliferation of the cells of the nucleated sheath of Schwann and the tumours have been called 'Schwannoma', 'neurilemmoma', and 'neurinoma'. The nerves are thickened and present elliptical bulges. The tumour may displace the nerve-fibres to one side so that it can be shelled out easily, or it may grow among the fibres so that extirpation of such a mass leads to a neurotmesis. The tumours are greyish yellow or grey and they may undergo cystic degeneration. Although neurilemmomas are usually a part of Von Recklinghausen's disease, they can be solitary. The generalized tumours are most commonly distributed on the arms, legs, chest, back, and neck. Changes in the skeleton occur in 7 per cent of cases of generalized disease, there being osteoporosis, hyperostosis, or subperiosteal cysts.

Clinical Features.—Tumours appear in childhood and are seldom present at birth, and the skin manifestations vary from coffee-coloured freckles (*tâche-au-lait*) to extensive pigmentation of a limb. The tumours tend to grow at puberty and increase in size only slowly in adult life. The swellings are elliptical or fusiform and their long diameter lies along the axis of the nerve. The tumour is usually freely movable laterally, but not mobile in the line of the nerve. The swellings are firm in consistency and painless, and anaesthesias and paralyses are absent, though if the tumours occur in a confined bony space they may give rise to facial pain, deafness, and anaesthesia of the face or paralysis of the muscles of mastication.

Treatment.—If the disease is generalized, excision of all the tumours is impractical and surgery should be confined to selected tumours which are causing symptoms or are particularly unsightly.

2. Plexiform Neurofibromatosis.—Half of the cases of plexiform neurofibromatosis are associated with the generalized form of the disease. In this condition anastomosing branches of one or more contiguous nerves or plexus of nerves are thickened, fusiform, and beaded to form a dense mass which may be confined to the soft tissue or invade muscle. The neck, head, and extremities are commonly affected and the swelling may be large and pendulous (pachydermatocele). When it affects the scalp it may hang down over the face like an apron. The tumour may involve the face producing a hemifacial hypertrophy, and this may close the eye, block the external auditory meatus, and produce an enormous soft-tissue swelling of the face. When the condition occurs in the mouth the teeth may be covered.

Treatment.—Treatment is by surgical excision, though the mass will probably recur.

3. Cutaneous Neurofibromatosis.—Multiple soft fibrous swellings occur on the face and in the mouth. They never occur on the palms of the hands or soles of the feet.

Treatment.—Treatment is by surgical excision of unsightly or inconvenient tumours.

4. Elephantiasis Neuromatosa.—This variety of neurofibromatosis becomes apparent at puberty or, if already present, undergoes a growth spurt at this time. The cutaneous tissues of the scalp undergo a massive increase in size, become pendulous, and may require surgical excision. Bones in the affected part may be either enlarged or thinner and more delicate than normal. The enlarged bones are involved by the neurofibromatous process and are greatly thickened. Knobbly outgrowths may be formed. The bony trabeculae are irregularly arranged and the condition may be mistaken for fibrous dysplasia of bone, although the bone is more radio-opaque than that found in the latter condition.

5. Solitary Neurofibroma.—These tumours are histologically similar to those found in the generalized form of the disease. They are rare in childhood and usually arise after 20 years of age. They arise anywhere in the body. It is an uncommon oral lesion, and Bhaskar (1966) found only 26 cases recorded in the files of the United States Army Institute of Dental Research. He described 2 further cases occurring in the palate.

Treatment.—Treatment is by surgical excision if the lesion in the mouth is interfering with mastication or the fitting of a denture.

6. Neurofibrosarcoma.—Neurofibrosarcoma may develop as malignant degeneration in a pre-existent neurofibroma of either the local or generalized form and the incidence is in the region of 8–15 per cent.

Appearances in the Mouth.—Neurofibromas may present as soft, pedunculated swellings of cheek, tongue, or palate with sessile masses on the gum. Deeper lesions produce a fusiform swelling, often soft and lobulated, in the substance of the cheek, tongue, or palate. In the first two sites they may be mistaken for lipomas because of their softness. Plexiform masses which involve the gingivae can prevent the eruption of teeth and when neuromas affect the inferior dental or infra-orbital nerves, the canals are enlarged. If the bone of the jaws is involved, there may be a uniform or lobulated enlargement. The overlying skin may be pigmented.

LIPOMA

The lipoma is a benign tumour composed of mature fat cells. The fat cells are histologically similar to normal fat cells but metabolically dissimilar, for on a starvation diet fat is not lost from a lipoma.

They are commonly found in the subcutaneous tissues, but are extremely rare in the mouth. Bernier (1947), in a review of 1822 benign swellings of the mouth, recorded only 3 lipomas and 1 fibrolipoma. Geshickter (1934) found only 3 oral tumours in a series of 490 lipomata. The oral lipoma is a sessile or pedunculated, painless, slowly-growing mass arising from the submucous connective tissues of the cheek, buccal sulcus, floor of the mouth, and lips. They are very soft and may exhibit pseudo-fluctuation. The lipoma is yellowish in colour and feels freely mobile within the tissues when palpated. Lipomas may be single or multiple and the patient may also have multiple lipomas distributed over the subcutaneous tissues of the limbs and trunk. Gray (1961) reported a case of a man with multiple lipomas in various parts of the body including one in the cheek. Myxomatous degeneration and calcification sometimes occur in lipomata of long duration, but although this is seldom seen in the mouth, occasional cases are reported. Lipomas of the cheek must be distinguished from herniation of the buccal pad of fat through the buccinator.

Treatment.—Treatment is by excision and, owing to its definite capsule and comparative avascularity, this is usually easy. If the excised tumour is sectioned it has a characteristic bright yellow colour.

GRANULAR-CELL MYOBLASTOMA

In 1926 Abrikossoff described a series of 5 cases presenting with lesions on the tongue which he called 'myoblastic myoma' in the belief that the granular cells in the tumour were adult striated muscle-fibres which were degenerating as a result of trauma or inflammation. In 1931 he discarded this concept and suggested that the tumour cells were derived from myoblasts, a view previously suggested by Klinge (1928). Similar single lesions had previously been reported as rhabdomyoma and xanthoma, but it was Abrikossoff's series of 5 cases which established the connexion with striated muscle. The exact histogenesis of these tumours is not established and this has resulted in a multiplicity of synonyms such as 'Abrikossoff's tumour', 'congenital epulis', 'granular-cell myoblastoma', 'myoblastic myoma', 'uniform myoblastoma', and 'embryonal rhabdomyoma'.

Incidence.—It is a comparatively rare tumour. Crane and Trenblay (1945) collected 157 cases from the literature and Kerr (1949) added a further 35. Simon (1947) reported 6 cases, Powell (1946) published a further 3, and Bernier (1947) reported 17 cases. Kerr (1949) reported 9 cases and Bret-Day (1964) described 5 cases. Most of the reports in the literature, however, refer to single examples of the tumour.

Clinical Features.—Two clinical types are observed: the so-called congenital epulis in the neonate and infant. These produce pedunculated or sessile lumps on the alveolar process which are usually large in proportion to the size of the mouth. In the adult the lesion lies usually within the substance of the part. The tumours are most frequent in the third, fourth, and fifth decades but may occur at any age. The highest incidence is on the tongue, alveolar process, and skin, although they can arise on any part of the body. They are often small, elevated tumours with a greyish-white smooth surface and are usually symptomless. On palpation they are found to be firm and non-tender and may show an increase in size. They may be identified clinically by their pallor when they occur subepithelially. The tumours are usually benign, but malignant varieties have been reported. The overlying epithelium may show marked downgrowths of the rete pegs which must not be mistaken for carcinoma in a biopsy.

Treatment.—Treatment is by local excision and recurrences have been reported when removal was incomplete.

MELANOTIC NEUROECTODERMAL TUMOUR OF INFANCY

Histogenesis.—Krompecher (1918) is reported to have been the first to draw attention to this tumour which he regarded as a 'congenital melano-carcinoma'. Other writers have preferred to call the condition 'melanotic epithelial odontome' (Mummery and Pitts, 1925), 'retinal anlage tumour' (Halpert and Patzer, 1947), 'pigmented congenital epulis' (MacDonald and White, 1954), and 'melanotic neuroectodermal progonoma' (Stowens, 1957), since these names accord more closely with the respective authors' concept of their aetiology.

Stowens (1957) and Willis (1958) present evidence against the tumour cells being either neural cells or neuroglia, and argue convincingly against an origin from the retinal anlage. Willis goes on to show in the material that he examined parts of the dental lamina and proliferating strands of odontogenic epithelium. The latter was identified as such by the formation in parts of columnar cells and by the production of a stellate reticulum arrangement. From this odontogenic epithelium sprouts of pigmented epithelium arose which were continuous with that seen in the neoplasm. He thus confirms similar observations made previously by both Krompecher (1918) and Mummery and Pitts (1925). Willis was also successful in demonstrating dendritic pigmented cells between the tumour epithelium.

Kerr and Pullon (1964) reviewed previous cases in detail, added new cases and supported their odontogenic origin. Pontius (1965) also contended that in his case neoplastic cells originated directly from an enamel organ.

Borello and Gorlin (1966) again reviewed the literature and presented a case in which some 6–8 times the normal amount of vanilmandelic acid was being excreted in the urine. When the tumour was removed the urinary level of this substance fell to normal. Since other tumours with which vanilmandelic acid in excessive amounts is excreted in the urine include neuroblastomas, ganglioneuroblastoma and phaeochromocytoma these authors suggest an origin from neural crest cells. They also accepted that certain tumours found in sites outside the jaws were histologically the same. Such tumours have been found in the anterior fontanelle (Clarke and Parsons, 1951), the shoulder (Blanc, Rosenblatt, and Wolff, 1958), the epididymis (Eaton and Ferguson, 1956), and the mediastinum (Misugi and others, 1965).

Both Neustein (1967) and Hayward, Fickling, and Lucas (1969) exam-ined histological material in detail including the electron microscopical appearances of the cells. They could not support the contention that some of the tumour cells were epithelial. Further, Koudstaal and co-workers (1968) compared the enzyme pattern of the cells with that of malignant melanoblastoma, paragangliomas and phaeochromocytomas and that of the small tumour cells with neuroblastoma cells. They concluded that both types of tumour cell in the melanotic jaw tumour were of neural crest origin.

The current view is therefore that these tumours are of neural crest origin and the preferred name is melanotic neurectodermal tumour of infancy. The odontogenic epithelium found in the jaw tumours, but not in those from other sites, is considered to be from the normal dental lamina and included secondarily in the tumour mass as it grows.

What remains to be considered are the accounts of multicentric tumours like those of Jones and Williams (1960) where each appeared to be related to a separate tooth germ and that of Pontius (1965) where it seems two separate lesions were seen. Should these be discounted as recurrences of incompletely removed tumours, or should the relationship to the tooth germs be considered fortuitous? It should perhaps be remembered that by far the majority of these lesions occur in the jaws—more in the maxilla than the mandible—and that neural crest cells appear to contribute to the development of the teeth. They probably induce the overlying epithelium to form enamel organs and may themselves form odontoblasts and pulp cells. Indeed Langdon (1970) has noted a relationship between conical teeth, absent teeth and delayed eruption with Rieger's syndrome and incontinentia pigmentosa—two developmental defects affecting neural crest. The relationship with the jaws and with the tooth germs may not therefore be entirely fortuitous.

Clinical Findings.—Infants within the first year to 18 months of life are affected often within the first six months and maxillary lesions are more common than mandibular ones. There is an expansion of the alveolar ridge which can increase in size quite rapidly. After a while the pigmented nature of the lesion can be appreciated through the overlying mucosa. Radiography reveals a rounded cavity expanding the jaw and containing or displacing a developing tooth or teeth.

At operation a grey to black soft or firm tumour mass is found. Mostly it lies in a smooth bony cavity, but may be more firmly attached in places. In some circumstances the overlying bone, often subperiosteal new bone, is pigmented, indicating invasion by the growth. In other cases finger-like processes of tumour penetrate the adjacent medullary bone. Because it is pigmented the tumour tissue can be identified and curetted out.

Histology.—Large cuboidal cells with a vesicular nucleus form groups and strands through the mass. The abundant cytoplasm is heavily pigmented. Smaller cells with deeply staining nuclei form similar groups, and sheets of elongated and stellate cells form arrangements which were mistaken for neuronal and neuroglial elements.

Some of the cuboidal cells outline irregular cystic spaces several of which contain small darkly staining cells. The whole is in a poorly vascularized fibrous stroma. In serial sections of jaw lesions the elements of dental lamina described by Willis and others may be discovered. Invasion of adjacent medullary bone spaces is to be seen.

Treatment.—Careful enucleation is the treatment required. While care should be taken to remove heavily involved bone and any pockets of tumour, a conservative approach should be followed. Any marked damage to the jaw at this age will, of course, produce a disfiguring deformity as the child grows up. Any tooth germs present within the lesion will be included in the specimen, often along with the successional germ. Adjacent teeth, however, should be spared.

Prognosis.—In spite of the poor prognosis normally associated with invasive and pigmented neoplasms, with this particular variety the prognosis is good. In some instances, there may be a single local recurrence which results from a failure to remove a pocket of tumour, but further enucleation and curettage is all that is required to effect control. Even where invaded bone must have been left behind, a good result has been obtained. In a case described by Battle, Hovell, and Spencer (1952) a melanotic tumour was seen involving the right body of the mandible in a child of 6 weeks of age. It was enucleated but recurred 6 months later. The mass then was so large the situation was considered hopeless and no further treatment was given. The patient was seen at the age of 6 when only a localized mass in the 3| region was present. This was removed and the continued presence of the tumour confirmed. It seems, therefore, that this condition may regress spontaneously, but it would be taking unnecessary risks to treat all cases expectantly as by its enlargement the tumour damages adjacent structures.

HAEMANGIOMAS

Haemangiomas are developed as proliferations of the embryonic vascular network and are congenital in origin. They are red or bluish in colour and all exhibit the characteristic physical sign of emptying on pressure. This physical sign is best demonstrated by pressure with a glass slide when they are seen to blanch. They may occur anywhere in the body and the most common sites in the mouth are the lips, tongue, buccal mucosa, and palate. They can be divided into capillary and cavernous types.

Capillary Haemangioma

These include the capillary haemangioma, the telangiectasis, the port wine stain, and the spider naevus.

1. Capillary Haemangioma.—The capillary haemangioma of skin is also known as the 'cutaneous naevus', 'haemangioma simplex', or 'salmon patch', and consists of a red network of small capillaries radiating from a central punctum which is the artery supplying the tumour. It lies flat with the surrounding skin and may occur on any skin surface. The lesion may be multiple and varies in size, but it is usually strictly unilateral. The strawberry patch is a capillary haemangioma which is raised above the surface. It is bright red, lobulated, and often grows rapidly. This variety often ulcerates.

Telangiectasis.—Telangiectasis is a dilatation of normal capillaries rather than a developmental anomaly and it includes the spider naevus. These are single or multiple bright red lesions about the size of a pinhead with several tiny thread-like arteries radiating away from them. They are often seen in patients with liver insufficiency. They are found in the immediate periphery of scarring of the skin which has followed irradiation. Spider naevi disappear on death (Aird, 1957).

Hereditary haemorrhagic telangiectasia (H.H.T.) (*Fig.* 7) is not a true intrinsic bleeding state and in affected persons it is usual to find that the currently recognized haemostatic factors are present at normal levels. The disease, which is known to involve cutaneous, mucosal, and visceral structures, is characterized by its familial occurrence and is transmitted as an autosomal dominant affecting both sexes equally. The diagnosis of the disorder is made on the basis of the clinical triad of characteristic telangiectatic lesions, hereditary incidence, and haemorrhagic diathesis. Nevertheless, a positive family history is not always forthcoming. The

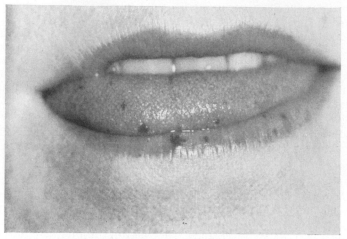

Fig. 7.—Hereditary haemorrhagic telangiectasia.

angiomatous skin or mucous membrane lesions pathognomonic of this malady fall into three types—punctiform, spider-like, and nodular—all of which tend to bleed when traumatized. The nodular type is tumour-like and may reach 2–3 cm. in diameter. There is, of course, a wide visceral distribution of the telangiectases.

Occasionally bleeding from the mouth may be severe, and alarming incidents including a fatality have been reported following the use of a toothbrush on the gingival tissues. If the gingivae are involved, the patient should be warned of the extra need for care during oral hygiene, but it is patently obvious that in the absence of a correct diagnosis bleeding may be wrongly attributed to periodontal disease. Regular conservation treatment will prevent injury to adjoining oral lesions from sharp, abraded carious teeth, but dental surgeons must be circumspect during the preparation and restoration of teeth and when using other instruments in the mouth to avoid damage to the oral mucosa. Conservative management for dental bleeding includes the topical application of haemostatic agents (e.g., gelatin sponge), diathermy, and the use of pressure packs. Blood transfusion is essential in cases of severe blood-loss and iron replacement therapy is indicated to correct anaemia produced by chronic bleeding.

Port Wine Stain.—Port wine stain is a pink, blue, or purple haemangioma of the skin produced by a generalized telangiectasis of the capillaries. These lesions are often seen on the face and in the mouth. Clinically there are two varieties—the smooth and the lumpy—depending whether the surface is heaped up. They often involve the entire side of the face and extend posteriorly to involve the palate and other areas of the mouth. Sometimes these ipsilateral tumours extend backwards to involve the leptomeninges over the posterior parietal and occipital lobes, which later in life may become calcified, producing at first a focal (Jacksonian) epilepsy and later a hemiparesis. This is known as the 'Sturge-Weber syndrome' or 'encephalofacial angiomatosis'.

Campbell de Morgan Spot.—The Campbell de Morgan spot is a bright red capillary naevus about 2 mm. in diameter. It develops on the trunk in middle age and was at one time wrongly associated with cancer.

Treatment.—Small haemangiomas can be treated by touching them with a stick dipped in trichloracetic acid or by electrocautery or cryotherapy. It is impractical to treat multiple spider naevi due to liver insufficiency, but they disappear if the liver condition can be corrected. Many of the extensive capillary haemangiomas present at birth tend to improve with age and some disappear entirely. Such lesions should therefore be kept under observation and treatment carried out only when further improvement appears unlikely, or in the rare event of the tumour enlarging. Capillary haemangiomas of the skin of the face are best disguised with a cosmetic cream such as Covermark and with such treatment the facial lesions are almost undetectable. For this reason treatments such as radiotherapy should be avoided as they spoil the texture of the surface and render subsequent treatment with disguising creams less effective. The 'lumpy' capillary haemangioma cannot be treated by camouflage with creams, and the area must be excised and grafted with skin.

The small lesions in the mouth in hereditary haemorrhagic telangiectasia are often inadvertently traumatized during routine dental treatment and occasionally they are responsible for a severe spontaneous haemorrhage from the mouth. It is impractical to excise all such lesions, but troublesome areas can be satisfactorily extirpated by cautery. The 'strawberry patch' lesions are best treated by injecting them with a bland sclerosing solution such as boiling saline solution. Capillary haemangiomas in the mouth may involve the alveolus and severe haemorrhage may occur as a result of tooth extraction. Cautery to the bleeding surface is the best way of dealing with this problem.

Haemangiomas may be treated also by cryosurgery. Large lesions should be treated by multiple sessions. Small lesions within the oral cavity can be dealt with by one or two freeze/thaw cycles on one occasion. Capillary haemangiomas of the skin are best dealt with by multiple short (10-second) freezes at fortnightly intervals so as to avoid scarring (Leopard and Poswillo, 1974). Pressure on feeding vessels to reduce the blood-flow and injections of vasoconstrictor can be used to potentiate the effect of the freeze.

Cavernous Haemangioma

The cavernous haemangioma is a raised red or bluish lesion which can be of any size, and it can occur anywhere on the body. It empties on pressure. On the face and in the mouth they are often very extensive and involve, for example, the entire tongue (*Fig.* 8). These hamartomas may undergo thrombosis and become swollen and painful during an actual episode of thrombosis. In these circumstances a lesion in the cheek may be mistaken for an inflammatory swelling but it must be recognized for what it is and not incised. Subsequently calcification in the thrombi produces phleboliths which can be mistaken for salivary calculi. Tumours present at birth have a tendency to regress in size and, therefore, no immediate treatment is indicated. The child should be kept under observation, and fortunately in some instances the haemangioma will disappear more or less

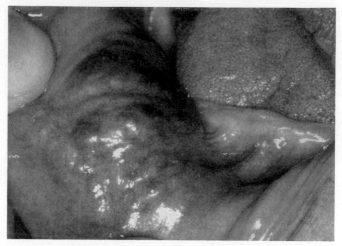

Fig. 8.—Cavernous haemangioma of lip.

completely. In other cases the lesion may remain stationary in size or in rare instances they may become larger.

Treatment.—When the lesion remains unchanged and no further improvement can be anticipated, or if it tends to enlarge, treatment should be advocated. Very small cavernous haemangiomas may be excised or treated by cautery, but the larger lesions should be injected with a sclerosing solution; the safest solution to use is near-boiling normal saline. It may be necessary to inject the haemangioma on more than one occasion, but the final result is usually quite satisfactory. Treatment with radiotherapy has been used in the past, but there is danger of adjacent growth centres in the bone being affected, leading to a growth failure. If the teeth are irradiated during the formative period they will be deformed and stunted, while there is the further possibility of the treated soft-tissue area breaking down at a later date through infection.

Traumatic Haemangioma.—As a result of a bite and damage to a vessel in the cheek or lip a haematoma forms. The haematoma cavity becomes lined with vascular endothelium to form a small localized cavernous haemangioma. It should be noted that there is no increased vascularity in the surrounding tissues. If unsightly, or if it is bitten again and bleeds, it may be excised quite simply and safely.

Central Haemangiomas.—Cavernous haemangiomas may be central in the mandible and maxilla and may present as destructive bone lesions with a radiographical appearance resembling that of a benign cyst. Surgical interference may lead to severe blood-loss and even death from exsanguination. Broderick and Round (1933) reported a case of fatal haemorrhage after tooth extractions in a patient with a cavernous haemangioma of the maxilla. Kroh (1926) described a patient who bled to death minutes after extraction of a loose tooth and at autopsy a cavernous haemangioma of the mandible was found. Smith (1959) summarized the literature up to 1959 and in a series of 20 cases of central haemangioma of the mandible described 3 in which the haemorrhage was fatal. Central cavernous haemangiomas are rare. Shira and Guernsey (1965) found only 41 cases recorded in the literature.

Diagnosis.—Diagnosis of a central haemangioma of the jaw prior to surgery is obviously of paramount importance and aspiration biopsy should be carried out when there is the slightest doubt concerning the exact nature of a radiolucent area in the mandible or maxilla. In some such lesions there is an arteriovenous shunt and a bruit may be heard on auscultation over the area. This physical sign was present in the case recorded by Shira and Guernsey (1965). A transmitted pulsation in a loose tooth is suggestive of an arteriovenous communication. Many cavernous haemangiomas of the mandible are particularly extensive and the entire jaw may be occupied by a multicystic radiolucent lesion having a soap-bubble or trabeculated appearance. Carotid angiography with hypaque is useful to demonstrate arteriovenous shunts into central haemangiomas of the jaws. Often, though not always, the blood-vessels in the overlying tissues are dilated and increased in number.

Mode of Presentation.—Most cases of central cavernous haemangioma are diagnosed as a result of investigation of an atypical radiolucent area in the jaws found during routine radiography. There is usually little expansion of the bone, but occasionally a pulsatile swelling may be present in the overlying soft tissues. The case described by Davies (1964) had a small pulsating mass behind the lower right 2nd molar. The clinical features may include a pulsating type of pain in the jaw. Spontaneous haemorrhage may occur in some instances and occasionally patients have experienced several haemorrhagic episodes. Davies (1964) described the bleeding as 'spurting' rather than a general ooze. Profuse haemorrhage following dental extraction is another obvious mode of presentation. The haemorrhage is of the character of that from a large vein. It is like water running from a tap and quite unlike the normal bleeding socket.

Radiology.—There are usually multilocular areas of bone resorption which produce either a soap-bubble or trabeculated appearance. Adjacent medullary spaces and vascular canals are widened so that the irregular outline has an indefinite border which blends into the normal architecture of the bone.

Treatment.—Treatment is required if spontaneous haemorrhage occurs or if teeth in relation to the haemangioma require extraction. The presence of a pulsatile soft-tissue tumour due to penetration of the bone also constitutes a potential hazard to the patient, and is a further indication for treatment. The lesions vary in their degree of vascularity: some appear to be capillary in nature, others solid in that the vascular channels are closed, and yet others are partially occluded with clot. It is lesions such as these which have been biopsied or treated by local surgery without danger. The dangerous ones are composed of venous sinusoidal vessels or arterio-venous malformations.

Some central cavernous haemangiomas respond favourably to radio-therapy and this may be carried out prior to surgical extirpation of the lesion. The latter is always a hazardous procedure. Unilateral clamping of the external carotid artery with arterial nooses or bulldog clamps may be indicated prior to operation, but this measure does not necessarily control the jaw haemorrhage (Moose, 1957; Packard and Baxter, 1960; Davies, 1964; and Shira and Guernsey, 1965). Bilateral ligation should not be practised since this leads to atrophy of the tongue. Resection of the affected portion of the jaw may be indicated and Shira and Guernsey (1965) successfully resected an extensive cavernous haemangioma of the mandible. Haemorrhage from the bone-ends was eventually controlled with bone wax.

Most of the cases in the literature have been treated either by radical surgery, which usually involves hemimandibulectomy, or by radiation.

Should a tooth be extracted, unknowingly, from a jaw affected by a central haemangioma, the operator will be in no doubt as to what has happened. The haemorrhage is torrential and requires rapid action if the patient is not to die. Appropriate pressure will control all haemorrhage. Clean gauze is packed into the socket until sufficient pressure can be applied so that the haemorrhage is controlled. An acquaintance of the author tells of packing 15 feet of 1-inch ribbon gauze (4·5 metres of 2·5 cm.) through a molar socket to arrest haemorrhage in a case he encountered.

OSTEOMA

This benign neoplasm may consist of compact or cancellous bone and is either endosteal or periosteal in location. True osteomas should show persistent growth and enlargement. The periosteal compact or ivory osteoma is a smooth, hard, painless lump which is usually sessile but may occasionally be pedunculated. The cancellous osteoma is composed of trabeculae of lamellar bone and covered with a thin layer of subperiosteal bone. They can occur anywhere on the jaws and may be single or multiple. Favoured sites are the angle of the mandible, the mental tubercle region, and the canine fossa. Radiologically they appear as a well-circumscribed dense radio-opaque mass.

Treatment.—If the osteoma is cosmetically unacceptable or if it inter-feres with the satisfactory construction of a denture it should be removed. Such a case was reported by Seward (1965). Pedunculated osteomas are easily removed by severing the base of the pedicle but the sessile osteoma can either be separated from the underlying bone or, if this would leave an unacceptable defect in the bone, the osteoma can be pared down and the normal jaw contours re-established. The latter treatment should be reserved for tumours which show little tendency to enlarge.

In the event of recurrence and with osteomas which have shown a tendency to enlarge, the tumour together with a small area of adjacent bone should be removed with a chisel or bur.

Torus Palatinus.—The torus palatinus, a developmental anomaly, is a slow-growing sessile compact exostosis which occurs in the midline of the hard palate and when it becomes large it tends to become lobulated. It is comparatively common and, when large, interferes with the satisfactory construction of a full upper denture and should be removed. This is carried out following a surgical approach through a midline incision from behind forwards which in the incisor area diverges on each side to form a Y. The mass can also be exposed through an incision made round the crest of the upper ridge which allows a large palatal flap to be reflected. The torus palatinus is of dense compact bone and is best sectioned with a bur and then removed with a vulcanite bur. Following excision the area is smoothed with a large round bur. Attempts to remove the torus with a chisel may result in fracture of the hard palate.

Incidentally, *exostosis* is a reactive hyperplasia or local enlargement, or an abnormal enlargement of a normal anatomical excrescence. Growth is not usually progressive particularly if the stimulus is removed. The term 'exostosis' should not be confused with *endostosis*. The latter is a reactive sclerosis within the bone which is not encapsulated and which ceases to enlarge after a time.

Periosteal Cancellous Osteoma.—The periosteal cancellous osteoma may also occur anywhere around the jaws and it is often pedunculated. Radiographs show a cancellous mass surrounded by a thin layer of compact bone. Its removal is facilitated by the fact that it is easily sectioned with a chisel.

Torus Mandibularis.—The torus mandibularis is a cancellous exostosis found on the lingual side of the mandible in the region of the premolars. Like the torus palatinus, it varies in size and shape but is usually bilateral. It constitutes a formidable impediment to the construction of a lower denture and is easily removed by chisel or bur through an incision of suitable length made along the crest of the lower ridge.

Endosteal Osteoma.—The endosteal osteoma is usually located in the mandible and may attain a considerable size. The so-called 'endosteal osteoma' of the nasal sinuses (Rawlins, 1938) is of course subperiosteal in origin, although occurring within the sinus cavity. Small osteomas are usually symptomless and are discovered as an incidental finding on routine radiography. However, when they increase in size they extrude from the mandible and large osteomas of this type have been reported by Fickling (1951), Gilbert (1954), Uhler (1957), and Cooke (1957). Treatment is by surgical removal and, following adequate surgery, recurrence is rare. Endosteal osteoma must be differentiated from reactive bone sclerosis and the gigantic type of cementoma.

Multiple Osteomas.—In 1943 Fitzgerald reported the case of a woman with bony exostoses, desmoids, and multiple polyposis of the colon, and in 1936 Thoma reported the case of a patient with bony tumours of the jaws and fibroids of the skin. Unaware of these earlier reports, Gardner and co-workers (1953; 1962) described a family with multiple osteomas especially of the facial bones, together with epidermoid and sebaceous cysts of the skin, multiple polyposis of the large bowel, and desmoids or fibromas of the skin, and they established the condition as a syndrome. Gorlin and Chaudhry (1960) suggested that the syndrome might be a heritable disorder of connective tissue and it is now considered to have an autosomal dominant pattern.

The multiple intestinal polyposis of the colon and rectum, which has a marked tendency to undergo rapid malignant degeneration, is characteristic of the syndrome, but the condition differs from the Peutz-Jegher's syndrome in that there is no circumoral or intra-oral pigmentation and the polyps which are mainly restricted to the large bowel often become malignant. Multiple osteomas may be scattered through the calvarium and facial skeleton. They first appear at about the time of puberty and similar lesions may be seen in the long bones. In the case reported by

Rayne (1968) a ten-year follow-up radiological examination showed no increase in the size of the oral osteomas. Lucas (1964) states that it is unknown whether the peripheral osteoma is a neoplasm or a developmental anomaly. He also states that the osteoma does not recur after removal and it would therefore appear logical to suggest surgery to remove particularly unsightly or prosthetically inconvenient osteomas in patients with this condition. Dental anomalies including odontomas and multiple unerupted supernumerary and permanent teeth have been reported and bear comparison with those found in cleidocranial dyostosis, while the presence of many epithelial anomalies such as polyps, adenocarcinomas, sebaceous cysts, and odontomas may imply that there is an ancillary growth disorder of epithelium.

REFERENCES

ABRIKOSSOFF, A. (1926), 'Ueber Myome ausgehend von quergestreifter willkürlicher Muskulatur', *Virchows Arch. path. Anat. Physiol.*, **260**, 215.
— — (1931), 'Weitere Untersuchungen über Myoblastermyome', *Ibid.*, **280**, 731.
AIRD, I. (1957), *A Companion to Surgical Studies*, 2nd ed. Edinburgh: Livingstone.
AXHAUSEN, G. (1940), *Die allgemeine chirurgie in der zahn, mund-u-kieferheil-kunde*, p. 355. Munich: Lehmann.
BARKER, D. S., and LUCAS, R. B. (1967), 'Localised Fibrous Overgrowths of the Oral Mucosa', *Br. J. oral Surg.*, **5**, 86.
BATTLE, R. J. V., HOVELL, J. H., and SPENCER, H. (1952), 'Pigmented Adamantinoma', *Br. J. Surg.*, **39**, 368–370.
BERNIER, J. L. (1946), 'Myoblastoma', *J. dent. Res.*, **25**, 253.
— — (1947), 'Myoblastoma', *Am. J. Orthod.*, **33**, 548.
BHASKAR, S. N. (1966), 'Periapical Lesions: Types, Incidence and Clinical Features', *Oral Surg.*, **21**, 657.
BLANC, W. A., ROSENBLATT, P., and WOLFF, J. A. (1958), 'Melanotic Proponoma (Retinal Anlage Tumour) of the Shoulder in an Infant', *Cancer*, **11**, 959–962.
BORELLO, E. D., and GORLIN, R. J. (1966), 'Melanotic Neurectodermal Tumour of Infancy', *Ibid.*, **19**, 196–206.
BRET-DAY, R. C. (1964), 'Granular Cell Myoblastoma', *Br. J. oral Surg.*, **2**, 65.
BRODERICK, R. A., and ROUND, H. (1933), 'Cavernous Haemangioma', *Lancet*, **2**, 13.
BUCHNER, H. J. (1937), 'Diffuse Fibroma of the Gums', *J. Am. dent. Ass.*, **24**, 2003.
CLARKE, B. E., and PARSONS, H. (1951), 'An Embryological Tumour of Retinal Anlage involving the Skull', *Cancer*, **4**, 78–85.
COOK, T. J. (1950), 'Fibroma of the Tuberosity of the Palate', *Oral Surg.*, **3**, 33.
COOKE, B. E. D. (1957), 'Benign Fibro-osseous Enlargements of the Jaw', *Br. dent. J.* **102**, 55.
CRANE, A. R., and TRENBLAY, R. G. (1945), 'Myoblastoma', *Am. J. Path.*, **21**, 357.
DAVIES, D. (1964), 'Cavernous Haemangioma of Mandible', *Dent. Abstr., Chicago*, **9**, 501.
EATON, W. L., and FERGUSON, J. P. (1956), 'A Retinoblastic Teratoma of the Epididymis', *Cancer*, **9**, 718–720.
FICKLING, B. W. (1951), 'Osteoma of the Mandible', *Proc. R. Soc. Med.*, **44**, 56.
FITZGERALD, G. M. (1943), 'Multiple Composite Odontomes Coincidental with other Tumerous Conditions', *J. Am. dent. Ass.*, **30**, 1408.
FOGH-ANDERSEN, P. (1943), 'Fibroma symmetrica gingivalis', *Tandlaegebladet*, **47**, 145–149.
FREEMAN, M. J., and STANDISH, S. M. (1965), 'Facial and Oral Manifestations of Familial Disseminated Neurofibromatosis', *Oral Surg.*, **19**, 52.
GARDNER, E. J. (1962), 'Follow-up Study of a Family Group exhibiting Dominant Inheritance for a Syndrome including Intestinal Polyposis, Osteomas, Fibromas and Epidermal Cysts', *Am. J. hum. Genet.*, **14**, 376.
— — and RICHARDS, R. C. (1953), 'Multiple Cutaneous and Subcutaneous Lesions occurring Simultaneously with Hereditary Polyposis and Osteomatosis', *Ibid.*, **5**, 139.

GESHICKTER, C. F. (1934), 'Diagnosis and Treatment of the More Common Diseases of the Oral Mucous Membrane', *Il Dent.*, **8**, 96.
GILBERT, R. K. (1954), 'A Case of a Peripheral Ivory Osteoma of the Mandible', *Br. dent. J.*, **96**, 15.
GORLIN, R. J., and CHAUDHRY, A. P. (1960), 'Oral Manifestations of the Fitzgerald-Gardiner Syndromes', *Oral Surg.*, **13**, 1233.
GRAY, W. (1961), 'Oral Lipoma', *Br. dent. J.*, **110**, 55.
HALPERT, B. and PATZER, R. (1947), 'Maxillary Tumour of Retinal Anlage', *Surgery*, **22**, 837.
HAYWARD, A. F., FICKLING, B. W., and LUCAS, R. B. (1969), 'An Electron Microscopic Study of a Pigmented Tumour of the Jaw of Infants', *Br. J. Cancer*, **23**, 702–705.
HEARD, G. (1962), 'Nerve Sheath Tumours and Von Recklinghausen's Disease of the Nervous System', *Ann. R. Coll. Surg.*, **31**, 229.
HIEBERT, A. E., and BROOKS, H. W. (1950), 'Fibroma of the Palate', *Plastic reconstr. Surg.*, **5**, 532.
JONES, P., and WILLIAMS, A. (1960), 'A Case of Multicentric Melanotic Adamantinoma', *Br. J. Surg.*, **48**, 282.
KERR, D. A. (1949), 'Myoblastic Myoma', *Oral Surg.*, **2**, 41.
—— and PULLON, P. S. (1964), 'A Study of the Pigmented Tumours of the Jaws of Infants', *Ibid.*, **18**, 759–772.
KLINGE, F. (1928), 'Ueber die sogenannten unreifen nicht guergestenmyome myoblasten-myome', *Verh. dt. path. Ges.*, **23**, 376.
KOUDSTAAL, J., OLDHOFF, J., PONDERS, A. K., and HARDORK, M. J. (1968), 'Melanotic Neurectodermal Tumor of Infancy', *Cancer*, **22**, 151–161.
KROH, F. (1926), 'A Cavernous Angioma in Mandible', *Br. Dent. J.*, **47**, 566.
KROMPECHER, E. (1918), 'Zur Histogenese und Morphologie der Adamantinome und sonstiger Kiefergeschwalste', *Beitr. Pathol. Anat.*, **64**, 165.
LANGDON, J. D. (1970), 'Rieger's Syndrome', *Oral Surg.*, **30**, 758–795.
LEOPARD, P. L., and POSWILLO, D. E. (1974), 'Practical Cryosurgery for Oral Lesions', *Br. dent. J.*, **136**, 185–196.
LINDERMAN, A. G. (1941), *Die chirurgie des gesichtes der mundhohle under der luftwege.* Berlin-Wien, 71–72.
LUCAS, R. B. (1964), *Pathology of Tumours of the Oral Tissues.* London: Churchill.
MACDONALD, A. M., and WHITE, M. (1954), 'Pigmented Congenital Epulides of Neuro-epithelial Origin', *Br. J. Surg.*, **41**, 610.
MISUGI, K., OKAJIMA, H., NEWTON, W. A., KENETZ, D. P., and LORIMER, A. A. (1965), 'Mediastinal Origin of a Melanotic Progonoma in Retinal Anlage Tumour—Ultrastructural Evidence for Neural Crest Origin', *Cancer*, **18**, 477–484.
MOOSE, S. M. (1957), 'Sinusoidal Aneurism of the Mandible', *J. oral Surg.*, **15**, 245.
MORRISON, D. BEERS (1953), 'Bilateral Fibroma of the Palate', *Ibid.*, **11**, 330.
MUMMERY, J. A., and PITTS, A. T. (1925), 'Melanotic Epithelial Odontome in Child'. *Proc. R. Soc. Med.*, **19**, 11 (Reprinted *Br. dent. J.*, **47**, 121).
NEUSTEIN, H. B. (1967), 'Fine Structure of a Melanotic Progonoma or Retinal Anlage Tumor of the Anterior Fontanel', *Exp. Mol. Pathol.*, **6**, 131–142.
PACKARD, H. R., and BAXTER, W. F. (1960), 'Aneurism of the Right Maxilla', *J. oral Surg.*, **18**, 71.
PONTIUS, E. E. (1965), 'Multicentric Melanoameloblastoma of the Maxilla', *Cancer*, **18**, 381–387.
POWELL, A. (1946), 'Granular Cell Myoblastoma', *Archs Path.*, **42**, 517.
RAHB, H. (1936), *Dt. Zahn- Mund- u. Kieferheilk.*, **3**, 555.
RAWLINS, A. G. (1938), 'Osteoma', *Ann. Otol. Rhinol. Lar.*, **47**, 735.
RAYNE, J. (1968), 'Gardiner's Syndrome', *Br. J. oral Surg.*, **6**, 11.
RUSHTON, M. A. (1957), 'Hereditary or Idiopathic Hyperplasia of the Gums', *Dent. Practnr dent. Rec.*, **7**, 136.
SEWARD, M. H. (1965), 'An Osteoma of the Maxilla', *Br dent J*, **118**, 27.
SHIRA, R. B., and GUERNSEY, L. H. (1965), 'Central Cavernous Haemangioma of the Mandible', *J. oral Surg.*, **23**, 636.
SIMON, A. (1947), 'Granular Cell Myoblastoma', *Am. J. clin. Path,.* **17**, 302.
SMITH, W. H. (1959), Haemangioma of the Jaws', *Arch Otolar.*, **70**, 579.
STOWENS, D. (1957), 'A Pigmented Tumour of Infancy: The Melanotic Progonoma', *J. Pathol. Bact.*, **73**, 43.
STRAITH, F. E. (1942), 'Fibroma of the Palatal Tuberosity', *Am. J. Orthod.*, **28**, 434.

THOMA, K. H. (1936), 'Osteodysplasia with Multiple Mesenchymal Tumours: Fibroma, Exotoses and Osteomas', *Orthodontia*, **22**, 1177.
UHLER, I. V. (1957), 'Massive Osteoma of the Mandible', *Oral Surg.*, **10**, 243.
WILLIS, R. A. (1958), 'Histogenesis of Pigmented Epulis in Infancy', *J. Pathol. Bact.*, **73**, 89.

CHAPTER VIII

BENIGN SOFT-TISSUE CYSTS

DERMOID CYSTS OF THE FLOOR OF THE MOUTH AND TONGUE

DERMOID cysts may be found in the midline of the floor of the mouth, in the midline of the tongue, and laterally in the gutter between the hyoglossus and mylohyoid muscles.

Midline Dermoid Cysts of the Floor of the Mouth.—In childhood midline dermoid cysts of the floor of the mouth may be found as small, yellowish spheres lying in the connective tissue beneath the lingual fraenum and just posterior to the mandible. As they increase in size they push apart the genioglossus muscles, moving deeper into the floor of the mouth and backwards into the tongue. They may be forced into this position by the tongue itself since the tongue occupies most of the space within the dental arches when the mouth is closed. (*Figs.* 9, 10.) Such cysts bulge

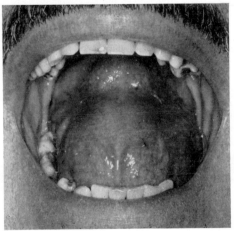

Fig. 9.—A median dermoid cyst of the floor of the mouth. The cyst is deeper in than the ranula, more firm to touch, and symmetrically disposed about the midline.

upwards and forwards towards the oral cavity as the mouth is opened and the mylohyoid and digastrics contract. When the mouth is closed they are displaced in the opposite direction producing a swelling in the submental region which the patient may mistake for a 'double chin'. A few cysts may develop rather more deeply in the tissues, that is between the genioglossl since they do not form the characteristic oral swelling.

Irrespective of their clinical presentation all median dermoid cysts of the floor of the mouth lie relatively close below the mucous membrane. As they increase still further in size, they pass downwards and backwards to the hyoid and epiglottis and separate the geniohyoid muscles to reach the mylohyoid. Some pass lateral to one of the geniohyoid muscles. A few squeeze part of their mass through the perforations in the mylohyoid muscles traversed by anastomotic branches between the submandibular and sublingual arteries. If they are left in situ beyond this stage they will cause an increase in size of the lower dental arch and then proclination of the lower incisors. Eventually it will prove impossible for the patient to close the mouth.

The lining epithelium may be plain, stratified, squamous epithelium (epidermoid type), or it may contain sebaceous glands and hair follicles (dermoid type). Some may have a small or substantial part of the lining composed of mucus-secreting and ciliated epithelium suggesting an endodermal origin. The dermal and epidermal varieties are filled with a

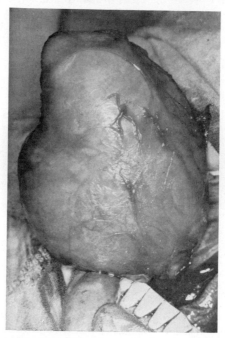

Fig. 10.—The same cyst at operation demonstrating the size of cyst which can be accommodated in the tissues at this site.

pultaceous mass of desquamated epithelial cells. The endodermal types are fluctuant and contain mucus. Because of the character of their lining epithelium, these lesions must arise close to the junction between ectoderm and endoderm and possibly between the paired contribution from the mandibular arch to the anterior two-thirds of the tongue.

Their removal is accomplished through an incision in the free edge of the lingual fraenum, from just behind the tip of the tongue down to its attachment to the mandible. A plane of cleavage is established between the cyst and the surrounding tissues. Any sizeable vessels crossing to the cyst are diathermized. Very large cysts must be opened once the dissection has progressed as far as possible around the periphery. The contents are aspirated and a finger inserted into the cavity so that the remainder can be separated in the same way as the sac of an inguinal hernia. That is, one finger is inserted into the cavity and indicates the site of the wall of the cyst while traction is applied to the lesion with the other fingers. It is then possible to separate the outside of the sac from the adjacent tissue with scissors without risk of tearing the sac or damage to adjacent structures. The wound is closed with vacuum drainage.

Dermoid Cysts of the Tongue.—Dermoid cysts occur as a rare entity in the midline of the tongue. They are, for the most part, of the epidermal type (Goldberg, 1965), but may have mucus-secreting, ciliated, or even gastric epithelium forming part of their lining indicating a mixed ecto-dermal and endodermal origin for the epithelium. Cysts in other locations about the tongue and floor of mouth with gastric and intestinal mucosa in the lining are described by Gorlin and Jirasek (1970). Treatment is by enucleation.

Lateral Dermoid Cysts of the Floor of the Mouth.—Lateral dermoid cysts arise in the gutter between the hyoglossus, geniohyoid, and genio-glossus which lie medially, and the mylohyoid which lies laterally. They are positioned deep to the submandibular duct and lingual nerve and anterior to the stylohyoid ligament. Thus, they may arise from the ventral end of either the first pharyngeal pouch, or the first branchial cleft (Seward, 1965). Most lateral dermoids are lined by stratified squamous epithelium which may come either from ectoderm or endoderm, while some may be lined by ciliated, columnar epithelium which implies an endodermal origin. A few contain hairs (Cook, 1950; Duvergey, 1907) suggesting an origin from the first branchial cleft. Gold (1962) has described an example with a subepidermal lymphatic infiltration as is found in second-cleft branchial cysts, but this is exceptional.

When they are small, these cysts produce a fullness laterally in the sub-lingual sulcus and anteriorly in the submandibular region. At this stage they are deep in the tissues and not particularly close to either surface. Later they emerge behind the posterior end of the mylohyoid and displace the submandibular salivary gland to present as a prominent swelling in the neck. If left, they can push backwards medial to the mandible, up to the tonsil, and downwards to the sternomastoid muscle and the internal jugular vein.

Small cysts may be removed through an incision in the floor of the mouth lateral to the tongue after careful identification of the lingual nerve and submandibular duct. Larger cysts should be removed through a submandibular incision so that adjacent blood-vessels can be formally exposed.

BRANCHIAL CYST

Branchial cysts may be found at the site of the second branchial cleft and pharyngeal pouch. Some more rare cysts found about the pharynx and neck may be related to the first and second pouches, the third and the fourth pouch (Wilson, 1955). The majority are lined by stratified squamous epithelium, but some of the deeper ones are lined by columnar epithelium. All have a subepithelial infiltration with lymphocytes.

Those developing from the second pharyngeal pouch present towards the back of the upper pole of the tonsil. Those developing from the second branchial cleft produce oval, fluctuant swellings emerging from beneath the anterior border of the sternomastoid, just below the angle of the mandible. In this situation they must be distinguished from a tuberculous abscess. Cautious aspiration through an oblique needle track may help to establish the diagnosis. Branchial cyst fluid often contains cholesterol crystals and tuberculous pus can be cultured or inoculated into guinea-pigs.

The treatment is excision.

MUCOUS EXTRAVASATION AND RETENTION CYSTS

These occur in two clinical forms about the mouth: small mucoceles or mucous cysts of the lips, cheeks, undersurface of tongue, and floor of mouth and the larger ranula.

Mucocele.—

*Aetiology.—*Formerly it was thought that these were all retention cysts resulting from the obstruction of the duct of one of the minor mucous salivary glands. Attempts to produce retention cysts by ligation of the duct of a salivary gland did not, however, result in the production of a cyst since acinar atrophy followed (Bhaskar, Bolden, and Weinmann, 1956; Standish and Shafer, 1957). In 1957, Standish and Shafer showed that the majority of mucous cysts did not have an epithelial lining, but that a mucus-filled cavity in the connective tissue communicated with a breach in the wall of the duct of an adjacent mucous gland. Other observers have confirmed these observations. Further experiments, in which the duct of a salivary gland was divided so that the secretions escaped into the tissues, resulted in the formation of similar cysts (Bhaskar and others 1956; Chaudhry and others, 1960). The majority of these lesions, therefore, result from damage to, or rupture of, the duct of a minor salivary gland such that mucus can escape into the tissues.

More recently Sela and Ulmansky (1969) have described small epithelium-lined cysts of minor salivary glands. These appear to constitute a dilatation, or saccular out-pouching, of the duct, and serial sections have revealed calculi within the duct. It seems, therefore, that with complete obstruction, pressure within the duct rises to a point where further secretion is prevented and acinar atrophy occurs. With incomplete obstruction, as by a calculus, secretion continues and dilatation of the duct eventually results.

*Clinical Appearances.—*Mucous cysts are usually superficial and only occasionally do they occur deep in the tissues. Superficial cysts appear as a circumscribed swelling which seldom exceeds 1–2 cm. in diameter. They form a tense or slightly flaccid swelling which has a bluish, greenish, or orange-yellow colour. The tense swelling is often inadvertently punctured by the patient's teeth, whereupon it bursts and discharges a gelatinous material. The lesion then subsides completely, only to fill up again over a period of time. Some patients deliberately bite, or puncture the cyst with a needle in order to get rid of it for a while. Deeply-placed mucous cysts are covered by normal mucosa, are more difficult to diagnose, and may be mistaken for a pleomorphic adenoma. Occasionally after rupture of the cyst, a sinus forms with a polyp of granulation tissue at the entrance. This is usually mistaken for a small fibro-epithelial polyp. Excision of the pedunculated swelling is invariably followed by its rapid recurrence. If, however, the cause of such a lesion is known, or the sinus closed by surgery and the reformed cyst observed before it can rupture again, then the correct diagnosis may be made. Provided that the causative mucous gland is then excised, a cure will result.

Histology.—The mucus extravasation cyst, in the early stages, is composed of pools of mucus lying in the connective tissue adjacent to a breach in the duct of a minor salivary gland. Granulation tissue is provoked and forms the first lining of the cyst. Some phagocytosis occurs both of the mucus and of some debris composed of desquamated epithelial cells from the duct. In time the granulations mature to form a fibrous capsule. The majority of such cysts remain without an epithelial lining, but in some cases epithelium from the duct migrates to line the wall partially. In others, flattened fibroblasts on the inner surface of the capsule may be mistaken for epithelial cells. The mucus retention cyst of Sela and Ulmansky is lined by a complete layer of duct epithelium.

Treatment.—The treatment is drainage of the mucus and excision of the salivary gland which is secreting the mucus. It is usual to remove the mucus by attempting to excise the entire cyst sac, but this is by no means easy. As has been seen in many cases, there is no definite sac, only pools of mucus, some of which may lie just beneath the mucous membrane of the mouth. Only the mature fibrous and epithelium-lined sacs can be removed, and these only provided that technical care is exercised. An incision is made in the mucosa to one side of the maximum eminence of the cyst and the cyst separated by gentle dissection with blunt-ended, fine scissors. A mixture of sharp and blunt dissection is necessary. The offending gland comes into view as the operation proceeds and is removed with the cyst. The resulting cavity is obliterated by the sutures as the wound is closed.

Ingenious operations in which alginate impression material is injected into the cyst cavity, or the cavity packed with ribbon gauze to facilitate marsupialization, are clearly unnecessary. Indeed, marsupialization is illogical since the majority of cysts are not epithelium-lined. Only if a fistula forms between the breach in the duct and the surface will the technique succeed, and this is usually prevented from happening by contraction and granulation of the connective tissue-lined cavity.

The Ranula.—The ranula is a thin-walled, bluish, transparent cyst which specifically occurs in the floor of the mouth beneath the tongue, blood-vessels in the mucous membrane course over the surface. The name arose because of the resemblance of the fully blown lesion to a frog's belly. (*Fig.* 11.)

It grows slowly and forms a painless, soft, fluctuant swelling, which usually occurs to one side of the midline, but may cross the midline as it enlarges. It is then constricted by the fraenum and may assume an hour glass shape. At first it is covered by mucosa of normal colour, but as it enlarges it takes on the classic appearance. Sometimes these cysts become sufficiently large to raise the tongue and if inadvertently punctured by the teeth or hard food they collapse with a discharge of mucoid material into the mouth. The ranula reforms when the puncture wound heals and it gradually refills with mucoid material. The stretched mucosa is always freely movable over the cyst. In some patients the submandibular duct passes over the surface of the ranula like a white cord.

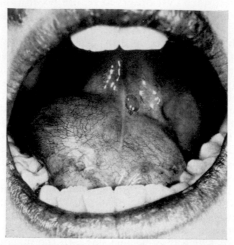

Fig. 11.—A typical ranula passing submucosally from right to left across the floor of the mouth. Note the dilated vessels which give the appearance resembling a frog's belly.

Two clinical forms of ranula are described: one is confined to the floor of the mouth and the other, the plunging ranula, passes back through the submandibular region and then down into the neck. In extreme cases it may almost reach the mediastinum.

Aetiology.—In the past there has been considerable controversy concerning the origin of these cysts. Obstruction of the duct of a salivary gland, inflammation or myxomatous degeneration of the sublingual salivary glands or the glands of Blandin and Nuhn were popular theories. A failure to understand their origin together with the incorrect notion that they were lined with epithelium led to many ineffective treatments and consequently recurrence was common.

Recently it has been realized that the ranula is an extravasation cyst, like the majority of the smaller mucoceles found on the lips and cheek. The only difference is that a larger gland, one of the sublingual glands, is involved and hence the volume of mucus saliva produced is greater. The anterior sublingual glands, either Bartholin's major sublingual or one of the minor sublingual glands, produce the ranula on the floor of the mouth. The posterior sublingual is the causative gland for the plunging ranula.

Histological Features.—These are similar to those of the mucocele. If a portion of the cyst sac is recovered it will be found to be composed of a thin layer of fibrous tissue. Not uncommonly a layer of cuboidal cells is seen, one cell thick on its inner surface. It is these which were mistaken for epithelial cells. Closer inspection shows them to be macrophages.

Treatment.—As long ago as 1897, Von Hipple advocated excision of the ranula complete with the sublingual gland and since then a number of authors have recognized this relationship to the sublingual gland. Crile (1957), for example, thought that excision of the cyst wall without removal of the gland resulted in recurrence and advocated simple drainage of plunging ranulas followed by excision of the appropriate sublingual gland. Whitlock and Summersgill (1962) eventually dealt successfully with a recurrent plunging ranula by excision of the sublingual gland and without a further attack on the cyst itself. Catone, Merrill, and Henny (1969) advocate formal exposure and removal of the sublingual gland.

A vasoconstrictor-containing solution is used to infiltrate the floor of the mouth and an incision made towards the lingual side of the plica sublingualis. As a first step the submandibular duct is identified and isolated. It is followed backwards and the lingual nerve found where it passes beneath the duct and a tape passed around it. Provided that the tissue lingual to the duct is not entered, the sublingual veins are not disturbed, and that the dissection is not carried deep to the submandibular duct and lingual nerve, neither the sublingual artery nor the hypoglossal nerve should be encountered.

The mucosal flap lateral to the incision is separated from the upper surface of the sublingual gland mass which can then be rolled medially off the surface of the mylohyoid muscle. Where the deep part of the submandibular gland is large, the lingual nerve tends to pass between the deep part and the duct as it travels forwards. Where the deep part is small, the posterior sublingual gland may be large and the nerve will pass obliquely under its posterior end from lateral to medial and will come into view again as the gland is rolled medially.

Final separation of the gland is from before backwards, lifting the anterior end out of the wound and completing the separation with a blunt dissector made by rolling cotton-wool pads tightly round the ends of closed artery forceps. Small vessels supplying the sublingual gland from the sublingual and submandibular arteries will be encountered and can be diathermized with care. The mucosa is then closed with few loose sutures.

The ranula itself is frequently ruptured and virtually vanishes at an early stage in the procedure, but this does not matter. If it does not do so, the sac can be separated and removed together with the gland.

RETENTION CYST OF SUBMANDIBULAR DUCT

Complete obstruction of the submandibular duct, as for example by ligation, results in atrophy of the submandibular gland or, should the duct rupture at or behind the ligature, the production of a salivary fistula into the mouth or into the tissues. However, a case of congenital occlusion of the duct has been described which resulted in a cystic swelling in the floor of the baby's mouth (Beke, Tomaro, and Stein, 1963).

ECTOPIC ORAL TONSILS

Knapp (1970) describes in some detail the appearances produced by oral tonsillar tissue. He describes round, oval, or bean-shaped elevations up to 1 cm. in length. Some are smooth and rounded, some flat plaques, and others nodular elevations. A few form yellowish globules which may discharge their contents on pressure.

The nodular lesions are hyperplastic lymphoid tissue around a tonsillar crypt. If the crypt becomes obstructed, keratin collects within to form a pseudocyst: the yellow globular lesion. Where the tonsils are traumatized they may be inflamed and hyperaemic, forming reddish elevations. Oral tonsils can be found on the soft palate, the tongue, and the floor of the mouth, either singly or in groups.

No treatment is required unless pseudocysts are formed which become infected. These may be either drained or excised.

OTHER ENTITIES

Lymphangiomas should not be mistaken for ranulas, since they often involve the dorsum of the tongue, are brownish and nodular, like the back of a warty toad rather than a frog's belly. Cystic hygroma may rarely involve the floor of the mouth, but involves the neck at the same time and is seen in the young infant. Curiously, although Fordyce's spots are common, sebaceous cysts are not seen. Even sebaceous adenomas of the buccal mucosa are rare, but Miller and McCrea (1968) have recorded such an occurrence.

REFERENCES

BEKE, A. L., TOMARO, A. J., and STEIN, M. (1963), 'Congenital Atresia of Sublingual Duct with Ranula', *J. oral Surg.*, **21,** 427.

BHASKAR, S. N., BOLDEN, T. E., and WEINMANN, J. P. (1956), 'Experimental Obstructive Adenitis in the Mouse', *J. dent. Res.*, **35,** 852.

CATONE, G. A., MERRILL, R. G., and HENNY, F. A. (1969), 'Sublingual Gland Mucus-escape Phenomenon: Treatment by Excision of Sub-lingual Gland', *J. oral Surg.*, **27,** 774.

CHAUDHRY, A. P., and others (1960), 'Clinical and Experimental Study of Mucocele (Retention Cyst)', *J. dent. Res.*, **39,** 1253.

COOK, J. T. (1950), 'Dermoid Cyst', *Oral Surg.*, **3,** 740.

CRILE, G. (1957), 'Ranulas with Extension into the Neck: So-called Plunging Ranulas', *Surgery, St Louis*, **42,** 819.

DUVERGEY, J. (1907), *Ann. Chir.*, **20,** 368.

GOLD, C. (1962), *Oral Surg.*, **15,** 1118.

GOLDBERG, A. F. (1965), 'Dermoid Cyst of the Tongue', *J. oral Surg.*, **23,** 649.

GORLIN, R. J., and JIRASEK, J. E. (1970), 'Oral Cysts containing Gastric or Intestinal Mucosa', *Ibid.*, **28,** 9.

KNAPP, M. J. (1970), 'Pathology of Oral Tonsil', *Oral Surg.*, **29,** 295.

MILLER, A. S., and McCREA, M. W. (1968), 'Sebaceous Gland Adenoma of the Buccal Mucosa', *J. oral Surg.*, **26,** 593.

SELA, J., and ULMANSKY, M. (1969), 'Mucous Retention Cyst of Salivary Glands', *Ibid.*, **27,** 619.

SEWARD, G. R. (1965), 'Dermoid Cysts of the Floor of the Mouth', *Br. J. oral Surg.*, **3,** 36.

STANDISH, S. M., and SHAFER, W. C. (1957), 'Serial Histologic Effects of Rat Sub-maxillary and Sub-lingual Salivary Gland Duct and Blood Vessel Ligation', *J. dent. Res.*, **36,** 866.

VON HIPPLE, R. (1897), 'Ueber Bau und Wesen der Ranula', *Arch. klin. Chir.*, **55,** 164.

WHITLOCK, R. I., and SUMMERSGILL, G. B. (1962), 'Ranula with Cervical Extension', *Oral Surg.*, **15,** 1163.

WILSON, C. P. (1955), 'Lateral Cysts and Fistulae of the Neck of Developmental Origin', *Ann. R. Coll. Surg.*, **17,** 1.

CHAPTER IX

GIANT-CELL LESIONS OF THE JAWS

THE CENTRAL GIANT-CELL GRANULOMA

THE term 'giant-cell reparative granuloma' was coined by Jaffe in 1953, for the central, giant-cell lesion of the jaws, although the term has since been applied by others to the giant-cell epulis as well.

In order to understand Jaffe's concept of the giant-cell reparative granuloma, it is necessary to review the way in which it arose. Jaffe, Lichtenstein, and Portis and then Jaffe made a study of the giant-cell tumours of bone and noted that there was a marked difference in the behaviour of the lesions of long bones and those of the jaws. They noted that the long bone osteoclastoma was a treacherous lesion which often recurred and could metastasize. By comparison the jaw tumours were benign. When Jaffe investigated the two groups he found further differences. The long bone tumours tended to occur between 20 and 55 years of age, whereas the maximum incidence for the jaw lesion was between 10 and 25 years of age. Further, in histological sections from long bone lesions there were many giant cells evenly distributed throughout the tumour and varying degrees of atypicality of the stromal cells. In general there was no new bone formation. Sections from the jaw tumours showed a focal distribution of the giant cells and spicules of woven bone were frequent.

Because of its behaviour, Jaffe felt that the jaw condition was dysplastic rather than neoplastic and looked upon it as an abnormal granulation tissue, or tissue of repair. Hence, he coined the name 'giant-cell reparative granuloma'.

Since Jaffe's papers in 1953, our concept of this lesion has undergone further modifications. Most people agree that the term 'reparative' was unfortunate and could imply, to those who did not know the context in which Jaffe used it, that the natural history of the condition was biased towards repair. In fact, it seems to remain destructive and few would be courageous enough to observe one in the hope of spontaneous cure. Thus, mostly they are now called 'giant-cell granulomas', and the word 'reparative' has been dropped.

In support of the non-neoplastic nature of the condition is the realization that incomplete removal can result in a cure. The periphery is complex and even after careful enucleation small pockets of abnormal tissue can be left behind. These do not necessarily lead to recurrence. Further, it can be shown histologically that the marrow spaces adjacent to the major bone cavity are involved and these are not touched by simple surgery, yet a successful outcome is not affected. On occasions a generous biopsy has been known to stimulate healing. None of this is compatible with the natural history of even a benign neoplasm.

Jaffe's concept of the age of incidence has had also to be modified. Quite a number of cases of giant-cell granuloma have been observed in the age-group 25–40 years and some in patients as young as $2\frac{1}{2}$–3 years and as old as 63 years.

Because a similar histological appearance is shared by a number of diseases of bone, the concept has grown up that they are all disturbances of the tissue which resorbs bone. Disturbances of a tissue which features multinucleated giant cells, thin-walled blood-vessels, a proliferation of a cellular, skeletal connective tissue, and histiocytes. Thus, the giant-cell granuloma can be looked upon as a dysplasia of the resorptive tissue of bone.

At various times it has been postulated that haemorrhage is the stimulus that incites the appearance of the giant cells. It is true that red cells are frequently seen in sections of surgical specimens and biopsies, but these are obviously spilt at the time of removal. It is also true that blood pigments can be found in the histiocytes, but even this is not surprising since the blood-vessels are so thin-walled. Indeed, in places the wall of a capillary may be replaced by a giant cell which 'collars' it, so that some leakage of red corpuscles in life could easily occur. There is, however, no evidence of appreciable phagocytosis of red blood corpuscles by the giant cell, nor are giant cells produced in other body tissues to deal with extravasated red cells.

There is, unfortunately, no histochemical difference between osteoclasts and foreign-body giant cells, but the constant association of the whole group of these lesions with bone makes it likely that these particular giant cells are osteoclasts.

It has been pointed out that the giant-cell granuloma favours the tooth-bearing part of the jaws and in particular regions which have supported primary teeth. This may be of diagnostic and possibly aetiological significance.

Females are said to be affected more often than males and the mandible more often than the maxilla. From their radiological appearances, central giant-cell granulomas can be subdivided into two types: those which appear to start in the medullary cavity and those which start subperiosteally.

The Central Medullary Type occurs almost exclusively in the tooth-bearing part of the jaws and produces an oval, or loculated, cavity in the bone. Marked resorption of the cortical plates takes place at an early stage in their development so that the transverse diameter of the lesion is often only a little less than its anteroposterior diameter. A thin layer of subperiosteal new bone covers the parts which have bulged beyond the original cortex. An important radiological characteristic of the sub-periosteal bone is that it is polyarcuate in outline as seen on occlusal radiographs.

Histologically the giant-cell granuloma consists of zones of the charac-teristic tissue, separated by septa rich in collagen fibres in which, in older lesions, woven bone is deposited. It is this lobulated structure, together with a marked ability to cause the resorption of adjacent bone and teeth, which accounts for its radiological features.

The lobulated surface results in a varying degree of ridging of the inner aspect of the bone cavity. In radiographs this produces a multilocular or cross-hatched appearance, particularly in the maxilla. New bone is laid down to form short, incomplete septa which run inwards from the indentations in the subperiosteal new bone. Where laterally directed X-rays pass tangential to these septa, linear shadows are produced in the periapical and oblique lateral jaw films which add to the multilocular appearance.

In the mandible early destruction of cortical bone results in dark, well-defined images in the lateral views which again can increase the appearance of loculation. Especially is this so if the subperiosteal new bone bulges laterally almost at right angles to the jaw surface so that a thin white linear image is cast, outlining the edge of the dark image.

In occlusal radiographs a Codman's triangle of new bone is seen at the junction of the subperiosteal sheet of bone with the old cortex. In some occlusal radiographs the raised periosteum appears to cover a greater area than the cortical perforation, though this could be a projection effect. Spicules of new bone other than those forming septa are often seen within that part of the lesion which bulges outside the original outline of the jaw.

Because little bone substance is removed by the intramedullary part of the cavity, the increased radiolucency which results in small and a well-marked periphery is seen only if the margin has a large radius of curvature.

Resorption of the roots of adjacent teeth is a frequent feature and where the surface of the lesion is lobulated several aspects of a root may be affected. Some giant-cell granulomas displace teeth as they increase in size while others loop up between the roots and come to surround them.

The Subperiosteal Type of giant-cell granuloma has the larger part of its bulk external to the normal contours of the jaw, but this does not preclude the involvement of the underlying bone to a considerable depth, especially

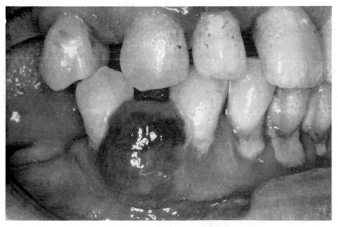

Fig. 12.—Subperiosteal giant-cell granuloma.

in the maxilla. Careful radiography will demonstrate a layer of subperiosteal new bone over at least part of the surface of the mass, though it may be less obvious than the subperiosteal bone formed over the extra-cortical expansions of the intramedullary type. (*See Fig.* 12.)

Because the cortex is attacked from the beginning, and often up to the greatest diameter of the tumour, the lesion has a dark, punched-out appearance in radiographs. When seen in profile, fern-like or tufted arrangements of new bone trabeculae penetrate into the radiolucent centre of the mass.

A variant of the subperiosteal type occurs at the time at which the primary teeth are shed.

There is an excavation in the surface of the alveolar crest which may penetrate between and around the crowns of the permanent teeth. The alveolar process is bulged laterally on one or both aspects and a layer of subperiosteal new bone covers the lesion at these points.

The place where the primary teeth have been lost appears at first sight to be ulcerated. In fact, the tumour is covered by a thin epithelium, but the colour here contrasts with the pale mucoperiosteum on the lateral aspect. Apart from the expansion of the alveolar ridge only the presence of dilated, small vessels on the surface indicates the extent of the condition.

In some instances the permanent teeth erupt around the side of the mass and are further displaced and separated by it as it grows.

Radiographs are generally disappointing, give a poor indication of the size of the lesion, and may reveal few helpful diagnostic features. With care the successional teeth can be conserved, but a cautious prognosis is in order preoperatively, because of the difficulty in judging the extent of the process from the films. It is, of course, tempting to attribute the origin of these particular giant-cell granulomas to the tissue which is responsible for resorbing the deciduous teeth.

Treatment.—The treatment of the central giant-cell granuloma consists of enucleation of the lesion following adequate surgical exposure of the area and this can usually be effected through an intra-oral incision. Following removal of the mass the underlying bony walls and bed of the resulting cavity should be carefully curetted with a sharp Volkmann's scoop. Alternatively, a large rosehead bur can be used, skimming the surface to a depth of 0·5 mm. If this is done small pockets of lesional tissue will be uncovered and removed. These lie in irregular outpouchings of the bony cavity and are left behind as the main mass is removed. Neither important neurovascular bundles nor adjacent teeth should be unnecessarily hazarded by this procedure. Neither electrocoagulation as recommended by Kruger (1959) or thermal or chemical cauterization as suggested by Archer (1956) and Thoma (1962) is necessary, and are to be deprecated since they damage an unpredictable layer of bone which subsequently must be resorbed or sequestrated. If for a particular lesion it is felt that a margin of tissue should be removed, this should be outlined at the beginning, so that the mass is removed intact together with the appropriate margin.

Radiotherapy should not be used for giant-cell granulomas. In a small proportion of cases it is true that radiotherapy will destroy the lesional tissue, but curiously bony healing of the bony cavity does not occur. What is observed is that the margins and any septa become more distinct in the radiographs. Then after some years the lesion starts to grow again. One is then faced with the problem of treating a lesion lying in irradiated bone. Furthermore, radiotherapy should not, in general, be used for the treatment of benign conditions, particularly in the young and especially for tumours of bone where such treatment carries a risk of osteogenic sarcoma arising in 20–25 years.

THE OSTEOCLASTOMA

The term osteoclastoma is now commonly reserved for the malignant neoplasm in this group of lesions. Presumably a benign neoplasm, the benign osteoclastoma, may also exist but there are, at the moment, no criteria by which it can be distinguished from the dysplastic giant-cell granuloma.

Only by their aggressive behaviour and, to some extent, by their histology, can neoplastic osteoclastomas be distinguished from giant-cell granulomas when they occur in the jaws. Indeed, the number of recorded cases which fulfil modern criteria for an osteoclastoma is small. Judging by these reports rapid growth, a poorly defined periphery in the radiographs, little evidence of new bone within the lesion, and little or no subperiosteal new bone over it are sinister features. The value of morphological differentiation between the neoplasm and granuloma is questionable, but certain histological features have been stressed. For instance, the giant cells in the osteoclastoma are stated to be more numerous and more evenly distributed in the spindle-cell stroma. These cells are also said to be of larger size than those of the granuloma, i.e., 50–100 µ, and contain 20–40 centrally placed nuclei. The nuclei may be vesicular or pyknotic and resemble those of the spindle cells. However, most of these characteristics are related to speed of growth and it is worth remembering that giant-cell granulomas can grow rapidly at times, particularly in the young and in pregnant women (McGowan, 1970).

Probably the most valuable criteria to look for are the usual histological characteristics of malignancy: increased nuclear-to-cytoplasm ratio, hyperchronic nuclei, variations in cell and nuclear size and abnormal mitoses.

Perhaps the most frequent malignant giant-cell lesion to involve the jaws is the giant-cell sarcoma seen in Paget's disease.

Treatment.—Once one becomes convinced that the lesion is a malignant osteoclastoma—that is, an aggressive neoplasm—then adequate radical surgery should be employed. The growth should be excised together with a wide margin. Radiotherapy may be necessary where palliative treatment is appropriate, or where tissue planes may have been contaminated by tumour cells during previous surgery.

THE PERIOSTEAL OSTEOCLASTOMA

This lesion has also been described variously as peripheral giant-cell reparative granuloma, peripheral giant-cell tumour, giant-cell epulis, periosteal osteoclastoma, myeloid epulis, and osteoclastoma. The multiplicity of the designations applied to the condition indicate the prevailing confusion concerning its nature and aetiology. It was originally considered to be a true neoplasm but more recently the view has been advanced that it represents an unusual proliferative response of the tissues to injury. Histologically it resembles the giant-cell granuloma.

Clinical Appearance.—The periosteal osteoclastoma almost always occurs on the buccal or labial aspect of the gingiva or alveolar process and appears to arise from the mucoperiosteum (*Fig.* 13). Though unencapsulated, it is not infiltrative. The majority are located in the canine-premolar region, that part of the jaw which has borne deciduous teeth. In the past, the

theory was advanced that a predilection for that site implied a proliferation of the osteoclasts which are normally involved in the shedding
of the deciduous predecessors during the transition from a primary to a
secondary dentition. However, this premise fails to explain the anomalous
occurrence of some of these lesions in the posterior region of the jaws.
The peripheral granuloma is sessile at an early stage, but later it becomes
pedunculated. Its colour is usually purplish, dark red, or haemorrhagic,
but its clinical appearance may vary and at times it may resemble a
fibroma or even a pyogenic granuloma. The maximum diameter rarely
exceeds 3 cm. and the consistency is soft or firm. Almost invariably the
swelling is painless, but rarely it may become ulcerated due to trauma
from opposing teeth or from the use of a toothbrush. When teeth are
present, the granuloma protrudes from an interdental space and may

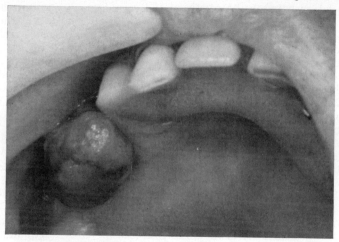

Fig. 13.—Periosteal osteoclastoma or giant-cell epulis; compare this lesion with
the prolapsed antral polyp in *Fig.* 4.

cause divarication of adjacent teeth. In the edentulous patient it usually
arises from the crest of the ridge. Increasing size of the lesion may cause
interference with sleep or mastication. According to Bernick (1948) females
are more commonly affected than males, but Cooke (1952) found that up
to the age of 15 years the sexes were equally involved, although from 20 to
45 years there was a preponderance of affected females which represented
42 per cent of his series. A survey by Killey and Kay (1965) indicated that
the mandible was more often involved than the maxilla.

Histology.—The lesion consists of a non-capsulated mass of tissue
consisting of delicate reticular and fibrillar connective tissue stroma
containing multinucleated giant cells. The latter are scarce and dispersed
in concentric arrangements around foci of haemorrhage. Numerous
capillaries are present and delicate trabeculae of osteoid or immature bone
may be conspicuous.

Radiological Appearance.—A radiological examination will not have
any specific value unless pressure resorption of the underlying bone has

occurred. In such cases, intra-oral radiographs will reveal a sauceriform depression in the surface of the alveolar process which may be well-defined or have an irregular contour.

Treatment.—Treatment is by excision through an incision around the base of the lesion. Unlike the fibroma an excision a few millimetres wide of the obvious periphery is necessary to avoid the possibility of a recurrence but the adjoining teeth should be preserved unless pocketing has occurred interdentally. The surface of the alveolar bone underlying the lesion should be curetted. If a relapse does take place, extraction of the teeth in immediate proximity to the mass must be seriously considered and a vulcanite bur should be run over the surface of the bone to ensure that all the lesional tissue has been removed. The raw area of bone left after the excision should be covered over with a pack of ribbon gauze soaked in Whitehead's varnish. This is left in situ for about ten days, after which the area will be found to have granulated. The site of the periosteal osteoclastoma should be kept under observation at regular intervals, for many months, for some of these lesions show a marked tendency to recur. The periosteal osteoclastoma is sometimes found in patients suffering from hyperparathyroidism and in all such cases a serum calcium and phosphorus estimation should be performed.

BROWN TUMOURS OR NODES

Peripheral or osteolytic central brown tumours or nodes occur in hyperparathyroidism and resemble the giant-cell granuloma both clinically and cytologically. Their incidence is difficult to assess from the literature, because most large published reviews of giant-cell lesions omit details of the proportion due to the endocrine disorder. In Killey and Kay's series of 23 cases, 3 were found to be central hyperparathyroid lesions. Dent (1962; 1966) recognizes three forms of hyperparathyroidism in addition to that due to carcinoma of the gland. These are primary, secondary and tertiary. Primary hyperparathyroidism is due to an adenoma or hyperplasia of the gland, secondary hyperparathyroidism is due to compensatory hyperplasia where there is phosphate retention or impaired calcium absorption, and tertiary hyperparathyroidism is due to an autonomous adenoma which arises in a case of secondary hyperparathyroidism. Secondary hyper-parathyroidism is worthy of special note because usually the serum calcium is not raised in this form of the disease, At one time it was thought that there were two parathyroid hormones: one producing severe bone disease, a high alkaline phosphatase, and renal damage, and the other a high plasma calcium, low plasma phosphorus and their associated systemic disturbances, but a low alkaline phosphatase and less overt bone damage. This is no longer thought to be likely. The possibility of latent hyperparathyroidism must always be considered when giant-cell granu-lomas are diagnosed and particularly if there is a recurrence of the lesion after adequate excision, even though initial laboratory reports reveal that the relevant investigations of blood and urine produce results that are within normal limits. From the limited evidence available, it does seem likely that the jaw lesions can presage the onset of manifest hyper-parathyroidism by a long period; in a case seen by the authors a time lag of one-and-a-half years occurred, and in another instance (Black and Ackerman, 1950) there was a lapse of thirteen years before the underlying parathyroid disease was detected.

Essential diagnostic blood determinations for hyperparathyroidism are the serum calcium, inorganic phosphorus, and alkaline phosphatase values. Excess calcium content in the urine can be determined by the Sulkowitch test which produces a cloudy reaction when positive, but some authorities are highly critical of this investigation, pointing out the high frequency of misleading results. Unfortunately, too, with localized skeletal manifestations of a parathyroid disorder, the alkaline phosphatase level is indecisive, often remaining at the upper limit of normal. McGeown (1961), however, has stressed that the serum calcium concentration is the most important single determination of parathyroid function, provided that the test is repeated three or four times, at intervals, in view of the observation that in hyperparathyroidism the serum calcium values fluctuate and often lie within normal limits. A small rise is significant, but as this can be concealed by increased inorganic phosphorus following exercise and a meal, the patient should be fasted overnight (Harris, 1966). Similarly, where there is a reduction in plasma protein, the loss of protein-bound calcium will also give a low figure. If the specific gravity of the plasma is less than 1·027, 0·25 mg. per cent is added to the calcium value for every unit by which the figure in third decimal place is less than seven, e.g., for a specific gravity of 1·023 add 1 mg. per cent. In contrast, venous stasis by raising the protein-bound calcium in the sample produces an artificially high value, so that a sphygmomanometer cuff must not be used in performing the venepuncture. Electrophoresis can also be employed to detect an abnormal protein picture.

Obviously early recognition of the disease is essential if irreversible renal damage is to be avoided in patients, and failure to identify a parathyroid abnormality in cases presenting with a peripheral granuloma is a well-known diagnostic pitfall. The clinical inquiry to assist in the exclusion or confirmation of hyperparathyroidism should be directed to the possibility of renal colic, lassitude, nausea, and vomiting.

Radiology.—The specific radiological signs of hyperparathyroidism may not even be present; only, in fact, an osteolytic area in the jaw identical in appearance to that of an endosteal giant-cell granuloma. Decreased definition of the bony trabeculae is supposed to be pathognomic and an inconstant dental sign of the disorder is partial loss or complete effacement of the lamina dura around the roots of the functioning teeth adjacent to the lesion. In X-ray films of the hands, subperiosteal resorption of the cortex of the phalanges is corroborative, and an abdominal projection is valuable in case of calcific changes in the kidneys. A lateral radiograph of the patella may also be helpful, for in hyperparathyroidism the softened patella appears to be wrapped round the femoral condyle. This phenomenon which is variously known as 'cloth cap patella' or 'Dixon's wrap-round sign', is due to a crush fracture in the bone produced by the pull of the quadriceps femoris.

Treatment.—Surgical removal of the over-active parathyroid tissue will allow the brown tumours to heal once the calcium metabolism is restored to normal.

CHERUBISM
(Disseminated Juvenile Fibrous Dysplasia, Familial Multilocular Cystic Disease of the Jaws, or Familial Fibrous Swelling of the Jaws)

Cherubism is the designation given to a familial giant-celled multicystic lesion of the jaws first described by Jones in 1933. The inheritance factor is an autosomal dominant gene and males appear to be affected twice as commonly as females. Thomas and Jones (1931) traced the condition back through five generations. At birth there is no evidence of this benign developmental abnormality and the facial deformity only becomes obvious at the age of about 2–4 years. This consists of a painless enlargement of both upper and lower jaws which develops rapidly up to the age of 7 years. The mandible is more frequently affected than the maxilla and the involvement is usually bilateral.

It is often dogmatically stated that the presence of bilateral changes is pathognomic of the condition, whereas, paradoxically, the youngest of Jones' original family was only affected on the left side. It is also pertinent to point out that the maxilla, too, may be only unilaterally enlarged. The extent of the lesions varies in size from changes restricted to the rami, tuberosities, and 3rd molar region to gross deformities of both jaws. A slower development of the deformity occurs between the age of 7 and puberty. The swellings in the jaws are firm and the mucosa overlying them becomes stretched and taut. Systemic manifestations are absent. After puberty the condition tends to regress with further maturation of the facial skeleton and eventually the cystic cavities are replaced with normal bone. Disappearance of the abnormality tends to occur at about the age of 22 years, but the authors have seen 2 patients aged 30 in whom there has been regression of the disease, but residual evidence of the original condition is still apparent on the radiographs. According to Jones (1965) enlargement of the local lymph-nodes is often present in early childhood. The lymphadenopathy regresses after the age of 5 years and has never been observed in adult patients either by Jones or by Caffey and Williams (1951). The enlargement is probably related to an upper respiratory tract infection.

The controversial matter of the 'heavenwards look' now appears to have been rationalized. Formerly, the extraordinary appearance of upturned eyes with exposed sclera between limbus and eyelid was attributed to the stretching of the skin overlying the expanded maxillary surface. It is now explained that this somewhat rare sign only occurs when the orbital floor is raised by a dome of dysplastic tissue which is continuous with the protuberant thickened anterior wall of the maxilla (Burland, 1962).

Intra-orally a diffuse swelling obscures the morphological distinction between the alveolus and body of the mandible. The palate may be almost obliterated by the gross enlargement of the tuberosities, and it is often narrowed in the anterior region. In places where the cortex is perforated, the swelling has a fleshy consistency. There is considerable interference with the normal development of both the deciduous and permanent teeth which may be absent due to premature exfoliation, displacement or failure to erupt. Agenesis of the 2nd and 3rd permanent molars is not uncommon, and McClendon, Anderson, and Cornelius (1962) reported supernumerary teeth in 1 of their patients and his paternal and maternal relatives. Ramon,

Berman, and Bubis (1967) reported a case complicated by gingival fibromatosis.

Radiographs demonstrate that the bones of the jaws are expanded and that there are multilocular radiolucencies especially in the ramus and body of the mandible and in the maxillary tuberosity. The antra may be completely obliterated and numerous unerupted teeth are seen. The radiolucent areas slowly fill in during the third decade, but some may persist until middle age. The lesions of this disorder are sometimes encountered in the long bones, metacarpals, and anterior ends of ribs. Some patients develop periosteal giant-cell lesions. There is no recognized abnormality of the serum calcium, phosphorus, or alkaline phosphatase levels.

Histology.—Histological examination of tissue from the lesions shows numerous giant cells arranged in groups around thin-walled blood-vessels in a fibrous tissue stroma. Epithelial remnants from developing teeth are sometimes seen scattered throughout the lesion and this may lead to an erroneous histological diagnosis of an odontogenic neoplasm.

Treatment and Prognosis.—It has been stressed that although the disease tends to progress rapidly in early childhood it tends to become static and even regress following puberty. Biopsy of the jaw lesions should be carried out to establish the diagnosis and if the condition is cosmetically unacceptable, surgical correction of the expanded jaw lesions can be carried out once the disease becomes quiescent.

REFERENCES

ARCHER, W. H. (1956), *Oral Surgery.* Philadelphia: Saunders.

BERNICK, S. (1948), 'Growths of the Gingiva and Palate. Connective Tissue Tumours', *Oral Surg.,* 1, 1098.

BLACK, B. K., and ACKERMAN, L. V. (1950), 'Tumours of the Parathyroid', *Cancer, N.Y.,* 3, 415.

BURLAND, J. G. (1962), 'Cherubism: Familial Bilateral Osseous Dysplasia of Jaws', *Oral Surg.,* 15, 43.

CAFFEY, J., and WILLIAMS, J. L. (1951), 'Familial Fibrous Swelling of Jaws', *Radiology,* 56, 1.

COOKE, B. E. D. (1952), 'The Giant Cell Epulis. Histogenesis and Natural History', *Br. dent. J.,* 93, 13.

DENT, C. E. (1962), 'Parathyroid Disease', *Trans. med. Soc. Lond.,* 77, 166.

—— (1966), 'Parathyroid Disease', *Ann. R. Coll. Surg.,* 39, No. 3, 150.

HARRIS, M. (1966), 'Cherubism and the Osteoclastoma', *Oral Surg.,* 25, 613.

JAFFE, H. L. (1953), 'Giant Cell Reparative Granuloma. Traumatic Bone Cyst and Fibrous (Fibro-osseous) Dysplasia of the Jaw Bones', *Ibid.,* 6, 159.

JONES, W.'A. (1933), 'Familial Multilocular Cystic Disease of Jaws', *Am. J. Cancer,* 17, 946.

—— (1965), 'Cherubism', *Oral Surg.,* 20, 648.

KILLEY, H. C., and KAY, L. W. (1965), 'Giant Cell Lesions of the Jaws', *J. int. Coll. Surg.,* 44, 262.

KRUGER, G. O. (1959), *Textbook of Oral Surgery.* St. Louis: Mosby.

McCLENDON, J. L., ANDERSON, D., and CORNELIUS, E. A. (1962), 'Cherubism— Hereditary Fibrous Dysplasia of the Jaws. Pathological Considerations', *Oral Surg.* 15, 17.

McGEOWN, M. G. (1961), 'Value of Special Tests o Parathyroid Function', *Proc. Ass. clin. Biochem.,* 1, 46.

McGOWAN, D. A. (1970), 'Central Giant Cell Tumour of the Mandible occurring in Pregnancy', *Br. J. oral Surg.,* 7, 131.

RAMON, Y., BERMAN, W., and BUBIS, J. J. (1967), 'Gingival Fibromatosis combined with Cherubism', *Oral Surg.,* 24, 435.

THOMA, K. H. (1962), 'Cherubism and Intraosseous Giant Cell Lesions', *Ibid.,* 15, 1.

THOMAS, P. J., and JONES, W. A. (1931), 'Further Observations regarding Familial Multilocular Cystic Disease of the Jaws', *Br. J. Radiol.,* 11, 227

Chapter X

THE ODONTOGENIC TUMOURS AND ODONTOMES

THE application of the term 'odontome' has varied considerably over the years. About 50 years ago it was used to cover all the abnormalities of the dental tissues whether developmental, inflammatory, or neoplastic. However, its present use is more restricted. Minor variations in size and number of the elements of a tooth are not now often described as odontomes, nor are the various odontogenic cysts, or those hamartomatous malformations and neoplasms which are largely composed of soft tissues. In general, the word is currently used for examples of the more extravagant variations in tooth morphology.

The term 'odontogenic tumour' is used for a group of lesions including the extreme morphological variants from the odontomes, together with the hamartomas and neoplasms of odontogenic tissues which have a large soft-tissue component to their structure. Some of these form cysts, but are separated from the other cystic odontogenic lesions for inclusion in this group because their epithelial component exhibits a growth and proliferation which is to a varying extent independent of the existence of a positive pressure within the cyst. Some other cystic lesions can be included because the lining is thick, the epithelium burrows extensively into the capsule of the cyst or induces odontoblasts to form.

Pindborg and Clausen (1958) proposed a classification of odontogenic tumours which recognized the inductive ability of odontogenic epithelium. This classification was used by Gorlin, Chaudhry, and Pindborg in their review article on the subject in 1961. The following classification is based on that of Gorlin, Chaudhry, and Pindborg.

ODONTOGENIC TUMOURS

Epithelial Odontogenic Tumours
With no inductive changes in the connective tissues
    Ameloblastoma
    Adeno-ameloblastoma
    Calcifying odontogenic epithelium tumour (Pindborg tumour)
With inductive changes in the connective tissues
    Ameloblastic fibroma
    Ameloblastic sarcoma
    Dentinoma (1) Fibro-ameloblastic type   (2) Mature type
    Calcifying odontogenic cyst
    Ameloblastic odontome
    Complex odontome
    Compound odontome
Mesodermal Odontogenic Tumours
    Odontogenic myxoma or fibromyxoma
    Cementifying fibroma.

The Epithelial Odontogenic Tumours

The Ameloblastoma.—

Origin.—The ameloblastoma seems almost certainly to be a neoplasm of odontogenic epithelium. Reasons for suggesting this are as follows:

1. No examples of this lesion have been reported from regions remote from the oral cavity. The so-called 'adamantinoma' of the tibia differs markedly from the condition found in the jaws, and only the craniopharyngioma resembles it histologically. Since the craniopharyngioma may arise from Rathke's pouch which derives from oral epithelium this latter similarity is consistent with the basic premise. A few have been reported in the soft tissue adjacent to the tooth-bearing parts of the jaws, but certain other odontogenic lesions are found in similar situations from time to time.

2. The epithelium bears a considerable histological similarity to that found in the bell stage of the enamel organ. The outer epithelium of the clumps is cylindrical and shows reversal of polarity like ameloblasts. The bulk of the rest of the cells resemble the stellate reticulum, but the innermost cells in the clumps of tumour cells have no counterpart in the normal structure. There are no cells resembling the stratum intermedium.

There are often sterile discussions as to whether this neoplasm should be regarded as benign or malignant. Some argue that it is not malignant since it virtually never metastasizes, unless subjected to repeated surgical trauma. It is suggested that as the ameloblastoma stems from odontogenic epithelium, which normally proliferates and penetrates into the jaws during odontogenesis, such behaviour is not necessarily that of a malignant neoplasm. However, it seems clear that a benign neoplasm should be encapsulated and readily enucleated and the ameloblastoma is not. Indeed, the degree to which it invades the tissues locally is such that recurrence is common, and eventual death of the patient from extension of the tumour into the skull a not uncommon occurrence.

The tumour normally arises centrally in the jaw, presumably from remnants of the tooth band. In some cases the lesion seems to stem from the alveolar epithelium, but since the tooth band developed originally from the oral epithelium this is quite reasonable. Fusion with the epithelium must, of course, be distinguished from origination.

As some examples have a dentigerous relationship to an unerupted tooth and may even form a unilocular cyst about the tooth, the suggestion is made that the ameloblastoma can arise from the epithelium lining a dentigerous cyst. In practice the validity of such claims can be difficult to assess. When the cells of an ameloblastoma are stretched over a large cyst they can closely resemble the epithelial cells which line simple odontogenic cysts. Only by careful comparison with the epithelium in the more solid part, the so-called 'mural ameloblastoma', will the observer realize that they also are ameloblastomatous. Another source of difficulty is the localized proliferations of odontogenic epithelium found from time to time within the capsule of dentigerous cysts. Should some of these take on a follicular form, it may require a pathologist of considerable experience to distinguish between innocent proliferation and an early ameloblastoma.

Incidence.—While there is no sex preference and no proved race incidence, there does seem to be a variation in the site most commonly involved in different races. In Europeans and North Americans over 70 per cent of lesions involve the molar and coronoid process region. In Nigerians, however, the anterior part of the lower jaw is the more commonly affected (Akinosi and Williams, 1968). The anterior part of the mandible is also rather more frequently affected in some Indians (Potdar, 1969). In all races maxillary lesions are the least frequent. It is not a particularly common neoplasm and the practising oral surgeon will see many more carcinomas than ameloblastomas.

When first seen, the patient is usually between 20 and 50 years, but children of 8 years and upwards and elderly people too may also be affected. It is difficult to gauge the age at onset, for although there is some variation in rate of growth, this is usually slow and sizeable tumours may have been present for many years.

Radiology.—The typical ameloblastoma is a truly multilocular lesion. That is, it is composed of several cystic compartments. The cysts vary in size and inspection of the periphery mesially, distally, buccally, and lingually reveals evidence of many small loculations in the periphery. Sonesson (1950) lays stress on the significance of a patchy sclerosis of the periphery and bony septa of an ameloblastoma. In some cases the lesion is composed of many comparatively small cysts, the microcystic or honeycomb variety of Worth (1938). These, particularly, exhibit considerable sclerosis of the adjacent bone.

Others have but one bony cavity and so may resemble simple cysts and encapsulated tumours. Differentiation on radiographical grounds is then most difficult. Such ameloblastomas may be composed of one large cyst with a more solid part somewhere in the periphery, or the entire bony cavity may be filled with tumour. Differentiation into solid and cystic forms is, however, not helpful, since most lesions have histologically detectable cysts and the number and size of the cysts seem to be related to age.

Differential radiographic diagnosis mainly involves the consideration of dentigerous and residual apical periodontal cysts, primordial cysts, fibromyxomas, and giant-cell granulomas. As has been said, unilocular lesions are difficult to differentiate. Some stress resorption of the roots of adjacent teeth, but while ameloblastomas tend to induce such resorption so do about one-third of sizeable simple cysts. Primordial cysts may be multilocular and the individual cysts are often of different size, but there are generally fewer locules than is the case with multilocular ameloblastomas. Sclerosis is not seen about the periphery of primordial cysts.

Both fibromyxomas and giant-cell granulomas create a single cavity with ridged walls and incomplete septa. The ridges and septa form straighter images than the walls of cysts and the periphery is lobulated but without the daughter cysts of the ameloblastoma. The fibromyxoma tends to produce a well-defined polyarcuate periphery and the giant-cell granuloma a less well-defined periphery. Resorption of tooth roots is common in relation to a giant-cell lesion.

Clinical Appearances.—The most frequent mode of presentation is an enlargement of the mandible. Multilocular examples may produce a knobbly enlargement and there is a tendency for the transverse diameter to be greater in proportion to the length than with simple cysts. Larger examples will produce a pale pink tumour mass with a granular surface, which bulges into the mouth. If it ulcerates the ulcer is dusky red and fleshy while the cut surface varies from pink to creamy white with sectioned cystic cavities.

Biopsy and Histology.—A biopsy must always be made to establish the diagnosis. Enough has been said about some of the difficulties which can arise in some cases and the opinion of a pathologist with experience of these lesions should be sought. In taking the specimen for histological examination the same rules as apply to the biopsy of malignant lesions should be followed. Representative samples from the more solid and non-ulcerated parts should be chosen if possible. Where an intra-bony lesion must be opened it should be approached by the shortest route, preferably through attached mucoperiosteum and through a wound which can be excised in toto should the subsequent diagnosis suggest that this is advisable. In particular, the wound must not widely open up tissue planes into which fragments of tissue or cyst fluid can escape. All surrounding tissues are copiously irrigated and aspirated dry with a clean sucker before the wound is closed.

Most ameloblastomas are composed of interlacing sheets and strands of epithelial cells surrounded by a fibrous stroma. Columnar cells showing reversal of polarity line the periphery of the strands and in the thicker parts the cells are joined only by the intercellular bridges so as to form a stellate reticulum-like arrangement. Where the network arrangement of tumour cell strands is predominant the appearance is described as 'plexiform' and where the cell masses are larger with a prominent stellate central mass of cells the pattern is described as 'follicular'. In the thicker masses squamous cell clumps may form, a few of which exhibit keratinization, parakeratinization, and ghostcell degeneration. In some otherwise typical neoplasms granular cells are to be found and a muco-epidermoid variant has been described by Hodson (1957). A few have a very vascular stroma and are described as haemangio-ameloblastomas. Both epithelium-lined and stromal cysts are formed.

Treatment.—In the past attempts have been made to approach the excision in a conservative manner. While in some cases this policy has been justified, it has resulted in far too high a recurrence rate for a neoplasm of this character. When recurrence does occur the neoplasm may remain undetected for many years, particularly if it is sited in the soft tissue planes. Incisions into the tumour and fragmentation of the mass during the operation predispose to seeding in the adjacent tissue planes. A proportion of recurrences are therefore inaccessible to further surgery and, after a protracted period of many years of increasing disability, result in death from intracranial extension, respiratory obstruction, or in cases where dissemination into the lungs has occurred, respiratory insufficiency.

Kramer (1963) provides the key to correct treatment. He has shown that the ameloblastoma can readily penetrate medullary spaces, but invades cortical bone with difficulty. It can also invade subperiosteal new bone. Thus, the tumour should be removed with a margin of approximately 1 cm. of cancellous bone where the periphery is in cancellous bone. Where original cortex survives, a subperiosteal excision is permissible;

but where the original cortex has been penetrated an extra-periosteal excision is necessary and where little or no bone remains over the tumour an adequate margin of soft tissues should be included.

In some patients a satisfactory removal will involve a partial thickness excision, in others a complete segment of jaw must be taken. If a high standard of repair is aimed at, few functional or cosmetic deficits should result. For the rare maxillary cases resection of the appropriate amount of maxilla is necessary. Since the periosteum contains large tumours within it for a considerable period of time, a successful *en bloc* removal may be possible, even where the lesion bulges into the pterygoid space, provided that the Crockett (1963) operation is employed. The lesion is radio-resistant and attempts to treat it by irradiation have produced some disastrous results. Follow-up should be for a minimum of 20 years, because the majority of recurrences do not manifest themselves until 10–15 years after surgery. Indeed, recurrences as late as 25 years after treatment are not unknown. If there is to be a hope of further successful treatment, recurrence must be detected early.

The Adeno-ameloblastoma.—The adeno-ameloblastoma is a benign encapsulated lesion which arises from odontogenic epithelium. Usually it has a central cavity and forms a thick-walled cyst, although occasional solid ones have been described. A dentigerous relationship to an anterior tooth is commonly observed. Most patients are less than 26 years of age, but examples in older age-groups are reported from time to time.

The lesion may be mistaken for a dentigerous cyst unless the calcified bodies in the lining are noted in the radiograph (*Fig.* 14). These form a layer of radio-dense spicules, at a distance internal to the margin of the

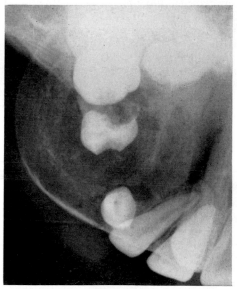

Fig. 14.—A lateral true occlusal radiograph of an adeno-ameloblastoma showing the calcified spicules distributed parallel to the periphery of the bony cavity.

bony cavity. This distance is uniform and represents the cyst capsule. In other cases the correct diagnosis may be suspected for the first time when an unusually thick cyst lining is found, perhaps with an eccentrically placed cavity. Approximately 2 cases have been described in females to every 1 in males.

Histology.—Great whorled masses of polyhedral epithelial cells accumulate and push into the capsule. A delicate vascular connective tissue penetrates between the masses. The epithelial cells separate to form a stellate reticulum. Within the masses columnar cells appear which surround small cystic spaces or form double rows of cells with an interval between. Some double rows are bent into an ox-bow shape. These cells show reversal of polarity characteristic of ameloblastomas and an eosinophilic material associated with reticulin fibres is formed within the lumen of the rings. Calcified globules, both single and in clumps, form in the epithelial masses and are the spicules seen in radiographs.

Treatment.—Simple enucleation is all that is required for this lesion which must not be confused with the ameloblastoma proper.

The Calcifying Odontogenic Epithelium Tumour (Pindborg Tumour).— Now that this neoplasm is more widely known, more frequent case reports are appearing, but it still remains a rare lesion. It arises usually from the reduced enamel epithelium of an unerupted tooth. The first indication of its presence, therefore, is a widening of the follicular space and a failure of the involved tooth to erupt. Where an unerupted tooth is not involved, it probably arises from remnants of the tooth band. While there is still a preponderance of examples from the mandible, the percentage of maxillary cases has increased.

Initially a circumscribed unilocular lesion is formed and at this stage enucleation is adequate treatment. Later a lobulated, or multilocular radiographic appearance is produced. Densely calcified spicules form clusters in the older parts of the lesion while the periphery is radiolucent. (*Fig.* 15.)

Histology.—Sheets of polyhedral epithelial cells are seen which invade the adjacent medullary bone and soft tissues. There is the usual fibrous stroma. In the older parts of the tumour eosinophilic globules appear and increase in size. They are concentrically laminated and soon become calcified. Adjacent globules fuse into a single mass and more material is added peripherally. The uncalcified material stains in a similar manner to ameloid (Ranløv and Pindborg, 1966), but is clearly related to the epithelial cells. It resembles globules found in relation to odontogenic epithelium in other locations and may be an aprismatic form of enamel (Seward and Duckworth, 1967a, b).

Treatment.—Enucleation is adequate for clearly circumscribed early lesions, but excision with a margin is required for advanced, multilocular lesions and those which exhibit invasive tendencies.

Ameloblastic Fibroma.—This comparatively uncommon odontogenic tumour is found during the first three decades of life. It is slowly growing and usually forms a unilocular cavity of simple outline, but may form a lobulated cavity with incomplete septa and so resemble the myxofibroma.

Histological examination reveals an encapsulated, dense, fibroma-like lesion in which strands and sheets of epithelial cells ramify. These are two

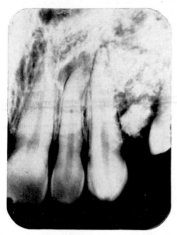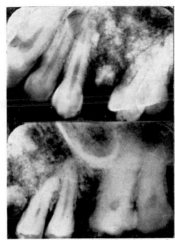

Fig. 15.—The clumped calcified spicules of high radiographic density and the irregular radiolucent margin of a calcifying odontogenic epithelium tumour.

cells thick for the most part and of a cuboidal or columnar shape. Terminal 'buds' may form on some of the strands where the cells increase in thickness and the central ones take on a stellate appearance. A cell-free zone occurs in the connective tissue adjacent to the epithelium.

Enucleation is adequate treatment, provided that care is taken to remove any outpouching of tumour if the periphery is irregular in shape.

Ameloblastic Fibrosarcoma.—The ameloblastic fibrosarcoma is a very rare odontogenic tumour composed of islands and strands of odontogenic epithelium in a cell-rich mesodermal stroma, the cells of which exhibit the histological features of a fibrosarcoma. The epithelium is indistinguishable from that in ameloblastic fibroma or ameloblastoma and it is probably a malignant variety of the ameloblastic fibroma. Most recorded cases have arisen in the mandible and the tumour is characterized by rapid growth and pain. An important diagnostic feature is that the pain has preceded the swelling in many instances and this has led to tooth extraction after which the tumour has extruded from the socket. Though the disease extends locally, despite surgical excision there are no recorded cases of the tumour metastasizing. This rare neoplasm is similar in histological appearance to the ameloblastic fibroma except that the fibrous tissue component is represented by a fibrosarcoma. The way in which this neoplasm should be fitted into the present classification is not clear If the basic neoplastic process is represented by the odontogenic epithelium and the fibromatous element the result of an inductive influence of the epithelium then it is not easy to see why it should undergo a malignant transformation. Alternative concepts are that the sarcoma is the definitive neoplasm, or that both elements are neoplastic. If the lesion is basically a fibrosarcoma arising within the alveolar process then it is conceivable that its presence could stimulate rests of odontogenic epithelium to proliferate. But should they proliferate to the degree seen in this particular neoplasm? If both elements are neoplastic then this is a 'mixed' tumour; a state of affairs which is contrary to the general philosophy of the classification. Another concept is that this is a collision neoplasm between two separate neoplasms. If this is so what happens to the stroma in which the odontogenic epithelium was proliferating? The treatment is radical surgery or radiotherapy depending on the particular case.

Dentinoma.—Two types of dentinoma are recognized by Gorlin, Chaudhry, and Pindborg (1961). The first resembles the ameloblastic fibroma save that odontoblasts are induced at the periphery of some of the sheets of epithelium. In some instances a stratum-intermedium-like layer is seen in the thicker bud-like parts of the epithelial cords. A tubule-free dentine or dentinoid is laid down by the odontoblast.

The second or mature type of dentinoma is composed of a laminated mass of dentinoid in parts of which some irregular dentinal tubules and enclosed odontoblasts may be found. The mass is usually opposed to the crown of an unerupted tooth in a similar fashion to certain complex odontomes. It is separated from the enamel of the tooth by the reduced enamel epithelium. Since odontoblasts cannot be formed without the inductive influence of epithelium, it is postulated that irregular, burrowing, cords of odontogenic epithelium initiated the dentinogenesis, perhaps originating from the external enamel epithelium of the enamel organ or from the adjacent tooth band. As the masses of dentine were deposited the epithelium was separated from any source of nutrition and died out. The mass of dentine therefore strangled the epithelium and stopped its proliferation in a manner resembling that seen in the complex odontome. Indeed, this type of dentinoma could be looked upon as a complex odontome in which the ameloblasts underwent sufficient histodifferentiation to induce the formation of odontoblasts, but not sufficient to lay down enamel or enameloid.

Both forms of dentinoma are very rare, are benign, and are treated by enucleation.

Calcifying Odontogenic Cyst.—Gorlin, Pindborg, Clausen, and Vickers (1962) and Gold (1963) independently drew attention to this entity. Certain odontogenic cysts have an epithelium forming the lining which has a basal layer of cuboidal or columnar cells. Some of the taller columnar cells exhibit reversal of nuclear polarity. In parts the epithelium increases markedly in thickness and undergoes the ghost cell type of degeneration. The ghost cells may subsequently calcify. Sometimes the ghost cell change can involve the full thickness of part of the epithelial lining. Where this happens the mass may be shed to leave an ulcerated surface. Should the degenerate mass remain in contact with the underlying connective tissue, it is invaded by granulation tissue and giant cells are formed which engulf the ghost cells. At other sites where the ghost cells come into contact with the connective tissue capsule, odontoblasts are induced and either an atubular dentinoid or tubular dentine is laid down.

Where no ghost cell change has occurred, the epithelium closely resembles that lining primordial cysts. The calcifying odontogenic cyst may therefore be related to the keratocysts since they can occur without a relationship to a formed tooth, or with a dentigerous or extra-follicular relationship to the crown of a tooth. Some may arise near the surface of the jaw so that only part of their circumference involves the bone or they may be found entirely in the soft tissues.

Again, like the primordial cyst some examples show some penetration of strands of epithelium into the capsule of the cyst, but this is comparatively uncommon. Occasional specimens, like that described by Duckworth and Seward (1965), are multilocular with some of the cysts having a very thick wall with deep penetration of large amounts of odontogenic epithelium into the fibrous capsule. The central cells in follicular expansions of these epithelial cords undergo both the ghost cell degeneration and calcification. Some of the cords of epithelium have a ring of early inductive changes in the adjacent connective tissue such as is seen in the ameloblastic fibroma. Both an atubular dentinoid and tubular dentine are induced. Enamel is not formed. It is such behaviour which can earn the calcifying odontogenic cyst a place in a classification of odontogenic tumours. A further matter of interest is the reports of two cases (Lurie, 1961; Duckworth and Seward, 1965) in which melanocytes were to be found in the tumours.

These lesions, like the adeno-ameloblastoma, should be suspected if dense calcified flecks or masses are detected forming an inner ring parallel with the inner surface of a bone cavity. A partially or completely extra-bony lesion showing such calcifications is almost diagnostic. Simple enucleation cures.

Ameloblastic Odontome.—In 1952 Cahn and Blum postulated that soft odontomes which were left undisturbed might subsequently calcify to become complex odontomes. It is a fact that tumours can be found in young people which are largely composed of soft tissues and which pursue this course, but these would now be recognized as immature complex composite odontomes. The ameloblastic odontome can be clearly separated from these lesions (Seward and Duckworth, 1967a).

It is the diversity of histological and morphological differentiation of the dental tissues which characterizes the ameloblastic odontome. In places, normal tooth follicles and teeth of varying size and form are produced. Elsewhere tubular dentine and prismatic enamel are to be found in featureless masses characteristic of the complex odontome. Between these more highly differentiated tissues, masses of polyhedral epithelial cells are seen in a fibrous tissue stroma. Some parts of these develop the ring-like structures and swirled cell masses seen in the adeno-ameloblastoma. Elsewhere calcified globules appear in relation to the epithelial cells and are quickly fused into masses by further material which is formed in layers on their surfaces. Dentinoid or dentine with scanty tubules appears in large quantities near the original calcified material, which seems to be a form of enamel. The dentine increases in amount until it traps the epithelial cells which subsequently die.

In other sections, the proliferating epithelium has a resemblance to that seen in the plexiform and follicular types of ameloblastoma, and both epithelium-lined and stromal cysts may develop. All these are to be found within the mass irrespective of the patient's age and the size of the lesion and this again is of diagnostic importance.

Generally these tumours are encapsulated and can be enucleated, but in one or two cases a recurrence has been recorded. While the recurrences could be due to a failure to remove a pocket of tumour, it may be that in some examples the ameloblastic element is more aggressive and local invasion occurs.

On clinical grounds the ameloblastic odontome should be suspected where an otherwise radiolucent tumour contains large masses of calcified tooth substance. The appearance is particularly suggestive of this diagnosis if the patient is over 25 years of age—beyond the stage where an immature complex odontome might be found. (*Fig.* 16.)

Complex Odontome.—The complex odontome in its mature form is a conglomerate mass of dental tissues. The dentine is tubular dentine, however, and the enamel, prismatic enamel. Properly organized dental pulps and cementum are also formed. While by definition the mass does not in any way resemble a recognizable tooth morphologically, nevertheless the tissues may show some order. Regular plates of dentine and enamel are laid down and these may be arranged in a definite pattern. Common shapes are rectangular blocks of parallel plates, or a sphere of radially disposed plates.

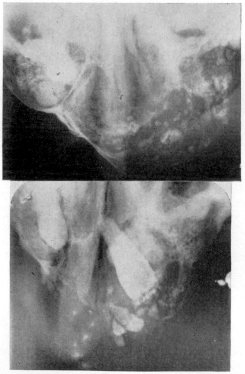

Fig. 16.—Radiographs of an ameloblastic odontome. Denticles, calcified masses, and calcified spicules lie in a mass of soft tissue. The bony cavity is well defined.

In its immature stage the lesion can be largely radiolucent and composed of a loose connective tissue penetrated by strands and sheets of odontogenic epithelium 2–3 cells thick and resembling those seen in the ameloblastic fibroma. However, when a follicular expansion is formed the epithelium rapidly differentiates into all the characteristic elements of an enamel organ and the normal stages of induction and odontogenesis occur. All that is lacking is a proper spatial arrangement such that a recognizable tooth is formed.

Some examples may continue to proliferate until past the normal time of tooth development, but all have ceased to grow by the early twenties. As the complex odontome ceases to grow, some consider it to be a hamartoma rather than a benign neoplasm. Others favour the neoplastic concept pointing out that the epithelium does not cease to proliferate of its own volition. It induces changes in the surrounding connective tissue so that calcified tissue is formed which traps the epithelium and prevents its further proliferation.

The dense laminated masses of the mature complex odontome are quite characteristic and easily recognized in radiographs. (*Fig.* 17.) Not infrequently they form over the crown of a developing tooth so that its eruption is prevented. Others appear to replace a tooth which is missing from the arch, and yet others occur in those parts of the jaw favoured by supernumeraries.

Their removal may present mechanical difficulties if they are large and if adjacent teeth are to be preserved, but there are no other problems with the mature tumour.

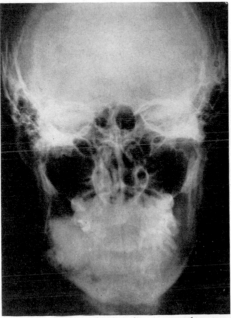

Fig. 17.—Postero-anterior radiograph showing a complex composite odontome.

If immature examples are removed, a limited recurrence can occur if part is overlooked, but as maturation and calcification take place its growth ceases and no great harm results.

Compound Odontome.—The compound odontome is somewhat similar to the complex odontome except that a higher degree of morphological differentiation is achieved and a number of denticles is formed. Surprisingly, large numbers may be found and it is not unusual to underestimate the number present from the radiograph. They vary greatly both in number and shape.

Careful removal of the denticles is in order, particularly if they are in a position to impede the eruption of a tooth of the normal series or to become infected. The usual precautions with regard to localization of the teeth and preservation of the adjacent normal teeth should be observed as in the removal of single supernumeraries.

THE MESODERMAL ODONTOGENIC TUMOURS

The Odontogenic Myxoma or Fibromyxoma.—

Aetiology.—If myxomatous change in other lesions such as chondromas, osteogenic fibromas, fibrous dysplasia, etc., is excluded there are virtually no records of fibromyxomas to be found at sites outside the jaws (Dahlin, 1957). Thus, while there is no positive evidence that these are odontogenic tumours some feel that this fact is sufficient to justify their place in the classification (Gorlin, Chaudhry, and Pindborg, 1961).

Histologically the tumour is composed of stellate cells with long processes which form a loose meshwork. A mucoid intercellular substance fills the spaces between the cells. Occasional strands of odontogenic epithelium may be found, but since these tumours occur in the jaws this may be a chance relationship. Similarly, too much cannot be made of the involvement of unerupted teeth, particularly wisdom teeth, since they often develop at a time when the 3rd molars are unerupted. Their growth is slow so that the most common age of presentation is the second and third decade.

It has been suggested that fibromyxoma of the jaws is an innocent tumour (Thoma and Goldman, 1947; Shear, 1959) and certainly it has a deceptively benign histological appearance, but its clinical behaviour is more suggestive of malignancy and its invasive nature has been recognized by Wawro and Reed (1950), Hayward (1955), Shafer and others (1963), and Killey and Kay (1964).

Clinical Features.—Fibromyxoma of the jaws is a rare tumour and it usually presents as a painless swelling of the bone or as an incidental radiological finding. It is alleged to arise more commonly in the second and third decades of life and to have a predilection for the posterior areas of the upper and lower jaws. It has a strong tendency to recur following operations such as local curettage and enucleation, but does not metastasize.

Radiological Features.—There are no diagnostic radiological features of the condition, but when it appears to be multilocular the straight septa divide the radiolucent image into square, rectangular, or triangular spaces, with a central portion traversed by fine, gracile trabeculations. This appearance has been likened by Sonesson (1950) to that of the strings of a tennis racket. As the tumour expands, the outer cortical plate first becomes a thin shell and finally it may be perforated.

Appearance at Operation.—The appearance of the fibromyxoma at operation is that of an ivory white tumour, which is firm in consistency with a smooth, lobulated, shiny surface. There is no evidence of encapsulation and prolongations of the tumour invade the surrounding bone and make dissection of the mass more or less impossible.

Differential Diagnosis.—Both clinical and radiological methods of examination sometimes fail to differentiate the fibromyxoma from such tumours as bone cysts, giant-cell granuloma, ameloblastoma, and fibrous dysplasia, and the only certain method of diagnosing the condition is by histological examination of the tissue.

Treatment.—In view of the fact that the behaviour of fibromyxoma is unpredictable and that it has a high recurrence rate even after local resection, it would seem prudent to avoid such treatment as local curettage or enucleation. Where the tumour is comparatively small and localized, a local resection of the tumour together with about 1 cm. of the normal surrounding bone may be carried out, after which a regular and careful follow-up should be instituted.

For the larger tumour a resection of the jaw is probably the only practical solution. There is no precise evidence concerning the response of fibromyxoma to radiotherapy. Shafer and others (1963) considered that the tumour was not radiosensitive, but Ackerman and Spjut (1963) suggested that fibromyxoma does, in fact, react to radiotherapy. However, Prossor (1963) feels that the prognosis can be improved by radiotherapy provided that it is carried out in conjunction with a wide surgical excision of the tumour, and this would appear to be the treatment of choice.

Cementifying Fibroma.—This condition is also known as multiple cementoma and periapical fibrous dysplasia. Although it was first recognized by Brophy in 1915 and described in detail by Stafne (1933, 1934, and 1943), by Ennis (1947), and by many others, knowledge of the condition still does not seem to be widespread. In its most common form periapical areas of bone destruction appear, presumably as a result of proliferation of the periodontal membrane. Any teeth may be involved, but anterior teeth are affected more than posterior and particularly the lower incisors.

After a while calcified spicules can be seen in radiographs in the centre of the radiolucencies. Histologically at this stage, the calcified tissues may have characteristics similar either to cementum or to woven bone. During these stages the lesions may be mistaken for inflammatory periapical lesions. In time the calcified masses increase and a radio-opaque mass is formed: either a knob of cementum attached to the root, a mass of cementum separated from the root by a reformed periodontal membrane, or even new trabeculae of bone so that only a slight alteration in bone pattern is to be seen. Obviously both difficulty in extraction of an involved tooth and infection of the socket are hazards associated with this condition.

Occasionally during the earlier stages one of these lesions will increase sufficiently in size to produce a deforming lump which requires surgical treatment.

The gigantic or gigantiform type of cementoma may be seen in two forms. In one form a large, relatively radiolucent lesion forms in which irregular masses of cementum are laid down. The condition is often mistaken for Paget's disease, but it should be noted that the cortex of the jaw remains normal: a state of affairs not found in Paget's disease. Following an extraction, infection sometimes supervenes, adding to the difficulties of reaching a correct diagnosis.

In the second form, large dense masses of cementum are to be found in the molar regions in each quadrant. There is a thin capsule about each mass separating it from the bone. When molar extractions are performed there is a considerable risk of the tumour becoming infected. If this happens, the whole lump must be removed. This can be a formidable undertaking since the knobbly surface indents the cortex of the jaw to such a degree that, in the mandible, undercut cavities are formed in the cortex. Releasing the mass by cutting away the bone may entail the removal of a considerable amount of mandibular bone at that site. Cutting up the mass itself is most difficult as it is immensely hard. In some cases resection of a length of jaw may be necessary. Typical cementoma lesions about the apices of the incisors may help in differentiating these masses from complex odontomes. Negroes seem particularly afflicted with the gigantiform cementoma.

ODONTOMES

As has been explained in the section on odontogenic tumours, the term 'odontome' has been variously applied. Minor variations in size and form are not now often referred to as odontomes and the hamartomas and neoplasms of dental tissues are usually grouped under the heading of odontogenic tumours. Only the more aberrant tooth forms, but ones in which prismatic enamel, tubular dentine, pulp, and cementum are formed and in which the structure reaches a finite size, are included under this heading. In this discussion the emphasis will be on points of surgical interest.

Gemination and Dichotomy.—In gemination two tooth elements which are separate at their coronal end subsequently become fused. Thus, there is at least a groove, or notch, marking the demarcation between the two occlusal surfaces or incisal edges. In some examples two separate crowns are supported on conjoined roots. Hitchin and Morris (1960) prefer the term 'connate' for these malformations and based their understanding of their formation on observations made on a strain of dogs in which connate incisors are common. They have shown that in these dogs stellate reticulum from adjacent enamel organs proliferates into the part of the tooth band which joins them so that one large enamel organ is formed.

Dichotomy is reduplication by division. A tooth germ splits into two parts during odontogenesis so that a single crown is supported on re-duplicate roots. Crudely put: in gemination there are two crowns on one root and in dichotomy one crown on two roots. However, with dichotomy the crown of the tooth is often excessively large and there is no clear evidence that a different mechanism is involved from that producing the connate tooth.

The surgical importance of these forms is the mechanical difficulties which they may pose if their extraction is required. Also in some instances of gemination a conical tooth form is fused to a crown of normal shape.

When such a tooth is partially erupted it may appear that a supernumerary tooth is adjacent to a tooth of the normal series and displacing it. Should the conical element be palatal or labial to the part of normal shape the site of union may be difficult to demonstrate radiographically. Only when an attempt is made to extract the supernumerary may the true state of affairs be discovered.

Such an arrangement is also bad from a periodontal point of view as well as an aesthetic or orthodontic one. Of course, if the tooth can be root-filled an attempt can be made to remove the extra part surgically, sealing the opening into the pulp cavity of the parent part with amalgam and replacing the flap tight against the tooth.

Invaginated Odontomes.—Because the area of attachment of the invagination to the tooth bud is small, the invagination probably results from the proliferation of comparatively few ameloblasts in the case of coronal invagination or epithelial cells of Hertwig's sheath in the case of a radicular one. Again, proliferation is probably the mechanism by which the invagination is formed because the large size achieved by some invaginations would be impossible by a mechanism of local growth arrest with continued growth of the rest of the epithelial component of the tooth germ around it.

The invagination may be small as in the case of the *cingulum invagination*, so frequently seen in upper lateral incisors and less commonly in other upper anterior teeth. If it is rather larger the tooth is deformed, or conical, but has a normal apex and a *dens in dente* is formed. These again are not uncommon in the upper incisor region, especially among supernumerary teeth. Some have a slit-like opening at the surface and produce an invagination to one side of a tooth which has a comparatively normal crown.

Where the invagination is larger still, it passes through the 'apex' and the pulp cavity forms a circular slit around the invagination. The external form of the tooth is altered and enlarged so that the lesion is described as a *dilated odontome*. Probably all invaginations have imperfect enamel and dentine at the bottom. The deeper varieties have only grossly deficient dentine or even an aperture at the fundus.

Invaginations in posterior teeth are most uncommon. Some coronal ones have a sizeable surface opening. Certain examples originate from Hertwig's sheath and involve only the root of the tooth and these are largely to be found in molar teeth. Multiple invaginations can occur so that the specimen superficially resembles a complex odontome. Invaginated odontomes are of importance mainly because organisms can penetrate the bottom of the invagination and either destroy the pulp of a *dens in dente* or cause a periapical infection directly in a dilated odontome. Root-canal treatment is always difficult and in some cases impossible so their extraction is usually required once infection has supervened. Dilated odontomes and root invaginations then present a problem because of their shape and must be removed by open surgery.

Compound and Complex Odontomes.—These odontomes have been discussed in the section on odontogenic tumours.

The Evaginated Odontome.—Evaginated, 'Leong's' or 'Tratman's' odontomes are small tubercles or extra cusps to be found on the occlusal surface of posterior teeth, palatally in the cingulum region of canines, and rarely on the palatal aspects of upper incisors (Leigh, 1925; Tratman, 1950; Oehlers, 1956).

On posterior teeth they are to be found in or close to the fissures and therefore in the centre of the crown. Premolar teeth are most often affected and mongoloid peoples, such as Chinese, Malays, and Eskimos, are almost exclusively the subjects of these anomalies.

The tubercle is covered by enamel and under a thin layer of dentine has a prolongation of the pulp. They can be taller than the adjacent cusps and are frequently worn away or fractured off. Caries of the fissure rapidly involves the pulp and cavity preparation is hazardous. Thus in many cases the pulps become infected, hence the oral surgical significance of this condition.

REFERENCES

ACKERMAN, L. V., and SPJUT, H. J. (1963), *Tumours of Bone and Cartilage*. Section 2—Fascicle 4. Armed Forces Institute of Pathology.

AKINOSI, J. O., and WILLIAMS, A. O. (1968), 'Adamantinoma in Ibadan, Nigeria', *W. Afr. med. J.*, **17**, 45.

BROPHY, T. W. (1915), *Oral Surgery: A Treatise on the Diseases, Injuries, and Malformations of the Mouth and Associated Parts*. Philadelphia: Blakistons.

CAHN, L. R., and BLUM, T. (1952), 'Ameloblastic Odontoma: Case Report critically analysed', *J. oral Surg.*, **10**, 169.

CROCKETT, D. J. (1963), 'Surgical Approach to the Back of the Maxilla', *Br. J. Surg.*, **50**, 819.

DAHLIN, D. C. (1957), *Bone Tumors: General Aspects and an Analysis of 2,276 Cases*. Springfield, Ill.: Thomas.

DUCKWORTH, R., and SEWARD, G. R. (1965), 'A Melanotic Ameloblastic Odontome', *Oral Surg.*, **19**, 73.

ENNIS, LeR. M. (1947), *Dental Roentgenology*, p. 368. London: Kimpton.

GOLD, L. (1963), 'The Keratinizing and Calcifying Odontogenic Cyst', *Oral Surg.*, **16**, 1414.

GORLIN, J. R., CHAUDHRY, A. P., and PINDBORG, J. J. (1961), 'Odontogenic Tumours', *Cancer, N.Y.*, **14**, 73.

— — PINDBORG, J. J., CLAUSEN, F., and VICKERS, R. A. (1962), 'The Calcifying Odontogenic Cyst: A Possible Analogue of the Cutaneous Calcifying Epithelioma of Malherbe', *Oral Surg.*, **15**, 1235.

HAYWARD, J. R. (1955), 'Odontogenic Myxofibroma of the Mandible', *J. oral Surg. Anesth. Hosp. dent. Serv.*, **13**, 149.

HITCHIN, A. D., and MORRIS, I. (1960), 'The Inheritance of Connate Incisors in the Dog', *J. dent. Res.*, **39**, 1101.

HODSON, J. J. (1957), 'Observations on Origin and Nature of Adamantinoma with Special Preference to Certain Muco-epidermoid Variations', *Br. J. plast. Surg.*, **10**, 38,

KILLEY, H. C., and KAY, L. W. (1964), 'Fibromyxomata of the Jaws', *Br. J. oral Surg.*, **2**, 124.

KRAMER, I. R. H. (1963), 'Ameloblastoma: A Clinicopathological Appraisal', *Ibid.*, **1**, 13.

LEIGH, R. W. (1925), 'Dental Pathology of the Eskimoes', *Dent. Cosmos*, **67**, 884.

LURIE, H. I. (1961), 'Congenital Melanocarcinoma, Melanotic Adamantinoma, Retinal Anlage Tumour, Progonoma and Pigmented Epulis of Infancy: Summary and Review of the Literature and Report of the First Case in an Adult', *Cancer*, **14**, 1090–1108.

OEHLERS, F. A. (1956), ' Tuberculated Premolar ', *Dent. Practnr dent. Rec.*, **6**, 144.

PINDBORG, J. J., and CLAUSEN, F. (1958), 'Classification of Odontogenic Tumours', *Acta odont. scand.*, **16**, 291.

POTDAR, G. G. (1969), 'Ameloblastoma of the Jaws as seen in Bombay, India', *Oral Surg.*, **28**, 297.

PROSSOR, T. M. (1963), personal communication.

RANLØV, P., and PINDBORG, J. J. (1966), 'The Amyloid Nature of the Homogeneous Substance in the Calcifying Epithelial Odontogenic Tumour', *Acta path. microbiol. scand.*, **68**, 169.

SEWARD, G. R., and DUCKWORTH, R. (1967a), 'A Review of the Pathology of the Calcifying Odontogenic Cysts and Tumours', *Dent. Practnr dent. Rec.*, **18**, 83.

— — — — (1967b), 'A Study of the Pathological Calcified Materials in the Calcifying Odontogenic Cysts and Tumours', *Ibid.*, **18**, 125.

SHAFER, W. G., HINE, M. K., and LEVY, D. M. (1963), *A Textbook of Oral Pathology*, 2nd ed. Philadelphia: Saunders.

SHEAR, M. (1959), 'Central Myxofibroma of the Mandible', *J. dent. Ass. S. Afr.*, **14**, 424.

SÖNESSON, A. (1950), 'Odontogenic Cysts and Cystic Tumours of Jaws: Roentgendiagnostic and Patho-anatomic Study', *Acta radiol.*, Suppl. **81**, 36.

STAFNE, E. C. (1933), 'Cementoma: Study of 35 Cases', *Dental Survey*, **9**, 27.

— — (1934), 'Periapical Osteofibrosis with Formation of Cementoma', *J. Am. dent. Ass.*, **21**, 1822.

— — (1943), 'Periapical Fibroma; Roentgenologic Observations', *Ibid.*, **30**, 688.

THOMA, K. H., and GOLDMAN, H. M. (1947), 'Central Myxoma of the Jaw', *Am. J. Orthod.*, **33**, 532.

TRATMAN, E. K. (1950), 'Indo-European Racial Stock with the Mongoloid Racial Stock', *Dent. Rec.*, **70**, 63.

WAWRO, N. W., and REED, J. (1950), 'Fibromyxoma of the Mandible: Report of 2 Cases', *Ann. Surg.*, **132**, 1138.

WORTH, H. M. (1938), 'Radiological Findings in some Less Common Jaw Affections', *Proc. R. Soc. Med.*, **32**, 331.

CHAPTER XI

HISTIOCYTOSIS 'X' AND MALIGNANT GRANULOMA

HISTIOCYTOSIS 'X'

'HISTIOCYTOSIS "X" ' is a term suggested by Lichenstein (1953) to describe a disease of unknown aetiology which is characterized by enlarging solitary or multiple destructive aggregations of proliferating histiocytes. The disease is not hereditary and there is no racial predilection. Males tend to be affected more often than females and Blevins and others (1959), who reviewed a series of 27 cases which involved the oral tissues, found that 20 males were affected. There are three clinically distinct variations of the disease, but all three syndromes are believed to be manifestations of the same pathological process. All three types of histiocytosis 'X' are rare, and in the first instance are characterized by a proliferation of histiocytes with secondary storage of cholesterol in them and finally by fibrosis and scarring. The disease may be localized or generalized and the generalized form of the condition is chronic or acute.

Localized Histiocytosis 'X'.—In the localized variety of the disease there is a lesion, often single, known as an 'eosinophilic granuloma' which is confined to the skeleton, usually the skull, vertebrae, pelvis, or extremities. Bone lesions of this type develop rapidly and are also found in the jaws, especially in the mandible. Jaw lesions are, however, rare. Blevins and others (1959) studied 600 cases at the Mayo Clinic and found oral involvement in only 27 cases. Occasionally there may be more than one bone involved and Schwartz (1965) reported a bilateral mandibular lesion. During the histiocytosis proliferation phase there is an accumulation of leucocytes. The condition tends to appear in young children mostly in the 4–6 year age-group. It presents as a local tumour of bone and the overlying soft tissues are often red, painful, and swollen. When it occurs in the jaws the radiograph shows an expansion of the bone surrounding an irregular radiolucent lesion.

In children two clinical types of eosinophil granuloma are seen and in some cases both varieties may affect the same child, but at different times. One appears to start in the cancellous bone and produces a highly irregular bony cavity. Radiographically the jaw has a worm-eaten appearance with enlargement due to the destruction of the original cortex and deposition of subperiosteal new bone.

The other type affects the gingival margin to produce a red or pink granulation tissue. The teeth become loose and the radiograph reveals severe destruction of the alveolar bone. Eventually the teeth are denuded of bone and 'float' in the lesional tissue. Radiographically they appear to be suspended in space.

In the adult; deep, foul, chronic periodontal pockets are found with considerable alveolar bone destruction. These may increase to such a size that almost all the medullary bone is involved. Once secondary infection has supervened chronic osteomyelitis is simulated. In other instances spherical cavities not unlike those of residual or periodontal cysts are seen in the radiographs. When these are opened granulation tissue or a mixture of granulation tissue and infected necrotic material is found.

Both curettage and a low therapeutic dose of irradiation will effect a cure but as far as possible irradiation should be avoided in the child because of the effect on growth of the tissues. In the adult the choice depends in part on the extent of the lesion. Occasionally apparently traumatic lesions or a denture granuloma of the sulcus or tongue may resemble eosinophil granuloma. Simple excision cures them and Bhaskar and Lilly (1964) have shown that experimental damage to the tongue in dogs can reproduce these lesions.

Treatment.—Treatment is by excision and curettage. At operation a layer of new bone is found covering an irregular cyst-like cavity containing deep purplish-red soft tissue which tends to bleed vigorously. Following removal of the contents of the cavity, the lesion tends to fill in with new bone. The condition should be kept under review, for in some instances the disease progresses to the chronic or acute variety.

The Chronic Variety.—The chronic variety of the disease is known as 'Hand-Schüller-Christian disease'. This is a chronic disseminated histiocytosis 'X' in which there are multiple skeletal and visceral lesions usually with the classic triad of skull defects, exophthalmos, and diabetes insipidus. The granulomatous lesions, which contain histiocytes, eosinophils, and foam cells, occur in many sites including particularly the lymph-nodes, spleen, liver, brain, and bones. The disease usually begins in the first five years of life but may occasionally occur later in life, even in middle age. Its onset is insidious with skull defects, diabetes insipidus, and exophthalmos, though often only one of this triad of symptoms is present. The diabetes insipidus is due to involvement of the region of the hypophysis at the base of the brain. There is a hepatosplenomegaly and often a maculopapular rash over the face and trunk. The granulomata often affect the jaws and there may be swelling and ulceration of the gums leading possibly to extrusion of the teeth. Scattered tubercle-like lesions may occur in the lungs and there may be bronchopneumonia. Radiographs show punched-out lesions in the bones and spontaneous fractures may occur.

Treatment.—Local radiotherapy to the lesions which are causing symptoms is effective, and remissions have been reported with courses of prednisone 2–4 mg. per kg. body-weight for 6–8 weeks, which is then tapered off over an 8–10 week period (Scott, 1966). The diabetes insipidus requires treatment with pituitary hormone. The disease is relatively benign and protracted, but may carry a mortality-rate of about 13 per cent.

The Acute Form of Histiocytosis 'X'.—The acute form of the disease is known as 'Letterer-Siwe's disease' and it is a diffuse, and rapidly progressive disease. It occurs in early infancy, often before the age of two years, and leads to death within a few weeks. The spleen, liver, lymph-nodes, skin, lungs, and bone-marrow are heavily infiltrated. There is generalized lymphadenopathy, hepatosplenomegaly, anaemia, and a tendency to haemorrhage.

Treatment.—The disease is usually rapidly fatal, but attempts to treat the condition with corticosteroids and ACTH are under evaluation.

MALIGNANT GRANULOMA AND WEGENER'S GRANULOMATOSIS

Malignant granuloma or lethal midline granuloma and Wegener's granulomatosis, according to Mills (1967), are one and the same disease. Where this rare disease is primarily localized to the midline of the palate and nose it is called 'malignant granuloma' while the generalized disease involving changes in the respiratory system (necrotizing granuloma), kidneys (necrotizing glomerulitis), liver, spleen, and skin is termed 'Wegener's granulomatosis'. Only the malignant granuloma is of interest to the oral surgeon, though occasionally oral manifestations occur in the generalized type of the disease. Morgan and O'Neil (1956) reported a case of Wegener's granulomatosis in which oral and cutaneous manifestations were predominant features. Several cases have been recorded in which the presenting sign of the disease was an ulcerative stomatitis or the failure of a socket to heal. More recently Clarke (1964) has described a case of Wegener's granulomatosis in which the patient presented with a single oral ulcer, and Brooke (1969) has mentioned the possibility that granular purplish-red gingival enlargement may be an important and even pathognomic manifestation of the disease. The course of the condition is usually rapid, progressing to death in a few weeks or months.

Malignant Granuloma.—Mills (1958) reviewed 86 cases of malignant granuloma; 55 were male and 31 female. In 67 of these cases the disease began in the nose and in 19 patients it arose in the paranasal sinuses. Mills points out that many had a preceding nasal or paranasal infection; he regards this as a sensitizing phase preparatory to a hypersensitivity reaction. As the disease process extends, there is a progressive destruction of the nose, face, and pharynx.

Aetiology.—Williams (1949) considers that malignant granuloma is due to a dysfunction of the immune mechanisms responsible for granuloma formation. This leads to a vascular allergy and either the Arthus phenomenon occurs in the case of capillaries or periarteritis nodosa if the arterioles are affected. The hyperimmune tissues become necrotic because of obstruction to the blood-supply.

Symptoms.—The symptoms depend on the site involved and usually the nose becomes stuffy and blocked and this leads on to a watery or serosanguineous discharge. This prodromal stage lasts for one or two months, but may persist for several years. Later a swelling develops on the side of the nose or the inner canthus. If secondary infection occurs the face and periorbital tissues are grossly swollen and painful. There may be diplopia and anaesthesia of the cheek. In spite of these symptoms the patient remains healthy, a fact which has been commented upon by several observers. The nasal mucosa is swollen and covered with crusts and on removing them masses of what appears to be simple granulation tissue is revealed. There may be exposure of bone. Ulcerations appear on the septum and conchae and as the condition progresses the hard palate is invaded with large spreading perforating ulcers. Small haemorrhages are frequent and involvement of a large vessel may result in a fatal termination. Cachexia is marked as a result of secondary infection and difficulty in obtaining adequate nutrition, and the patient may die of exhaustion or bronchopneumonia or from meningitis if the meninges are invaded. The course of the disease may last for years, but often it results in death within a year.

Blood Picture in Malignant Granuloma.—There may be a hypochromic microcytic anaemia due to toxic absorption, and in some cases there is an eosinophilia. Walton (1958) reported that 45·9 per cent of his 37 cases had an eosinophilia. However, a noticeable feature of the disease is the poor white-cell response associated with the extensive tissue destruction. Mills reported that the ESR was helpful in the diagnosis of malignant granuloma and was useful in monitoring the activity and progress of the disease. The very high ESR estimations are used as evidence for classifying these conditions as collagen disorders. There is a hypergammaglobulinaemia.

Urinary Changes.—There are no urinary changes in malignant granuloma, but urinalysis is valuable to exclude kidney involvement.

Bacteriology.—No specific organism has been found in either malignant granuloma or Wegener's granulomatosis.

Histology.—In the words of Stewart (1933) the main histological features of malignant granuloma are 'a chronic inflammatory process with proliferation of the endothelial cells, lymphocytes and plasma cells, and formation of granulation tissue at first cellular, but later becoming fibrous. As the disease progressed, fibrous tissue was laid down fairly loosely, just beneath the surface and more densely in the deeper parts with small, round-celled infiltrates still present among the fibrous tissue. The blood-vessels were proliferating in the early stages, but later had enormous thickening of their walls and endarteritis with hyaline changes'.

Differential Diagnosis.—A differentiation should be made between malignant granuloma and reticulum-cell sarcoma. At first sight this should not be difficult, but in practice it can be far from easy in some cases. Reticulum-cell sarcomas of the mouth or respiratory passages frequently become ulcerated and heavily infiltrated with acute and chronic inflammatory cells. In these circumstances it may take a skilled pathologist to spot the neoplastic cells. To add to the problem some reticulum-cell sarcomas die out in the older part of the lesion while continuing to invade and proliferate in the periphery. This actually results in healing of some parts of the ulcer and, of course, a biopsy from the older parts will be negative. Repeated biopsy may be needed to establish the correct diagnosis. It is possible that the cases of so-called 'malignant granuloma' which respond to irradiation are really reticulum-cell sarcomas of this type.

Treatment.—There is no specific treatment, but irradiation of the local lesion is effective in some cases of malignant granuloma. Antibiotic therapy is used to control secondary infection, but has no effect on the progress of the disease. More widespread disease is treated with cortisone, and to keep the disease in check the patient must be kept on a maintenance dose of steroids. The prognosis is very poor.

REFERENCES

BHASKAR, S. N., and LILLY, G. E. (1964), 'Traumatic Granuloma of the Tongue (Human and Experimental)', *Oral Surg.*, **18**, 206.

BLEVINS, C., DAHLIN, D., LOVESTEDT, S., and KENNEDY, R. (1959), 'Oral and Dental Manifestations of Histiocytosis "X"', *Ibid.*, **12**, 473.

BROOKE, R. I. (1969), 'Wegener's Granulomatosis involving the Gingivae', *Br. dent. J.*, **127**, 34.

CLARKE, P. B. (1964), 'Wegener's Granulomatosis', *Br. J. oral Surg.*, **1**, 205.

LICHENSTEIN, L. (1953), 'Histiocytosis "X" Integration of Eosinophilic Granuloma of Bone, Letterer-Siwi Disease and Schüller-Christian Disease as Related Manifestations of a Single Nosolytic Entity', *Archs Path.*, **56**, 84.

MILLS, C. P. (1958), 'Malignant Granulomas', *J. Lar. Otol.*, **72**, 849.

— — (1967), 'Malignant Granulomas and Wegener's Granulomatosis', *Hospital Med.*, **2**, 183.

MORGAN, A. D., and O'NEIL, R. (1956), 'Oral Complications of Polyarteritis, and Giant-cell Granulomatosis', *Oral Surg.*, **9**, 845.

SCHWARTZ, S. (1965), 'Bilateral Lesions of Eosinophilic Granuloma', *J. oral Surg.*, **23**, 172.

SCOTT, R. BODLEY (1966), *Price's Textbook of the Practice of Medicine.* London: Oxford University Press.

STEWART, J. P. (1933), 'Progressive Lethal Granulomatous Ulceration of the Nose', *J. Lar. Otol.*, **48**, 657.

WALTON, E. W. (1958), 'Giant-cell Granuloma of the Respiratory Tract (Wegener's Granulomatosis)', *Br. med. J.*, **2**, 265.

WILLIAMS, H. L. (1949), 'Lethal Granulomatous Ulceration involving the Midline Facial Tissues', *Ann. Otol. Rhinol. Lar.*, **58**, 1013.

CHAPTER XII

SOME PREMALIGNANT CONDITIONS OF THE ORAL CAVITY

LEUCOPLAKIA

LEUCOPLAKIA is regarded as a premalignant disease, but some care is required in defining exactly what is meant by the term. By definition, 'leucoplakia' means 'a white patch', but all chronic white lesions in the mouth are by no means premalignant. Pindborg, Renstrup, and others (1963) defined leucoplakia as a white patch that cannot be rubbed off, cannot be reversed by removing obvious irritants, and cannot be assigned to any other diagnostic category on the basis of clinical or microscopic features. This may be a satisfactory academic definition, but it is not particularly helpful to the clinically orientated oral surgeon, for not only is some difficulty experienced in differentiating the various white patches in the mouth clinically but similar difficulty is also found by the pathologists when the material is examined microscopically. In addition, some other white lesions not normally included under the term 'leucoplakia', such as lichen planus, can also undergo malignant change. Even when the pathologist can make a definite diagnosis in the case of a white patch, there is not, at present, any simple means of assessing whether it is likely to become malignant, though Kramer (1969) has suggested a most ingenious method of predicting a malignancy by computer analysis of a number of histological features of the lesion.

Incidence of Leucoplakia.—Pindborg and others (1965a) screened 10,000 patients in India and found 328 or 3·28 per cent had oral leucoplakia. Bruszt (1962), of Hungary, found a 3·6 per cent incidence in 5613 patients. In India, Mehta and others (1969) examined 4734 men and found a 3·4 per cent incidence of oral leucoplakia.

Types of White Patch.—Some of the chronic white patches in the mouth which may be premalignant are:—

1. *Leucoplakia of Developmental Origin or Developmental Epithelial Naevi.*—These chronic white lesions have been termed 'congenital', but they are not usually found in children and may not appear until middle age. Clinically there are two varieties:

a. A generalized irregular oedematous thickening of the superficial epithelium of the floor of the mouth or a symmetrical folded lesion on the insides of the cheeks. In some instances there is a family history and the condition may be inherited as an autosomal dominant. This condition is usually termed 'white sponge naevus'.

b. The other type can involve either side of the undersurface of the tongue. It has well-defined margins and a soft wrinkled surface. Although these two conditions are termed 'developmental', it does not necessarily imply that they always remain benign.

2. *Frictional Keratosis.*—If the oral mucosa is abraded by a broken tooth or denture, it may become hyperkeratinized. If the source of the irritation is removed the oral mucosa will revert to normal provided the source of local trauma is the only cause of the keratosis. Chronic mechanical irritation of the oral mucosa has long been regarded as a potential cause of oral carcinoma, but there is no experimental evidence to substantiate this view.

3. *Keratosis from Smoking.*—Keratosis of the palate with inflammation and swelling of the mucous glands can occur as a result of smoking, but even when the leucoplakia is severe, the condition may regress if the patient can be induced to give up smoking. The condition is often seen in the palate as a result of pipe smoking. However, the palate is an uncommon site for oral carcinoma. Heavy smoking has been implicated as a cause of carcinoma of the bronchus and it has been shown by Moore and Catlin (1967) that the main sites of oral carcinoma are in what they term the 'drainage area' of the mouth, i.e., the sides and underside of the tongue and the floor of the mouth extending back into the pharynx. Some 75 per cent of all oral carcinomas develop in this region which forms only 20 per cent of the total area of the mouth. It has been suggested by Cawson (1969) that if there is a relationship between smoking and oral cancer it could be due to carcinogens from the cigarettes becoming dissolved in the saliva which could then leak down and affect this drainage area. There is certainly a direct relationship between smoking and cancer of the lip and lesions on the lip associated with smoking clay pipes are well substantiated in the literature as well as carcinoma as a result of leaving a lighted stub of cigarette lying on the lip. The likelihood of a second carcinoma appearing in the oral cavity after successful treatment of the original lesion is materially increased if the patient continues to smoke (Silverman and Griffith, 1972).

4. *Syphilitic Leucoplakia.*—There is a strong association between syphilis and leucoplakia and Weisberger (1957) reported 14 patients with leucoplakia and positive serology for specific infection. Syphilis and candida are responsible for the only cases in which leucoplakia occurs as a result of an infection, and once the leucoplakia has reached a certain stage of development the condition is irreversible even though the causative infection has been eradicated. Patients with syphilitic leucoplakia have a marked tendency to develop oral carcinoma and a reduction in the incidence of syphilis may be responsible for a falling off in the number of cases of oral carcinoma. Recently there has been an increase in the incidence of new cases of syphilis, and it would seem logical that there should be a corresponding increase in oral leucoplakia of syphilitic origin. However, the condition usually arises in the tertiary stage of the disease and with the efficacy and availability of modern anti-syphilitic treatment, this should not necessarily occur.

5. *Chemical Leucoplakia.*—Various chemical irritants will produce hyperkeratotic lesions, although not in all subjects. Examples of such irritants are hot spices, ginger, and the betel nut quid. Carcinoma of the mouth in betel nut chewers is well known, but the activity of the various ingredients is not properly understood.

6. *Lichen Planus.*—Lichen planus is clinically distinguishable from

leucoplakia, but in a minority of cases the clinical and histopathological differential diagnosis may be difficult. Lichen planus is a generalized dermatological condition, the skin lesions appearing as small flat papules a few millimetres in diameter which coalesce into larger plaques covered with a fine glistening scale which shows tiny white radiating lines (striae of Wickham) across its surface. Early in the disease the lesions are red, but they soon become violaceous. The disease often manifests itself in the oral cavity before the appearance of the skin lesions and it may occur alone. In the mouth lichen planus usually appears as a series of radiating white or grey lines which cross over each other forming a reticular pattern. The buccal mucosa in the molar area is most commonly affected and the lesions often have a violaceous hue. The oral condition may be asymptomatic, but the patient sometimes complains of a burning sensation at the site of the lesion. Occasionally vesicle or bulla formation occurs, and this erosive form of lichen planus usually arises *de novo* and not as a progression from the non-erosive lesion. Lichen planus used to be regarded as a benign condition, but recently reports have appeared in the literature of carcinomatous changes in the lesions. Warin (1960) has referred to an incidence of 10 per cent which become malignant, while Altman and Perry (1961) reported the incidence to be 1 per cent. Andreasen and Pindborg (1963) reviewed 46 cases of carcinoma developing in patients with oral lichen planus, 16 of which occurred in patients with the erosive variety of the disease. However, 24 of the 46 patients had an additional predisposing cause of oral carcinoma, some of them suffering from syphilis. In the authors' experience likewise, patients with lichen planus who have developed carcinomas in the oral lesions have also been heavy smokers. Eggleston (1970) has reported a case in which both leucoplakia and lichen planus were present in the mouth of a patient, and in view of the unknown aetiology of both conditions and difficulty of distinguishing them clinically, the explanation may be that they are variants of the same condition.

7. *Leucoplakia of Unknown Aetiology.*—In a large number of cases of leucoplakia there is not an obvious aetiological factor and only a small number of these cases are dyskeratotic. Cooke (1963) pointed out that the presence of dyskeratosis cannot be judged from the clinical appearance. Pindborg and others (1963) found that the so-called 'speckled' leucoplakias, in which the surface is patchy red and white, were often dyskeratotic or were found to be carcinomatous. Carcinoma in situ is an unusual finding in the mouth and neither leucoplakia, dyskeratosis, nor carcinoma in situ is an inevitable precursor of invasive carcinoma. Verrucous carcinoma forms a grossly proliferative warty plaque which may at times be one of the intermediate stages between leucoplakia and carcinoma.

Patients with the Paterson-Kelly (Plummer-Vinson) syndrome, i.e., microchromic, microcytic anaemia, dysphagia, koilonychia, and smooth red tongue, have a high incidence of oral carcinoma. The tongue lesions are essentially hyperkeratotic with areas of desquamation. (*Figs.* 18, 19.) Patients with widespread leucoplakia are particularly at risk and may develop multiple primaries either serially or at about the same time.

Keratinizing Squamous-cell Carcinoma.—Early carcinoma can appear clinically as a white lesion and is on inspection indistinguishable from leucoplakia. Later, of course, the lesion will probably become ulcerated. Such cases are not leucoplakic patches undergoing malignant changes, but are primary carcinomas.

Candidiasis as a Form of Leucoplakia.—Invasion of the epithelium with Candida may cause hyperplasia and the progressive development of plaques in patients with long-standing candidal infection. Beyond a certain point this epithelial proliferation appears to be irreversible, even after the original infection has been eradicated, and in this respect it resembles the reaction in syphilitic leucoplakia. It has been suggested that

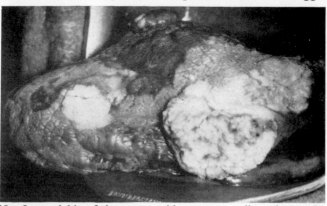

Fig. 18.—Leucoplakia of the tongue with squamous-cell carcinoma. There are two primary carcinomas; one arising in a fissure anteriorly and a fungating ulcer more posteriorly. There is also a fibro-epithelial polyp on the dorsum.

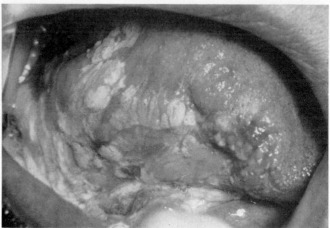

Fig. 19.—Leucoplakia of the floor of the mouth and side of the tongue with a squamous-cell carcinoma.

when candidal infection is found in association with leucoplakia it is a superimposed infection (Jepsen and Winther, 1965), but according to Cawson (1969) it is more likely that the candidal infection is itself the cause of the leucoplakia.

The Incidence of Carcinoma in Patients with Leucoplakia.—Einhorn and Wersall (1967) followed 782 patients with clinical leucoplakia for periods of 1–42 years and found that carcinoma developed in 2·4 per cent of cases within 10 years and 4 per cent in 20 years. Pindborg and others (1968), in a series of 214 patients, found malignant changes in 4·4 per cent in a period of 3·7 years. Cooke (1964) followed 50 cases of leucoplakia for varying periods of up to 10 years and reported an incidence of carcinoma of 12 per cent. This is a high figure, but the series is probably too small to be statistically significant. It is probable that about 5 per cent of cases of leucoplakia will develop malignant changes in a five-year period and this incidence is about 50–100 times the incidence in the normal mouth.

Treatment.—In view of the multiplicity of white patches which may occur in the mouth and the widely differing varieties which are clinically indistinguishable, it is essential to biopsy all white lesions in order to confirm or establish a diagnosis. If the lesion is small (i.e., up to 2 cm. across) an excision and biopsy will have the advantage of establishing the diagnosis and eliminating the lesion. It is also logical to remove leuco-plakic patches which are subject to friction from dentures, etc., in view of the possible increased risk of malignancy. The problem arises as to whether all leucoplakic patches should be excised. Arguments in favour of excision are that it eradicates the disease and avoids the possible development of malignancy. However, in leucoplakia of unknown aetiology the lesion may recur and there is not, at present, any long-term follow-up of leuco-plakic patches treated by excision. Indeed, Einhorn and Wersall (1967) found over a period of 15 years that the incidence of carcinoma was twice as high in those cases where excision had been carried out. In view of the available evidence that about 5 per cent of all leucoplakic patches become malignant, it follows that in 95 per cent of cases malignancy is unlikely to occur. It would therefore seem logical to adopt a more conservative approach to the treatment of leucoplakia and, therefore, after the diag-nosis has been established by biopsy the condition should be kept under review at a three-month review clinic. It should, of course, be impressed upon the patient that any alteration in the lesion which occurs between visits should be reported immediately. Evidence of malignant change usually takes the form of ulceration, fissuring, or nodularity, and any suspicious area in the leucoplakic patch should be biopsied immediately. If carcinoma is found to be present, it should be treated without delay.

There are, of course, other difficulties: patients often fail to attend after a period of follow-up. This fact tends to bias the clinician towards the excision of the lesion where this is easily accomplished. It does not, of course, mean that follow-up can then be abandoned, for further white patches may appear.

Where a patient has had one malignancy of the mouth treated, the clinician may be inclined to advise the excision of any as yet non-malignant white patches in the hope of avoiding a second primary. Some lesions, of course, appear 'unstable' on clinical grounds and these will be removed and all known irritants eliminated.

The problem comes with widespread lesions. It is impracticable to replace almost all the mucosa of the mouth and pharynx and in some patients this is the extent of the disease. The areas most likely to give trouble can, of course, be excised and grafted. Repeated biopsies and surgery can cause a patient to cease to attend for follow-up and then when they do re-appear it may be with a large carcinoma. To avoid this, other methods can be used to monitor the affected areas.

Various stains such as iodine can be applied to the mucous membrane. Early carcinomas will stain darkly. A dissecting microscope can be used to examine suspicious regions and serial photographs may help the clinician to spot a shape he would otherwise overlook. Epithelial scrapings can be spread on a slide, fixed and stained, and examined for hyper-keratotic and malignant cells. Such scrapings should be taken in a way that the area from which they come can be identified. If a positive report is received a biopsy is performed. Such an examination is called an 'exfoliative cytological examination', but as the cells have not yet exfoliated, the term is more correctly used for the examination of sputum, cavity washings, etc. 'A desquamated cytological examination' is probably a better term. An excellent paper on this aspect of diagnosis of oral carcinomas has been published by Spengos (1967).

BOWEN'S DISEASE

Bowen's disease is a precancerous epithelial skin lesion consisting of firm papules covered by a keratinized layer or crust. The lesion may persist for years and in approximately one-fifth of patients with Bowen's disease the lesions undergo malignant transformation. The lesions of Bowen's disease occur on the extremities, abdomen, and buttocks, but they may also occur in the oral cavity and in this situation they are usually multicentric. Bowen's disease represents a carcinoma in situ.

QUEYRAT'S ERYTHROPLASIA

Queyrat's erythroplasia is a rare precancerous lesion of unknown aetiology which takes the form of a bright red, velvety plaque and occurs on mucous membranes particularly the glans penis, prepuce, and vulva. Oral manifestations have been described on the buccal mucosa, tongue, and lips and histologically it appears as a squamous carcinoma in situ.

SUBMUCOUS FIBROSIS

Submucous fibrosis is a disease usually confined to patients of Asiatic descent and the majority of the reported cases have occurred in Indians. A few Europeans living in India have developed the disease and a recent case of an English woman married to a Pakistani, but living in Manchester, was reported by Simpson (1969). The condition arises only in the mouth and there is at first a progressive stiffening of the cheeks due to a proliferation of fibrous tissue and the fibrous replacement of muscle. As a result, fibrous bands are readily palpable in the cheeks and the condition may progress to involve the tongue, lips, faucial pillars, palate, and pharynx and all these structures become hard and lose their mobility. This leads to inability to open the mouth and dysphagia, and if the tongue or soft palate are affected there may be interference with speech. The mucosa tends to be pale in colour. Experimentally betel nut has failed to produce the lesion and it has been speculated that the consumption of chillies may play a part in the aetiology. Vesicles may appear at an early stage but are later followed by hypopigmentation or patches of irregularly mottled pigmentation. A burning sensation in the mouth is sometimes complained of.

Pindborg (1965b) and Pindborg and others (1967) found the incidence in India to be less than 1 per cent, but in 100 Indian patients with oral carcinoma the incidence of submucous fibrosis was 40 per cent. Of 50 cases of submucous fibrosis in Bombay, 2 per cent had oral carcinoma and of 51 cases seen in Lucknow, 9·8 per cent were affected. Lemmer and Shear (1968) reported 6 cases of submucous fibrosis which they examined histologically and one of these showed dyskeratosis with atypism.

Treatment.—None of the suggested treatments are very effective, but eradication of forms of chronic irritation, e.g., sharp, jagged teeth, should be carried out. Cutting of the fibrous bands only seems to lead to the production of more fibrous tissue, and the use of topical, local, or systemic corticosteroids is equally ineffective.

REFERENCES

ALTMAN, J., and PERRY, H. O. (1961), 'The Variations of the Cause of Lichen Planus', *Archs Derm.*, **84**, 179.

ANDREASEN, J. O., and PINDBORG, J. J. (1963), 'Development of Cancer in Oral Lichen Planus', *Nord. Med.*, **70**, 861.

BRUSZT, P. (1962), 'Stomato-oncological Screening Tests in 7 Villages of the Baja and Bacsalmas District', *Magy. Onkol.*, **6**, 28.

CAWSON, R. A. (1969), 'Leucoplakia and Oral Cancer', *Proc. R. Soc. Med.*, **62**, 610.

COOKE, B. E. D. (1963), 'Exfoliative Cytology in evaluating Oral Lesions', *J. dent. Res.*, **42**, 343.

— — (1964), 'Leucoplakia Buccalis', *Ann. R. Coll. Surg.*, **34**, 370.

EGGLESTON, D. J. (1970), 'Lichen Planus or Leukoplakia', *Oral Surg.*, **29**, 845.

EINHORN, J., and WERSALL, J. (1967), 'Incidence of Oral Carcinoma in Patients with Leukoplakia of the Oral Mucosa', *Cancer, N.Y.*, **20**, 2189.

JEPSEN, A., and WINTHER, J. E. (1965), 'Mycotic Infection in Oral Leukoplakia', *Acta odont. scand.*, **23**, 239.

KRAMER, I. R. H. (1969), 'Precancerous Conditions of the Oral Mucosa', *Ann. R. Coll. Surg.*, **45**, 340.

LEMMER, J., and SHEAR, M. (1968), 'Precancerous and Cancerous Lesions of the Mouth', *J. dent. Ass. S. Afr.*, **23**, 274.

MEHTA, E. S., PINDBORG, J. J., DAFTARY, D. K., and GUPTA, P. C. (1969), 'Oral Leukoplakia among Indian Villagers, the Association with Smoking Habits', *Br. dent. J.*, **127**, 73.

MOORE, C., and CATLIN, D. (1967), 'Anatomic Origins and Locations of Oral Cancer', *Am. J. Surg.*, **114**, 510.

PINDBORG, J. J., RENSTRUP, G., POULSEN, H. E., and SILVERMAN, S., jun. (1963), ' Studies in Oral Leukoplakias', *Acta odont. scand.*, **21**, 407.

— — and others (1965a), 'Frequency of Oral Leukoplakia and Related Conditions among 10,000 Bombayites', *J. all-India dent. Ass.*, **37**, 228.

— — and others (1965b), 'Clinical Aspects of Oral Submucous Fibrosis', *Acta odont. scand.*, **22**, 679.

— — and others (1967), 'Oral Epithelial Changes in Thirty Indians with Oral Cancer and Submucous Fibrosis', *Cancer, N.Y.*, **20**, 1141.

— — and others (1968), 'Studies in Oral Leucoplakia', *J. Am. dent. Ass.*, **76**, 767.

— — POULSEN, H. E., and ZACHARIAH, J. (1967), 'Oral Epithelial Changes in Thirty Indians with Oral Cancer and Submucous Fibrosis', *Cancer, N.Y.*, **20**, 1141.

SILVERMAN, S., and GRIFFITH, M. (1972), 'Smoking Characteristics of Patients with Oral Carcinoma and the Risk of Second Oral Primary Carcinoma', *J. Am. dent. Ass.*, **85**, 637.

SIMPSON, W, (1969), 'Submucous Fibrosis', *Br. J. oral Surg.*, **6**, 196.

SPENGOS, M. N. (1967), 'Dental Diagnosis of Oral Carcinoma. Early Detection Cytology', *Dent. Radiogr. Photogr.*, **40**, 51.

WARIN, R. P. (1960), 'Epithelioma following Lichen Planus of the Mouth', *Br. J. Derm.*, **72**, 288.

WEISBERGER, D. (1957), 'Precancerous Lesions', *J. Am. dent. Ass.*, **54**, 507.

CHAPTER XIII

THE CLINICAL DIAGNOSIS OF ORAL MALIGNANCY

THE clinical diagnosis of malignancy of the oral cavity, an area which includes the lips, tongue, floor of the mouth, cheeks, and pillars of the fauces, presents few diagnostic difficulties and, provided that the clinician carries out a systematic examination of the oral cavity, there is little chance of a malignant lesion being overlooked. Difficulty can only arise if the lesion is exceptionally small or if it lies in an anatomically inaccessible area. However, the diagnosis of malignant neoplasm arising within the mandible or the maxillae is more difficult in the early stages of the disease.

Table I.—MALIGNANT NEOPLASMS AFFECTING ORAL CAVITY

Primary Carcinomas:—	Of a surface.
	Of a gland—usually a salivary gland.
	The rare intra-bony of the jaws:—
	1. Arising in a cyst lining.
	2. *Krompecher* carcinoma arising from residual odontogenic epithelium.
Secondary Carcinomas:—	Centrally in the medullary cavity of the jaw bones.
	On the surface of the mucosa—malignant cell from sputum grafted on to raw area.
	In lymph-nodes from a head and neck primary.
Primary Sarcoma:—	Centrally in the tissues:—
	1. In the jaws osteogenic sarcoma,
	reticulum-cell sarcoma,
	Ewing's tumour,
	Lymphosarcoma.
	2. In the muscles
	Fibrosarcoma,
	Leiomyosarcoma,
	Rhabdomyosarcoma.
Reticuloses:—	Usually in the cheeks, sometimes centrally in the jaws
	Hodgkin's disease
	Leukaemic deposits, etc.

Symptoms of Carcinoma of the Oral Cavity.—The general symptoms vary according to the site of the carcinoma and as the lesions are always painless in the early stages they may be overlooked, especially when they are sited towards the back of the oral cavity. Carcinoma of the lip is usually noticed by the patient as a painless lump or ulcer on the lip, while carcinoma of the anterior part of the mouth may first be discovered by the patient's tongue probing the lesion. In the posterior part of the mouth symptoms are usually slight until the lesion has reached a diameter of 2–3 cm. or until it becomes infected, when pain and swelling supervene, which may cause difficulty in deglutition.

Pain and tenderness only develop when a malignant ulcer becomes secondarily infected or if the lesion involves a sensory nerve. Occasionally symptoms are absent until the tumour has metastasized to the regional lymph-nodes and the patient notices a hard lump in the neck. In such cases the primary growth may be merely a minute crack in the lip or in the region of the fauces and carcinoma of the nasopharynx often presents in this fashion.

Late Symptoms.—Late symptoms of carcinoma of the oral cavity are pain due to secondary infection or involvement of the nerves in the region, excessive salivation, difficulty in deglutition and speech and haemorrhage which usually manifests itself as blood-stained saliva.

Neoplasms arising within the Bone.—The early symptom of a neoplasm arising within the bone of the mandible or maxilla is a painless swelling which characteristically involves both the buccal and lingual or buccal and palatal sulci. If teeth are present they may become loose and painful and often the patient seeks aid because he thinks he has an acute alveolar abscess. If the patient is edentulous a previously satisfactory denture may no longer fit and may be displaced or it may cut into the soft tissues and produce a localized denture hyperplasia or granuloma. Anaesthesia of the upper or lower lip is quite common. The malignant conditions which may affect the mouth are classified in *Table I.*

Carcinoma of the Lip.—Carcinoma of the vermilion border is most common between the ages of 50 and 70 years and the majority of the patients are male. According to Aird (1957) it is most common among unskilled labourers and is a disease of the lower classes. The patients tend to have dirty, jagged, stained teeth and, indeed, sometimes the malignancy does arise at a site irritated by a jagged tooth. Common precipitating factors may be some form of irritation and leucoplakic change due to hot tobacco smoke caused by leaving a lighted cigarette stub lying on the lip. There is an increased incidence of carcinoma of the lip in occupations and countries where the patient is subjected to intense solar radiation. According to Rains and Capper (1969) 40 per cent of patients with carcinoma of the lip give a history of blistering cheilitis due to sunlight. Carcinoma of the lip is therefore more common in countries where there is protracted sunshine and among patients whose occupation causes them to be unduly exposed to the elements. The condition is known colloquially as 'countryman's lip'. The lower lip is affected in 93 per cent of cases and the upper lip in 5 per cent, while 2 per cent occur at the angle of the mouth. Sometimes a growth occurs on the upper lip at a point opposite the lower lip lesion, possibly due to direct implantation of cells. The tumour begins as a small, painless scabbing ulcer, which arises in the substance of the lip and if untreated spreads to the cheek, gum, and jaw. According to Aird (1957) 10 per cent of the patients with carcinoma of the lip develop metastases within a year and 36 per cent within two years and the lymph-nodes affected are the submental, submandibular, and upper jugular groups. Death eventually occurs from infection or aspiration pneumonia.

Differential Diagnosis.—Carcinoma of the lip must be distinguished from molluscum pseudo-carcinomatosum which also has a predilection for the lower lip and is clinically indistinguishable from carcinoma.

Carcinoma of the Tongue.—Carcinoma of the anterior two-thirds of the tongue affects males nine times more frequently than females. Cancer of the posterior third affects the sexes equally, and most of the patients are over 60 years of age. Females with cancer of the anterior two-thirds of the tongue are often found to be suffering from a Paterson-Kelly or Plummer-Vinson syndrome. The oral hygiene is usually bad in patients with carcinoma of the tongue. The disease is often associated with heavy drinking of alcohol and this may be correlated with a deficiency of vitamin B_1 which is known to produce a precancerous mucosal atrophy. Alcohol contains an adequate number of calories to sustain life without the necessity of eating an adequate diet, but unfortunately it does not contain vitamins. Twenty-five per cent of the patients have suffered from syphilis and 5 per cent have had leucoplakia. Other precancerous lesions include superficial glossitis, papilloma, fissures, and non-specific ulcers. The tumours lie near the lateral edge of the tongue in 58 per cent of cases and the dorsum of the tongue is involved in 2–4 per cent, the tip in 7–15 per cent, and the posterior third in 21–33 per cent. Carcinoma of the posterior third of the tongue is often overlooked by the patient and even the clinician. Alteration of the voice is often a presenting symptom in these cases. According to Aird (1957) there are five naked eye appearances of carcinoma of the tongue: (1) The ulcerative type, (2) Papillary, (3) The flat nodule, (4) A malignant fissure which is often a sequel of syphilitic fissuring, (5) Scirrhous or atrophic.

Clinical Features.—The earliest symptom is a painless swelling or an ulcer. Once the ulcer is established, pain is continuous and severe and may radiate to the ear. This is due to involvement of the lingual nerve and referred pain to auriculo-temporal region may occur. It is accompanied by excessive salivation and there is marked foetor oris, haemorrhage, and finally immobility of the tongue as it becomes fixed to the floor of the mouth. Before this stage is reached, the tongue becomes fixed on one side and when the patient protrudes the tongue it deviates towards the affected side. Dysarthria and dysphagia may also occur. The life expectancy of an untreated carcinoma of the tongue is about 16 months. Carcinoma of the tongue presents as an induration, ulceration, or fungation which spreads directly to the floor of the mouth and from there to the alveolar process. From the posterior third of the tongue the spread is to the fauces, valleculae, and epiglottis. Metastases are restricted to the regional glands. In the anterior two-thirds of the tongue metastases are ipsilateral and bilateral metastases only occur if the tumour extends to the midline of the tongue. The metastases from growths in the posterior third of the tongue are bilateral. In the untreated case death is inevitable and can occur as a result of inhalation bronchopneumonia, cachexia and starvation, haemorrhage (usually from a metastasis eroding a major artery), and asphyxia.

Carcinoma of the Mouth.—Carcinoma occurs in the floor of the mouth, cheek, palate, and faucial pillar. In the floor of the mouth it is usually a typical malignant ulcer extending to the alveolar process and tongue. The cheek lesion is often warty and proliferative. On the alveolar process the tumour may be warty, nodular, or proliferating. (*Fig.* 20.) Such neoplasms must be distinguished from the results of denture irritation and, where teeth are present, from a periodontal abscess. Carcinoma of the palate is often papillary or ulcerative and usually spreads extensively before it affects the bone. It is difficult to distinguish it from a carcinoma of the maxillary sinus which has spread to the palate.

Carcinomas of the soft palate and fauces are proliferative, fungating tumours, and carry a particularly poor prognosis. They spread to the base of the tongue and there is early involvement of the lymph-nodes bilaterally. Secondary infection causes pain and dysphagia, and death frequently occurs following erosion of the carotid artery.

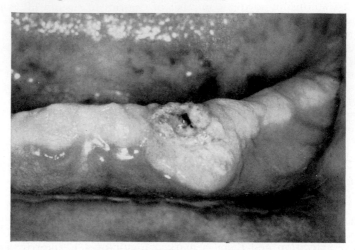

Fig. 20.—Proliferating squamous-cell carcinoma of the alveolus.

Malignant Neoplasms of the Maxillary Antrum.—The squamous-cell carcinoma accounts for between 90 and 95 per cent of antral malignancies. All degrees of differentiation are found, but many are anaplastic. The tumour infiltrates the soft tissues, destroys bone, and can ulcerate into the mouth, pharynx, and skin of the face. Lymphatic metastasis to the upper deep cervical nodes occurs and rarely lymphatic spread may take place to the retropharyngeal group of nodes. Other malignant growths arise in the maxillary sinus such as adenocarcinoma, lympho-epithelioma, and sarcoma, but their incidence is obviously small.

While confined to the bony walls of the antrum the neoplasm does not produce definite symptoms, but with extension certain clinical features develop and these specific signs and symptoms should be known to every dental surgeon to ensure prompt recognition of the disease.

The earliest presenting symptom is often a unilateral sero-sanguineous discharge or frank epistaxis. The possibility of a carcinoma of the maxillary sinus should always be considered when an elderly patient presents with epistaxis of recent origin. The established carcinoma of the maxillary sinus may produce unilateral swelling of the cheek, buccal sulcus, or palate. Intra-oral swelling may dislodge a denture which has up to that time fitted satisfactorily and, where the edge of the denture cuts into the soft tissue mass, there may be a denture hyperplasia or granuloma. If teeth are present in relation to the floor of the maxillary sinus they may become loose, painful, and periostitic. The patient may sometimes, in fact, present with an acute alveolar abscess. There may be anaesthesia of the cheek in the distribution of the infra-orbital nerve, or anaesthesia or paraesthesia of the palate due to involvement of the sphenopalatine ganglion. If the nasolacrimal duct is occluded due to medial spread, epiphora will ensue. The eye on the affected side may be proptosed and if the tumour has invaded the orbit and interfered with one or more of the orbital muscles or the nerves which innervate them, there will be strabismus, limitation of ocular movements and the patient will complain of diplopia. The pupillary level may be raised on the affected side and in very

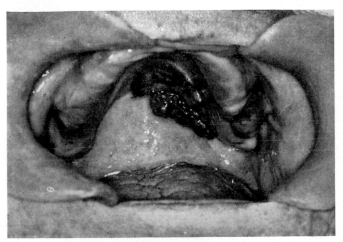

Fig. 21.—Malignant melanoma of the palate.

advanced cases there may be amblyopia. The nostril on the affected side may be blocked and on inspection with a nasal speculum the tumour mass can often be seen growing down the nostril. There is frequently a blood-stained discharge of pus from the nostril. Pain is sometimes due to secondary infection of the maxillary sinus and in extreme cases the swelling on the face bursts through the cheek and fungates. Trismus may occur due to encroachment upon the medial pterygoid.

The importance of the dental surgeon as a diagnostician in antral neoplasia is evident from the improved five-year cure rate prognosis for those with oral symptoms alone (Kay, 1970), but generally the outlook is poor, since at least 70 per cent of patients with malignancies occurring in or affecting the maxillary sinus will die from their disease (Harrison, 1971). It should be realized, however, that the characteristic radiographic changes of antral mucosal malignancy, i.e., destruction of bony walls, do not appear early, so the fact that an occipitomental view may show normal antral bony contours in a case which is suspicious on clinical grounds does not exclude the existence of serious disease.

Further Management.—A biopsy is essential to confirm the diagnosis and so that treatment is based on a proper knowledge of the nature of the lesion. Chest X-rays and/or radiographs of other bones and a careful general inquiry and physical examination are necessary, both to uncover any overt secondaries and to establish the degree of physical fitness of the patient. A haemoglobin estimation, blood-film examination, white-cell count, and blood group determination are other essential preliminary investigations.

More than in the treatment of most oral diseases, a careful social history and a discussion with relatives are necessary to understand fully the implication of the various forms of treatment.

Malignant Melanoma (*Fig.* 21).—Primary malignant melanoma of the oral cavity was first reported by Weber in 1859. It is a rare condition and Chaudhry, Hampel, and Gorlin (1958) reviewed 105 cases from the literature between 1859 and 1957. It is seen more frequently in men than in women and 75 per cent of the patients are 40 years of age or over. It presents as a raised, soft, vascular, dark brown or black mass, and bleeding and ulcerations are common. When it occurs in the mouth it destroys adjacent bone and loosens teeth in its vicinity. It has a tendency to invade blood-vessels and lymph channels and some 50 per cent of cases show involvement of the lymph-nodes when first seen. For this reason, a search of the body for a possible primary lesion should always be made when a melanoma is seen in the oral cavity. Cade (1961) believes that in many cases diagnosis can be made on clinical grounds alone and that biopsy is unnecessary. However, in view of the mutilating surgery required to treat the condition, histological evidence is usually required before embarking on treatment. Cade advocates a frozen section if biopsy is considered necessary. The prognosis of intra-oral melanoma is very poor.

REFERENCES

AIRD, I. (1957), *A Companion to Surgical Studies*, 2nd ed. Edinburgh: Livingstone.
CADE, S. (1961), 'Malignant Melanoma', *Ann. R. Coll. Surg.*, **28**, 331.
CHAUDHRY, A. P., HAMPEL, A., and GORLIN, R. (1958), 'Primary Malignant Melanoma of the Oral Cavity. A Review of 105 Cases', *Cancer, N.Y.*, **11**, 923.
HARRISON, D. F. N. (1971), Paper given at the 4th International Conference on Oral Surgery, held in Amsterdam, 17–21 May.
RAINS, A. J. H., and CAPPER, W. M., ed. (1968), *Bailey and Love's Short Practice of Surgery*, 14th ed. London: Lewis.
WEBER, C. O. (1859), *Chirurgische erfahrungen und untersuchungen reimer*. Berlin.

CHAPTER XIV

THE TREATMENT OF MALIGNANT NEOPLASMS

THE treatment of patients with malignant neoplasms involves a type of medicine which has been made almost redundant in many other fields by potent, effective, therapeutic agents which, by and large, have few, or tolerable, side effects. The treatment of malignant neoplasms means responsibility for the patient for the rest of his or her life. It means the making of judgements which affect the patient's survival, livelihood and social contacts. It involves a relationship with the patient and the relatives which is more emotionally charged than that experienced by oral surgeons in most other aspects of their work.

Treatment of oral malignant neoplasms starts properly with the general dental practitioner and the avoidance of premalignant conditions. Patients' mouths should be maintained in a healthy state, free from chronic sepsis and chronic irritation. Natural teeth and appliances should be kept smooth and in good repair. While there is no proper statistical evidence linking irritation from rough teeth and carcinoma, occasional highly-suggestive cases are seen and the fact remains, whatever the reason, that more lingual carcinomas are seen on the lateral borders of the tongue than on the tip or centre (unless the patient has leucoplakia of the tongue). Smoking, strong spices, strong spirits and the betel-nut quid, particularly if indulged in regularly and in excessive amounts, are known to produce premalignant lesions in a proportion of those who use them. Patients should be advised against such potentially harmful habits. The effective treatment of syphilis is important to avoid the precarcinomatous, leuco-plakic tongue which is a late sequela of this infection. Benign neoplasms or granulomatous swelling should be excised, particularly if they are subject to repeated trauma. Chapter XII deals more fully with premalignant conditions.

The successful treatment of malignant neoplasms depends much on early diagnosis and again the general dental practitioner has an important role to play with regular and careful examinations of the patient. The dental surgeon should have a healthy suspicion of the slightly unusual—for example, a deep 'periodontal pocket' with florid granulations and bone destruction in an otherwise healthy mouth, or a chronic ulcer, or fissure with no apparent cause.

Features which demand careful consideration are:

a. Chronic ulcers or fissures with no apparent cause or ones which do not respond promptly to simple treatment.

b. Swellings with no apparent cause, especially if there are dilated small vessels over the surface, but no marked oedema or redness.

c. Rapid and unexpected loosening of a group of teeth, irregular bone destruction seen radiographically, or unexpected fracture following minimal trauma *d.* Signs of infiltration, such as tethering of an organ or lump, or limitation of the normal movement of the part.

e. Signs of involvement of adjacent nerves producing persistent pain, anaesthesia of the part, or paralysis of muscles.

f. Signs of obstruction of related ducts such as salivary ducts, or obstruction of related veins with vascular engorgement.

g. Repeated, small haemorrhages from a particular location.

h. Enlarged lymph-nodes without surrounding oedema and no obvious simple cause.

i. An 'abscess' with no apparent cause which may be a necrotic neoplasm.

j. Anaemia with no obvious cause.

k. Sweating, malaise and toxicity not due to an obvious infection.

The clinician should not rely solely on the biopsy report for information about the type of neoplasm. The length of history, mode of presentation and clinical and radiographic appearances may give clues as to the type of tumour which is present. If a decision is made in this way on clinical ground the validity of the biopsy report can be better assessed, particularly where there is an element of doubt.

If a malignant neoplasm is discovered in the oral cavity, the next step is to consider whether it is the primary lesion, or a secondary deposit. An inquiry into the patient's general health may reveal symptoms suggestive of another lesion elsewhere. A careful, full, physical examination likewise may reveal a primary in another organ. Careful probing of the person's past history may uncover treatment of a previous malignancy, an incident which the patient is perhaps reluctant to recall, but which may be highly relevant under the circumstances. Patients sometimes 'censor' information about a system outside the field of the specialist they are consulting and regard it as no concern of his! X-rays of the chest may reveal a bronchial primary, or secondary deposits and films of the skull may reveal further metastatic lesions. The biopsy report may contain the clue to the organ of origin.

In general, no lesion should be treated as a malignant neoplasm until histological proof has been obtained by means of a biopsy. With few exceptions it is neither legally nor morally right to treat the patient for a malignant neoplasm until proper evidence of its nature has been obtained. Nor may proper advice be given to the patient and a prognosis to the relatives unless a histological diagnosis is forthcoming. Mostly malignant neoplasms in the region of the oral cavity and its associated parts are easily accessible for removal of a specimen for biopsy. Masses in some organs like the major salivary glands or in relatively inaccessible sites present special problems (*see* p. 229) and a primary exploratory operation may be proper. Should the tumour be judged benign beyond reasonable doubt and amenable to treatment which does not leave the patient with a major deficit, definitive surgery can be undertaken at the same time. Where there is any doubt as to the nature of the mass and particularly where a more aggressive neoplasm is suspected, then a specimen for frozen section should be taken, and the report seen before surgery is continued, assuming that this is the appropriate form of treatment. Should there still be a doubt as to the diagnosis, or the right course of action, then the wound should be closed and treatment delayed until paraffin sections are available. Precautions against spillage of cells into the wound may be necessary.

Once the clinician is sure he is dealing with a primary neoplasm the extent of its spread must be determined. Local spread is assessed by physical and radiological examination and lymphatic spread by careful palpation of the regional lymph-nodes. In the neck, displacement of the relaxed sternomastoid muscle first forwards and then backwards so that the palpating fingers can seek underneath is an important manoeuvre. A search for evidence of generalized spread involves radiographs of chest and bones, for example the cranial vault and spine, a blood film for evidence of leuco-erythroblastic anaemia and a general examination for other abnormal masses, or an enlarged liver and spleen, etc.

At this stage it is proper that an explanation should be given to the patient. How frank this is depends upon any direct questions that the patient asks, an assessment of the patient's personality, and an understanding of his or her responsibilities in the home and at work (Cade, 1963). No direct lies are permissible, but what is said and the way in which it is said should carry hope and increase the patient's confidence in his adviser. If possible the patient's morale should be increased and certainly not destroyed by what is said. Phrases such as 'a tumour', 'an ulcer' or 'a lump which needs treatment' can be used without recourse to emotive words like 'cancer'. However, patients know that extensive resections, or radiotherapy, are usually used for malignant lesions and hence come to understand the nature of their disease.

Few men have the breadth of skill and experience to advise properly on all aspects of the treatment of malignant neoplasms affecting the oral cavity and a consultation at a joint appointment is advisable at this point. If such cases are handled regularly a special combined clinic should be set up. A radiotherapist and a surgeon form the basic unit for such a consultation. The surgeon should be one who has a special interest in the pathology, natural history and management of neoplastic disease of this region. Because these tumours may well transgress the anatomical boundaries or skills of more than one surgical speciality, several surgeons with appropriate abilities may need on occasion to meet over the problem. Since anaesthetic difficulties and general disease are commonly met with in these patients, the advice of an anaesthetist, or a physician, may also be appropriate. Most radiotherapists include the use of cytotoxic drugs in their armamentarium, but for some conditions, such as the leukaemias, a physician such as a haematologist may be the local expert in this field.

When the nature of the treatment is explained, the clinician should say that with prompt and proper treatment there is every chance of a cure. The patient should then be given the opportunity to ask further questions, if he or she so wishes, and honest, but kindly, answers should be given.

The patient's relatives will usually wish an opportunity for a private interview. A clear, simple statement of what has been found, what must be done, and what may be the final outcome should be given. Frequently relatives, and indeed patients, misunderstood and any misinterpretations must be cleared up as soon as they are recognized. Their co-operation and support must be mobilized and are important for the patient's well-being. A letter giving full details of the results of the investigations, consultations and proposed treatment must be sent to the medical G.P. as well as the referring dental surgeon, for the patient's doctor must play a large part in the subsequent long-term care of the patient.

Treatment may be either curative or palliative. Curative treatment can be considered for primary tumours with no evidence of spread other than local spread, and for those tumours which have metastasized to the regional lymph-nodes, but where these are still moveable on adjacent vital structures or are amenable to radiotherapy, as in the case of a reticulosis. The means available for hopefully curative treatment are radiotherapy and/or surgery and the treatment for a particular patient is best decided by discussion at the joint clinic between surgeon and radiotherapist. Certain factors need to be borne in mind when such decisions are being made. Without doubt radiotherapy, if successful, will give far better functional and aesthetic results than radical surgery and for the common squamous-cell carcinoma in many sites there is little difference in success rates between the two methods of treatment. The only major disadvantages of radiotherapy are:

a. The loss of teeth which may be necessary as a prophylaxis against post-irradiation osteomyelitis.

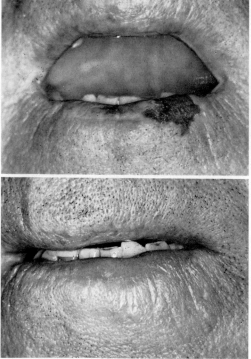

Fig. 22.—A small carcinoma of the lower lip (upper photograph) at the site where the patient habitually held a self-rolled cigarette. Lower photograph after treatment by radium needle implant; 4-year follow-up.

b. The risk of post-irradiation osteomyelitis itself.

c. A more remote risk of necrosis of the soft tissues, cartilage or bone due to local overdose.

d. Damage to the salivary glands and dryness of the mouth, which together with atrophy of the mucous membrane can make the wearing of dentures difficult.

e. Radiation cataract in the case of tumours which are close to, or involve, the eye although the latter is often excised at a subsequent operation.

f. And, occasionally, temporary depilation, or radiation fibrosis of muscles.

With modern treatment methods the risk that the patient will suffer any of these complications is materially smaller than in the past.

Small squamous-cell carcinomas of the anterior two-thirds of the tongue do at least as well with a radium or caesium needle implant as after surgery and the patient retains an intact tongue. Squamous carcinoma of the lower lip similarly may be treated with a substantial percentage of

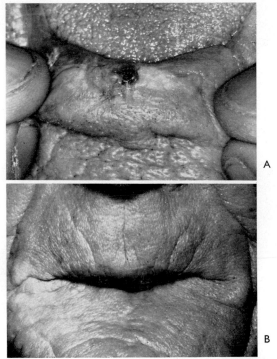

Fig. 23.—A, A patient had been treated 3 years previously for a squamous-cell carcinoma of the lower right alveolar process which had arisen in a zone of leuco-plakia involving the inside of both cheeks and the floor of the mouth. Treatment 6,500r by cobalt 60 irradiation. B, He then developed a squamous-cell carcinoma of the lip. He was a heavy smoker and an outdoor worker with solar keratosis of the lower lip. Treatment: a lip shave and wedge excision of the lower lip, closing with a Z-plasty to prevent a notched lower lip.

successful results by either method, but mostly is treated by radiotherapy using radioactive gold seeds, needles, or external DXT avoiding the wide, full-thickness resection necessary for surgical treatment (*Figs.* 22 and 23). Carcinoma of the cheek near the commissure does less well than carcinoma of this site more posteriorly situated, but again the alternative is wide, often full-thickness, surgical removal and repair (*Figs.* 24 and 25). Since many such patients have extensive premalignant changes of the oral mucous membrane on both sides of the mouth radiotherapy may be the first choice. Advanced carcinoma of the anterior two-thirds of the tongue can be treated by total glossectomy, but primary treatment by megavoltage radiotherapy gives a similar, even if poor, chance of survival without the difficulties created by complete loss of the tongue.

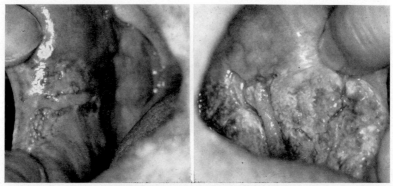

Fig. 24.—Bilateral carcinomas of the cheek, the left more extensive than the right. Treated by cobalt 60 external irradiation.

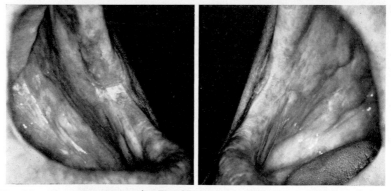

Fig. 25.—The same case as in *Fig.* 24: post-irradiation appearance at 3 years after treatment.

Where there is a choice of treatment, radiotherapy is usually employed first (Easson, 1963). If the blood-supply to the part is materially damaged by previous surgery, radiotherapy is less successful because the effectiveness of treatment is related to proper oxygenation of the tumour tissue. Again treatment planning for radiotherapy can be complicated by injudicious operative treatment. On the other hand, if radiotherapy appears not to be controlling the disease, there must be no delay in turning to surgical treatment. The treatable must not be permitted to become untreatable. There is unfortunately no way of predicting which patients will do well and which badly by a particular technique. Apart from the radiosensitivity of the neoplasm the immune response and resistance of the patient are important. Indeed, where a case does badly with radiotherapy the latter may be the reason, in which case surgery also will have a poor prognosis.

Both the histological type of neoplasm and its site affect its likely response to radiotherapy. Thus squamous-cell carcinomas tend to do well particularly if small and well differentiated—leastways, well in the context of malignant disease. Adenocarcinomas respond less well and sarcomas may melt away only to recur. Melanomas are usually unresponsive. Most authorities are now agreed that once a neoplasm involves the bone of the jaws, the chances of success with radiotherapy alone are reduced, so that subsequent surgery will be required.

Surgery is always mutilating in that sizeable blocks of tissue must be removed. Margins of apparently normal tissue of between 1 and 3 cm., depending on the type of neoplasm, must be removed, *en bloc*, from all aspects of the visible, radiographic and palpable limits of the lesion. This margin must be increased where spread is known to be facilitated in a particular direction. For example, if the posterior part of the mandible is involved the bone from anterior to the mental foramen to posterior to the mandibular foramen must be removed, irrespective of the size of the neoplasm, because of the risk of spread along the inferior dental canal.

Adenocystic carcinomas of salivary glands tend to permeate in the perineural tissues, some believe along the perineural lymphatics, so that the spread along adjacent nerves may be to a much greater distance than elsewhere. Some neoplasms will spread through medullary bone without inciting resorption of the adjacent trabeculae. The advancing edge may then be far removed from the radiographic limits of the disease. Again adenocystic carcinomas are notorious in this respect and the extent of the resection must be increased accordingly.

For some neoplasms and particularly where unpredictable, extensive, infiltration is a feature of their behaviour, experience teaches that surgical resection to the maximum extent feasible to reduce the volume of the neoplasm together with irradiation of the periphery of the surgical field gives the best chance of control of the disease. It should be stressed that such an excision should include a proper margin of tissue around the known limits of the disease. In other circumstances similar tactics will be dictated because the anatomical situation precludes the excision of an adequate margin, uniformly on all aspects.

Normally, when irradiation is used for the treatment of the primary tumour a radical neck dissection is performed only when suspicious mobile nodes are palpated. Since it is of the utmost importance that involved nodes should be detected promptly, regular follow-up visits *must* be maintained and a system of recall set up which checks on missed appointments. Initially, follow-up examinations will be at monthly intervals and this time will be extended only when the risk of the appearance of regional lymph-node metastases seems to be past—for example, after 1 year. Three-monthly and, later, 6-monthly appointments are then instituted. Since the primary neoplasm must be eradicated at the same time as, or before, a neck dissection is undertaken, radiotherapeutic treatment of the primary normally precedes neck dissection. To remove the filtering lymph-nodes before the primary has been dealt with, so permitting cells to pass further afield more readily, is obviously bad tactics. If lymph-node enlargement is noted before regression of the primary has been achieved then excision of the primary is combined with the neck dissection. In some cases a holding dose of irradiation can be delivered to the nodes to reduce the risk of further spread before the surgery is performed or to give the primary a chance to complete its resolution.

When surgical treatment is the method of choice there is greater divergence of opinion about the place of a simultaneous neck dissection (Freund, 1967). Several factors influence the decision. Adequate local surgery often involves the detachment of relevant muscles from the hyoid bone and clearance of the submandibular region, including the submandibular salivary gland and the adjacent lymph-nodes. Adhesions from such a dissection may make more difficult a subsequent neck dissection in the region of the upper deep cervical nodes—a point where adequate clearance is often most important. There is therefore good reason for doing the neck dissection as part of the initial procedure. Further, the main venous drainage is controlled before the primary tumour is handled, so reducing the systemic shower of cells. On the other hand the addition of a radical neck dissection adds to the amount of surgical trauma. Many patients with oral malignant neoplasms are elderly and may be in quite poor general condition as a result of chronic cardiovascular and pulmonary disease. Their ability to withstand the additional surgery must be considered. Furthermore, there is no convincing evidence that prophylactic block dissection improves the prognosis.

Primary neoplasms in some situations may metastasize to either or both sides of the neck (*Fig.* 26). Bilateral neck dissections have a materially more gloomy outlook in terms of survival and morbidity than the unilateral operation. Indeed the unilateral procedure occasions surprisingly little inconvenience to the patient once healing is complete.

For patients who have a primary at one of the sites susceptible to bilateral metastasis, such as lower lip and midline of floor of mouth, it is reasonable to delay a neck dissection until involved nodes are felt. If bilateral neck dissection becomes necessary, this may be performed as a staged procedure—performing the second side 3 weeks after the first. Even so, venous engorgement of the head may be seen and this is of course the major disability resulting from this treatment. Raised intracranial pressure due to venous engorgement may be treated by intravenous mannitol (Stell and Maran, 1972). Some surgeons suggest bilateral neck dissection with preservation of the internal jugular vein on one side, and this may be done. However, the fact that such a manoeuvre contravenes the principle of block removal of the tissues containing the lymph-nodes and lymphatics and takes the operator close to the malignant deposits must be recognized.

Suprahyoid block procedures are generally deprecated. However, a suprahyoid clearance almost inevitably forms a part of the local removal of neoplasms affecting the lower jaw, tongue or floor of mouth and may occasionally have a place where there is simultaneous involvement of submandibular nodes on both sides *without* detectable trouble in other groups of nodes (*Fig.* 26). By this means a bilateral full block may be avoided since if further metastatic nodes become apparent they may be on one side only.

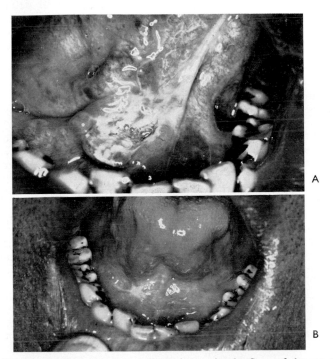

Fig. 26.—A, A small squamous-cell carcinoma in the floor of the mouth in a man of 28. Treated by a gold grain implant. B, The healed primary lesion.
He subsequently developed bilateral simultaneously-enlarged submandibular lymph-nodes which were adherent to the mandible. These were removed by a bilateral suprahyoid block which included the adjacent lower borders of the mandible. Four months postoperatively enlarged upper deep cervical nodes were noted on the right, and a right-side full neck dissection carried out. Since then (2 years) he has been free of further recurrence.

The seeding of viable cells into the operation wound from ulcerating surfaces or from accidental incisions closer than was intended to the tumour mass has given surgeons a good deal of food for thought. Thorough irrigation of the wound after resection is an important prophylaxis against local recurrence. Seeding by injudicious biopsy technique should be avoided, and the precept to remove part of the surrounding normal tissue to provide histological evidence of invasion is less strongly preached than in the past. Inadequate removal as a result of an attempted 'excision' biopsy is to be deprecated. The dissemination of cells via lymphatics or veins following the handling of the tumour also causes concern and severance of the venous drainage and lymphatic field before operative mobilization of the primary is good practice.

More recently an appreciation of the important role played by the patient's own immune mechanisms have tended to revise attitudes to accepted methods of treatment of malignancies. Most agents which attack malignant cells also damage the patient's immunological defences and the question of the degree to which these methods harm rather than help the patient is under debate. Thus cytotoxic drugs have fallen out of favour as a prophylaxis against metastatic spread as a result of cells shed at operation, because trials showed no benefit from this use of these agents. There are arguments against preoperative irradiation on the grounds that damage may be done to immune defences and spread of the neoplasm facilitated. Others (Lee and Wilson, 1973) advocate the use of preoperative radiotherapy so as to reduce the chance of successful growth of any cells shed at the operation.

Full therapeutic doses of irradiation undoubtedly reduce the vitality of the tissues in the treatment area. During the early post-irradiation period, haemorrhage at operation is increased and postoperative ooze is more persistent. Later, both soft tissues and bone withstand the trauma of surgery less well and the incidence of trouble with wound healing is increased. This particularly applies to the skin flaps over the neck. Four to 6 weeks after the completion of a full course of radiotherapy is the optimum time for surgery.

Palliative treatment covers a number of measures. Palliative radiotherapy alone is probably the best course of action. The primary neoplasm may be excised and pre- or post-operative irradiation given for a lesion where there is little hope of cure in the long term, but where such measures have been shown to give the patient a prolonged period of freedom from symptoms of his disease. Tumours which progress slowly, but which have already spread, or metastasized beyond the bounds of effective curative treatment, may be treated in this way. Pulmonary metastasis from muco-epidermoid or adenocystic carcinomas of salivary glands may increase in size very slowly and the patient may live for 3 to 6 years or more largely in ignorance of their presence.

Other primary neoplasms may be excised because their ultimate enlarge-ment, fungation and necrosis would cause the patient great distress before death supervened. If this is done the surgeon must be reasonably sure that the risk of local recurrence following his operation is small and that the surgically-created defect and deformity is less unpleasant for the patient than the anticipated course of the disease. The cryo-probe also may be used to destroy fungating masses and so improve patient comfort.

Radiotherapy to the primary, to involved lymph-nodes and to distant metastases may be used. Such treatment may reduce pain, cause tumour masses to disappear—or at least result in a reduction in their size, or may restrain for a while their further growth—and pathological fractures may be encouraged to heal. Radiotherapy is the principle palliative measure for oral malignancies.

Cytotoxic agents have had a chequered career. In the case of Burkitt's Lymphoma, and leukaemias, progress has been made towards their curative treatment by cytotoxic drugs, often by the use of several such agents at the same time. For most solid tumours they can play only a palliative role and their side effects can be quite unpleasant. Examples of such side effects are marrow depression, gastro-intestinal disturbances, alopecia and oral ulceration. However, new drugs are constantly being produced and this is a fruitful field of research. Bleomycin is currently used in the palliation of squamous cell carcinoma.

Techniques of hormonal control of metastases are now part of standard treatment, particularly for carcinoma of breast and prostate. On occasions the first metastases from these neoplasms to manifest themselves are in the jaws.

Attempts to improve the patient's own immune response are being made, particularly as some aspects of the patient's immune defences can be quantified (Cannell, 1973). By vaccinating patients and other manoeuvres, attempts have been made to affect the course of metastatic malignant melanoma and with some limited improvements in some patients. Unfortunately the presence of large tumour masses overwhelms the patient's immunity so presenting a major stumbling-block to this form of treatment.

In the oral cavity, general dental surgeons can do much to keep the mouth and any neoplastic masses reasonably clean and inoffensive. All carious lesions need treatment, for further extractions should be avoided in case intra-bony neoplasm fungates through the socket, or in case post-irradiation osteomyelitis should be precipitated.

Pain from infection should be controlled by treating the infection, but pain due to infiltration of peripheral nerves needs effective control to prevent demoralization of the patient. Alcohol nerve blocks or peripheral nerve section can have a part to play, and the dentists' skills in giving a local anaesthetic, or the oral surgeon's skill in finding a peripheral nerve, may be required.

Analgesics, narcotics and tranquillizers may be needed to relieve chronic intractable pain and depression. Adequate control in this way of pain which cannot be relieved by other means is essential (Saunders, 1963). By the more central division of pain pathways the neurosurgeon may be able to help at times.

The management of the dying patient is not a skill which most dental surgeons have, fortunately, to employ very often. Medical general practitioners, radiotherapists and general surgeons and physicians are more skilled in this art. District nurses, social workers and the patient's religious minister are all people whose help and advice can be enlisted in the case of the terminal patient. Not least, of course, is the family necessary at this time, but relatives may in their turn seek support from the clinician. The booklet *People and Cancer* by The British Cancer Council (Bennette, 1970) is recommended reading on this subject.

Once progress of the disease has been halted and if possible when a reasonable likelihood of a cure has been achieved, reconstruction and rehabilitation become important. If surgical excision has been undertaken substantial reconstruction should be attempted at the same operation. Broadly speaking primary reconstruction can lay emphasis on either the hard or the soft tissues. Repair of both at the same time is not easily possible with current techniques. Clear advice on the repair of the soft tissues is given by Lee and Wilson (1973) and by Conley (1970). Use of the forehead flap and the deltopectoral flap to reconstruct the oral cavity and the face and neck respectively provides a standard method of repair which gives first-class results in expert hands. An adequate bulk of vascular soft tissue and a sufficient surface of epithelium is thus made available to avoid the displacement of the remaining tissues which adds to the patient's disability. The contour of the face can be restored also by this technique. However, since a seal of the wound is not achieved where the pedicles of these flaps enter the defect, simultaneous bone grafting carries a risk of infection of the graft.

Subsequent reopening of the operation area is not easy and re-establishment of space for a bone-graft at any site, once healing has occurred, can be quite difficult.

Function even without a bone-graft can be good, but too much must not be expected of such a repair. The crippling distortion of the remaining lips, cheek and part of the tongue may be avoided but the connective and adipose tissues of the flaps can never replace the functioning muscles and nerves of the original tissues.

Prefabricated metal prostheses can have a part to play where extensive resection of the mandible is necessary (Bowerman and Conroy, 1969; Cook, 1969), but allelografts can be more demanding than bone-grafts in their requirements in terms of a suitable soft-tissue bed. They save the patient additional surgery at a time when extensive surgery is already necessary, but remain a buried foreign body and their eventual loss remains a permanent risk. Immediate bone-grafts too may fail since the conditions for their insertion are far from ideal, but once a successful take is achieved the chances of complications decrease and in this way they differ from allelografts.

Various temporary allelografts have been tried to provide stability of widely separated bone fragments. In particular prefabricated metal prostheses and temporary allelografts have a place where extensive removal of tissues and mandible from the centre of the lower jaw is necessary. The use of temporary allelografts may enable the best possible soft-tissue repair to be performed. Subsequently the prosthesis is removed through skin incisions, the graft bed enlarged and a bone-graft inserted, again with more favourable circumstances for survival of the graft. However, enlarging the channel for the graft and detaching the allelograft from the bone ends in the face of dense postoperative fibrosis and without entering the mouth can be difficult. A bone-graft placed immediately after the resection and at the same operation occupies the maximum space and produces the best possible contour that can be achieved. The problem is soft-tissue coverage. The wound must be closed in layers and local flaps may produce difficulties with feeding, speech and saliva control, particularly if tongue flaps are used, until such time as secondary soft-tissue repair is possible. The choice therefore is between primary skeletal repair and secondary soft-tissue repair on the one hand and primary soft-tissue repair and secondary bone replacement on the other.

It must be emphasized once more that careful follow-up of the patients for the rest of their life is important, to detect recurrences, to look for evidence of metastases, or for evidence of fresh malignant neoplasms in adjacent or other sites and to record accurately the results of treatment so that rational patient management can evolve.

Following treatment of the malignancy and any necessary surgical reconstruction, the patient frequently needs prosthetic treatment, speech therapy and rehabilitation into normal social life. The construction of dentures raises a problem, for frequently the denture bearing area is abnormal and offers little scope for a retentive appliance. Thin, atrophic mucous membrane which is easily ulcerated, and a dry mouth, add to the difficulties. For some patients with widespread premalignant mucosal changes it is advisable that dentures are withheld. Both speech therapy and support of friends and relatives during the patient's return to work and during the re-establishment of social contacts is important if life is to take on a worthwhile quality.

In the case of the upper jaw the skeletal replacement is by means of an obturator with replacement of cheek only by means of suitable flaps. Provided the cavity can be maintained as a pyramidal shape the obturator will be retained in place. The inner surface of the wound is lined with a split-skin-graft on a gutta-percha bung supported on a temporary obturator.

Details of operative procedures are outside the scope of this book but can be found in standard reference works and papers. References to a few helpful publications are included in the bibliography at the end of this chapter (Conley, 1970; Stell and Maran, 1972; Lee and Wilson, 1973; Lore, 1973).

While general advice on treatment is to be found in published work, more than in any field a special assessment must be made of each patient's problem. An open mind, a willingness to try the unorthodox, if this seems in the patient's best interest, and a willingness to debate the patient's problem with colleagues and with the patient himself are necessary ingredients for a proper decision.

REFERENCES

BENNETTE, G. (ed.) (1970), *People and Cancer*. London: The British Cancer Council.

BOWERMAN, J. E., and CONROY, B. (1969), 'A Universal Kit in Titanium for Immediate Replacement of the Resected Mandible', *Br. J. oral Surg.*, **6**, 223.

CADE, SIR S. (1963), 'Cancer: the Patients' Viewpoint and the Clinicians' Problem', *Proc. R. Soc. Med.*, **56**, 1.

CANNELL, H. (1973), 'Oral Cancer and Immunity', *Br. J. Oral Surg.*, **11**, 171.

COOK, H. P. (1969), 'Titanium in Mandibular Replacement', *Ibid.*, **7**, 108.

CONLEY, J. (1970), *Concepts in Head and Neck Surgery*, p. 139. Stuttgart: Georg Thieme Verlag.

EASSON, E. C. (1963), 'Radiotherapy in Oral Cancer 1932–62', *Br. dent. J.*, **115**, 139.

FREUND, H. R. (1967), *Principles of Head and Neck Surgery*, p. 94. London: Butterworth.

LEE, S., and WILSON, J. S. P. (1973), 'Carcinoma involving the Lower Alveolus', *Br. J. Surg.*, **60**, 7.

LORE, J. M. (1973), *An Atlas of Head and Neck Surgery*, Vols. I and II. Philadelphia: Saunders.

SAUNDERS, C. (1963), 'The Treatment of Intractable Pain in Terminal Cancer', *Proc. R. Soc. Med.*, **56**, 195.

STELL, P. M., and MARAN, A. G. D. (1972), *Head and Neck Surgery*, p. 107. London: Heinemann Medical.

Chapter XV

SOME METHODS USED IN THE SURGICAL CORRECTION OF THE JAWS IN CASES OF FACIAL DEFORMITY

The anomalies of the upper and lower jaws which constitute an unacceptable facial deformity in the patient's opinion and cause him or her to seek a surgical solution to the problem may be divided into the following categories:—

1. Patients with a receding chin.
2. Patients in whom there is a true or relative mandibular retrusion.
3. Patients in whom there is a true or relative mandibular protrusion.
4. Patients in whom the mandible deviates to one side or is otherwise asymmetrical.
5. Patients with a malocclusion unassociated with a gross skeletal malrelationship of the upper or lower jaw.

These abnormalities, the majority of which are simple growth aberrations, can be corrected surgically by means of onlays, inlays, osteotomies, and ostectomies with or without bone-grafts.

It should be appreciated that although the principal reason for an individual seeking corrective treatment is ugliness there are other problems which favour a surgical solution, such as masticatory difficulties, difficulty or the impossibility of providing prosthetic replacements for the natural teeth, speech defects, and soft-tissue trauma due to the malalinement of the teeth.

Age at which Operation should be performed.—It would seem logical in most cases to defer the operation for a jaw deformity until maturity is reached and maximum bone growth is achieved. If, however, a gross deformity of the jaws in a young patient is causing severe mental distress, a surgical correction should be performed, although the parents must be advised that a further operation may be necessary when facial growth is complete.

In cases of unilateral hyperplasia of the condyle leading to unilateral overgrowth of the mandible, operation at an early age will not only correct the deformity, but prevent further growth of the mandible. Condylectomy for this condition was first performed by Humphrey (1856) and has since become a recognized procedure (Rushton, 1946; Hovell, 1956; Taylor and Cook, 1958).

In cases of unilateral undergrowth of the mandible due to congenital causes, e.g., a first arch or other developmental defect or interference with the condylar growth centre from trauma or infection, the lack of mandibular growth gives rise to a secondary deformity of the maxilla on the affected side. In such cases serial bone-grafts between the bone-ends in the ramus following a vertical subsigmoid osteotomy will compensate for the lack of growth in the mandible and prevent the occurrence of secondary deformity of the maxilla. Possibly, in such a patient, two bone inlays may be required during the growth period of the facial skeleton.

1. THE RECEDING CHIN

Recession of the chin unassociated with micrognathia or retrognathism is uncommon, but moderate recession of the chin may occur as a hereditary characteristic in some families. It can also occur as a result of severe trauma to the chin, such as a comminuted fracture or where there has been bone loss, as in gunshot wounds of the lower jaw. It may also be the main complaint in patients who have a relative mandibular retrognathism and a small chin and in whom the dental abnormality has been treated orthodontically. The receding chin can be remedied surgically by: (*a*) Onlays on the mental prominence. (*b*) A sliding genioplasty. (*c*) A buccal inlay and prosthesis. (*d*) Bilateral osteotomy of the mandible followed by advancement of the anterior part of the mandible and bilateral bone-grafts to fill the resulting gaps.

a. Onlays to the chin may be in the form of: (i) Autografts, (ii) Homografts, (iii) Allelografts.

i. *Autograft Onlays.*—Onlay bone-grafts to the chin may be inserted from a submental or an intra-oral surgical approach (*Fig.* 27A). The submental approach has the disadvantage of leaving a scar beneath the chin, but by careful siting of the incision and closure of the wound, this scar can be made aesthetically acceptable. The intra-oral approach is made through an incision around the buccal side of the gingival margin of the anterior teeth or through an incision in the buccal sulcus. There is more risk of postoperative infection when the intra-oral route is used, but this risk is minimal when adequate doses of a suitable antibiotic are administered postoperatively. One of the problems of all onlay grafts of bone is that the graft may become resorbed in accordance with Wolf's law, through pressure of the overlying skin and tissue over the bone-graft. A chin which is built up with bone chips rapidly resumes its original contour through this mechanism and in order to overcome this tendency the tissue overlying the graft should have its tension on the graft reduced. This can be achieved by extensive undermining of the overlying skin and possibly the insertion of additional skin in the form of a graft beneath the chin. A slightly curved incision is made from one side of the mandible to the other beneath the chin with the convex aspect of the curve facing forward. The skin is undermined forwards over the chin so that tension over a graft will be relieved and then the defect beneath the mandible is grafted. This procedure has the disadvantage of leaving a skin deformity beneath the jaw.

A more simple and acceptable method is to use a block of iliac crest bone contoured with compact bone facing outwards against the overlying tissues. At operation a suitable bed is made in the bone of the mental prominence by removing cortical plate and exposing a cancellous bed. The cancellous underside of the bone onlay graft will then lie against cancellous tissue in the mandible. The compact bone of the outer aspect of the graft will resist the tissue pressures more satisfactorily than the chip grafts and will do this for a protracted period of time. Onlay blocks of bone-graft on the mental prominence are held in position by transosseous wiring at either end of the graft or with vitallium bone screws.

ii. *Homograft Onlays.*—Homograft onlays can be used to restore the mental prominence in a similar manner to the autograft onlays, but they

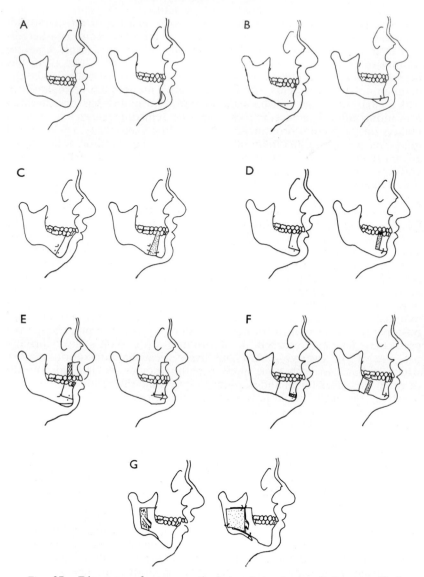

Fig. 27.—Diagrams of some methods used to treat relative mandibular retrognathism.

A, The chin onlay. B, The sliding genioplasty. C, Body osteotomy and block graft. D, Advancement of the lower incisor segment with the placement of a graft and bridge. E, The Wassmund procedure on the premaxilla combined with the Köle procedure on the mandible. F, Advancement of the mandible using a sagittal splitting procedure combined with lowering of the lower incisor region. G, Seward's modification of the Caldwell procedure whereby a vertical osteotomy is combined with a block graft to advance the mandible.

have the added disadvantage of being less reliable than the autograft and more liable to be lost through infection.

iii. *Allelograft Onlays.*—The restoration of the mental prominence by means of allelografts is most unsatisfactory in the long term. Various allelografts, such as tantalum, stainless-steel, chrome cobalt, acrylic, nylon, teflon, terylene, wool, silastic, etc., have been tried and they may be inserted from an extra-oral or intra-oral route and fixed in position when applicable with transosseous wires or screws. They all have the disadvantage that sooner or later the allelograft either becomes a focus of infection or the patient receives a knock on the chin and the graft becomes partially extruded. Should the patient become edentulous there is the added risk that infection may reach the implant via ulceration under the denture. Infection supervenes, the graft has to be removed, and there is a sudden change for the worse in the patient's appearance. As a general rule allelografts, to be successful, must be deeply buried in the tissues as in the hip-joint, or the overlying skin must be relatively immobile as in the case of the scalp. Neither of these conditions obtain at the chin and on the whole results with allelografts are extremely disappointing in the long term. This is unfortunate, for their insertion is simple and the immediate improvement in the patient's appearance is excellent. Even where successful implantation is achieved, resorption of the bone under the graft tends to occur with a regression towards the original contour of the chin (Robinson and Shuken, 1969).

b. The Sliding Genioplasty.—Obwegeser (1957, 1969a, b) and others have described a sliding osteotomy where the bone is sectioned backwards from the chin and the lower fragment advanced to create a mental prominence (*Fig.* 27B).

An incision is made from 1st molar round to 1st molar. The junction of attached and sulcus mucosa is followed in the premolar region, but the incision passes on to the lip side of the sulcus anteriorly. In this latter part a submucosal flap is raised towards the jaw, and then the muscle penetrated down on to the periosteum. After the mandible has been 'de-gloved' the periosteum is divided around the mental nerves and vessels and these structures released, outwards towards the lip. Any double chin is mobilized by dissection deep to the platysma, well into the neck, and a wrinkled chin smoothed out by cross-hatching the periosteum beneath it. The proposed bone cut is outlined with a bur and should extend from 1st molar to 1st molar region. It may be angled to adjust the final height of the chin and the section made with a Stryker saw. If necessary a median vertical cut is made and the advancement achieved by wiring the buccal cortex of the upper fragment to the lingual of the lower. The wound is closed in two layers with vacuum drainage and a pressure dressing applied.

c. The Buccal Inlay.—The buccal inlay is a relatively simple surgical procedure which, used in conjunction with a mandibular prosthesis, enables a very acceptable restoration of the chin to be achieved. This procedure is particularly useful where there has been gross loss of genial bone. First, a surgical pocket is created in the buccal sulcus. An incision is made in the buccal sulcus about $\frac{1}{4}$ in. from the gingival margin and is extended parallel to the gingival margin from about the 1st molar region on the one side to a similar position on the opposite side of the jaw. The incision is made down to but not through the periosteum, and then deepened towards the lower border of the mandible superficial to the periosteum. This creates a large pocket in the sulcus which is maintained by filling the pocket with a black gutta-percha mould which is held in place with a perforated German silver plate on its upper surface, the plate being in turn secured either to a silver copper alloy cap splint on the teeth or, if the patient is edentulous, to a lower plate held in position by two circumferential wires in the canine region. The raw area over the periosteum is grafted with a split skin-graft taken from the inside of the patient's arm or thigh, two areas which are not normally hair-bearing. The split skin-graft is draped over the gutta-percha bung with its raw surface, of course, facing the raw area over the periosteum and the gutta-percha mould, which is in turn fixed by the prosthesis, holds the skin-graft in place until it has healed over the raw periosteum. This part of the healing process takes about seven days, and at the end of this time the gutta-percha bung is removed and cleaned with soap and water and the graft is inspected. The buccal pocket is then gently irrigated with saline and the gutta-percha mould is replaced. For convenience, a screw device is attached to the splint or plate to enable the German silver plate which holds the bung in position to be removed and replaced easily. Skin-grafts in the mouth have a great tendency to shrink and only become stable after some months. In the early days after grafting, therefore, the gutta-percha bung should only be left out for short periods. After a few weeks the graft becomes more firmly established and the gutta-percha bung can then be replaced with an acrylic prosthesis.

Meticulous attention to oral hygiene must be paid in the first weeks after grafting, for infection can rapidly destroy the graft. Infection, when present, is usually caused by coliform-type organisms, and irrigation of the buccal pocket with warm 1 per cent eusol solution is most efficacious. Small areas of sprouting granulation tissue appearing in the graft should be touched with a silver nitrate stick. The patient should be taught to change the bung every three or four days once the graft has begun to settle. If the graft is of a considerable size, it may be desirable to carry out the first change under a short general anaesthetic. The gutta-percha bung is resilient and will not cause a pressure sore on the graft, provided that it has an even surface. To provide a uniformly smooth surface and create a bung without crevices which might harbour bacteria, the appliance should be made with sealed edges. This is achieved by taking a sheet of gutta-percha, which has been softened in boiling water and then folded in half. The free edges are then trimmed with a large pair of scissors. Cutting along the edges in this manner produces a perfect seal. The gutta-percha is then folded again and the process repeated with the scissors. When a bung of roughly the correct size is achieved final trimming is carried out with scissors and again a perfect seal is attained, so that the final mould has no crevices. As gutta-percha is impervious to fluids the temporary appliance will remain sanitary even after it has been in the mouth for several weeks. This is certainly not the case if crevices exist in the mould such as those which occur when the material is trimmed with a hot knife.

It is important to remember that as acrylic is hard and unresilient, if the final prosthesis to restore the chin is fitted too early, i.e., when the skin-graft still has a tendency to contract, it will cause pressure ulcers on the surface of the graft. This inevitably leads on to infection and partial or total loss of the graft. When the skin-graft is completely stable a prosthesis is constructed which restores the normal contour of the chin. It the patient is edentulous this can be incorporated in the lower denture, and takes the form of a downward projection of the anterior part of the lower denture, into the newly created 'pocket'. The buccal inlay and prosthesis is a most satisfactory method of restoring chin contour.

d. Bilateral Osteotomy of the Body of the Mandible with Advancement of the Anterior Fragment and Bilateral Bone-grafts to fill the Defect.—A vertical body osteotomy is made bilaterally at some convenient point between the canines and the 1st molars, if necessary after liberation of the inferior dental nerve. The soft tissues are widely undermined beneath the platysma, the periosteum divided along the line of the bone cuts, and the anterior fragment tilted to put the chin into its correct position. Carefully cut block iliac crest bone-grafts are inserted into the gaps so created and wired in place. The fragments are further supported by firm inter-maxillary fixation and this should be maintained for six weeks. Some trimming of the anterior fragment may be necessary to avoid a step in the lower border of the mandible. The technique lacks the bone-to-bone contact of the original jaw fragments which is achieved by other techniques and is technically weak on this account. It is essential, therefore, that the pull of the muscles attached to the anterior fragment should be resisted until firm union has been achieved (*Fig.* 27C).

2. Patients in whom there is a True or Relative Mandibular Retrusion

Micrognathia is seen in an extreme form in the Pierre-Robin syndrome, but moderate recession of the chin is found as a hereditary characteristic in some families. Marked micrognathia is also present in the rare pheno-menon of a bilateral 'first arch' defect and in such cases there is an associated deformity of the tragus of the ear with the presence of accessory auricles together with an anomaly of the malleus and incus on each side. In more severe cases there is almost complete absence of the middle and inner ears, hypoplasia of the soft tissues, skin scarring, hypoplasia of the nerves, macrostomia, and other disturbances suggesting a more wide-spread deficiency, possibly vascular in origin. Failure of growth of the mandible may also be caused by interference with the condylar growth centre of the mandible following trauma, infection, or irradiation. The more usual types of patient seeking correction of relative mandibular retrusion are those with an Angle's Class II malocclusion for whom orthodontic treatment has not been successful.

Bilateral osteotomy of the ramus above the level of the lingula for the correction of mandibular retrusion was originally described by Blair (1907), but experience has shown that following this operation there is a great tendency for the anterior fragment to relapse owing to muscular pull. A sliding step-like osteotomy was described by Nicolsky in which an L-shaped cut was made with the short arm of the L passing down vertically from the upper border in the 3rd molar region, and the long arm horizont-ally backwards. The anterior fragment was displaced forwards, the posterior border of the angle wired to the front of the posterior fragment. A Z-shaped osteotomy of the body of the mandible with the long arm passing horizontally forwards and the short arms passing up to the alveolar margin at the back and down to the lower border at the front was described by Eiselsberg in 1907. He wired the fragments end to end, but Pehrgadd (1965), who made the posterior vertical cut behind the last molar, wired the fragments after displacement across the long horizontal cut. The operation can be improved by working the horizontal cut through the bed of the inferior dental canal and thence vertically down to the lower border below the premolars (Dingman, 1948). Pichler (1948) makes a similar cut but with the vertical limbs at the opposite ends of the horizontal ones. After the mandible is sectioned, the anterior fragment is made to slide forwards to correct the mandibular recession. Owing to the slope of the long arm of the L osteotomy, bone contact is maintained. Firm, exact splinting is essential to ensure bony union with the anterior fragment in its new position since the muscle forces on the chin exert a strong downwards and backwards pull.

A bilateral body osteotomy with advancement of the anterior fragments and bone-grafting of the gap was advocated by Limberg (1928) and Axhausen (1939). In extreme cases it may be necessary to insert skin beneath the mandible by pedicle grafting in order to relieve the skin tension on the mental prominence in its new position. Correction of micrognathia by this procedure is an extensive surgical exercise, but can give a good cosmetic result when successfully completed, apart from submandibular scarring and some degree of residual anaesthesia of the lower lip.

Trauner and Obwegeser (1957) devised an L-shaped division of the ramus and inserted a bilateral bone-graft between the bone-ends. This operation is, of course, carried out through a submandibular incision. Caldwell and Amaral (1960) have described an operation for the correction of mandibular retrognathism which is a modification of a vertical subsigmoid osteotomy in the rami. The technique follows the usual pattern of vertical section of the rami. The bone-ends are decorticated, the body of the mandible is advanced to a predetermined functional relationship with the maxilla. An autogenous iliac bone-graft is cut and inserted so that it is inlayed both into the decorticated areas and into the gap created in the rami. Obwegeser (1964) has used his sagittal splitting osteotomy of the ramus to elongate the mandible and this technique has the advantage that neither skin incisions nor bone-grafts are required.

After discussing in general terms the treatment of retrognathism, it is important to mention the guiding principles used in selecting the treatment for individual types of cases.

1. Patients with a receding or small chin, but with a relatively normal articulation of the teeth as a result of orthodontic treatment. This condition is corrected by chin augmentation using one of the following alternatives: (a) Onlay graft, (b) Allelograft, (c) Sliding genioplasty (Fig. 27 A, B).

2. Patients with a post-normal occlusion. The two types are treated as follows:—

   a. Angle's Class II, division 1:—
      i. Where the mandible and chin are well formed (e.g., true maxillary

protrusion); by a Wassmund procedure reducing the prominence of the premaxilla (*Fig.* 27E).

    ii. Where the mandible is sizeable, but the chin small; by a Wassmund procedure on the premaxilla and a sliding genioplasty.

    iii. Where the mandible is sizeable and the chin prominent, by advancement of the canine and incisor alveolar segment only. Bone-grafts and bridges or a denture are used to fill the gaps in the alveolar process and dental arch (*Fig.* 27D).

    iv. Where there is obvious mandibular retrognathism, by an Obwegeser sagittal splitting osteotomy with advancement of the mandible. The lower incisor segment may be lowered and chin contour improved as necessary by a Köle procedure.

    b. Developmental.—Treatment often has a poor chance of success because soft-tissue deficiency and lack of muscle may accentuate the deformity particularly during movement.

    i. Serial bone-grafts in a ramus osteotomy.

    ii. Köle and oblique body slide and graft.

    iii. Grafts of growing bone-end, either fibula, rib, or clavicle.

Receding Chin (*Fig.* 27).—For some patients with mandibular retrognathism the complaint is mainly of a lack of chin prominence. It is frequently the case that orthodontics has been undertaken in childhood and an acceptable arrangement of the teeth achieved. Thus, not only would any alteration of jaw position need reversal of the orthodontic treatment, since without an incisal overjet mandibular advancement is impossible, but clearly such a course is unnecessary. A genioplasty is all that is required. Of the three types of procedure available for this, the sliding genioplasty is the one which is most successful, probably because the bone is mainly cortical bone and because the bulk of the mandible remains unaltered, merely changed in shape.

Maxillary Protrusion.—Certain cases of relative mandibular retrognathism due to such factors as maxillary protrusion, or a lower dental arch which is more posteriorly placed than usual on the mandible, may be successfully corrected, or disguised by procedures devised by Wassmund, Wunderer, and Köle. These techniques mobilize the premaxilla or the lower anterior alveolar segments. Where the patient has a mandible of normal or near normal size and a good chin prominence, a premaxillary osteotomy is indicated.

The original operation was described by Wassmund (1935), and variations of this procedure have been reported by Schuchardt (1954), Wunderer (1962), Murphy and Walker (1963), Cradock-Henry (1966), Straith and Lawson (1967), Matras (1967), and Markwell (1967). The operation should be considered in patients with marked maxillary protrusion and sound anterior teeth. An osteotomy is carried out in the upper 1st premolar area, after which the anterior fragment is repositioned. Sometimes a similar procedure has to be carried out in the lower incisor region if there is an associated deep overbite.

Operative Technique.—The upper 1st premolars, or other suitable teeth, are extracted and a slice of bone of predetermined width cut from the palate and the buccal sides of the maxillary alveolar process so as to include their sockets. Both the buccal and palatal bone cuts are made with suitable burs working from the buccal side; the soft tissues of the palate being tunnelled to a minimal extent sufficient to allow the insertion of a protective retractor. If better access to the middle of the palate is required a median incision can be made. In some cases a nasal re-fracture saw is suitable for making the palatal cuts. The buccal cuts are carried forwards horizontally above the apices of the teeth to the lateral margin of the anterior bony aperture of the nose. The anterior part of the nasal septum is approached through a vertical midline incision into the labial frenum. If it is necessary for the upper anterior segment to be widened to accommodate the lower arch after it has been repositioned, a vertical midline cut is made between the upper central incisors using thin burs and special small osteotomes. Alternatively, the inter-canine width can be increased preoperatively by orthodontic means. If the premaxilla is to be split this must be completed before the nasal septum is divided. The latter manœuvre is accomplished with an osteotome introduced above the anterior nasal spine. After the anterior fragment has been freed it is repositioned and held in its new position with splints or orthodontic bands and arch bars until bony union occurs. Both the height and angulation of the upper incisors can also be adjusted during the operation. One point which must be noted is the size of the nose. These patients may well have a large one, with an obvious hump, and the reduction in size of the maxilla will increase its prominence.

Alveolar ostectomy for maxillary protrusion may be performed as a two-stage procedure and this has been recommended by Schuchardt (1954), Cradock-Henry (1966) and Mohnac (1966), but according to Barton and Rayne (1969) the single stage operation does not prejudice the blood-supply to the anterior fragment. Indeed, the two-stage procedure is illogical since the blood-supply from the greater palatine artery is damaged during the first operation and the healed wound will not compensate for this before the second stage must be performed.

Choice of Operation for Maxillary Protrusion.—If the patient's upper incisors and canines are carious, heavily filled, root filled, crowned, or in other ways unsightly, it may be more satisfactory to extract them and carry out an intra-septal alveolotomy so that they may be replaced by a denture. If the patient has an excellent set of anterior teeth the alveolar ostectomy is usually the treatment of choice, but as with other osteotomies there should be a full discussion with the patient about what is involved.

Retrusion of the Lower Dental Arch.—If the patient has a mandible of normal length and a good chin, but the lower dental arch is too far back, advancement of the lower anterior segment of the mandible will produce the required result (*Fig.* 27D). Sometimes a concurrent operation on the premaxilla will be necessary to adjust the angulation of the upper incisors.

Mandibular Retrognathism.—Treatment of the Angle's Class II, division 1 malocclusion with mandibular retrognathism requires a more elaborate sequence of treatment. In the preparatory phase the inter-canine and inter-premolar width of the maxillary arch is expanded orthodontically if this is necessary to accommodate the mandible in the new position. At the same time the inclination of the upper incisors is reduced, the spaces between them closed, and the lower incisors slightly depressed. It is useful to over-expand the inter-premolar and canine width a little, but excessive retraction of the incisors must be avoided, or adequate advancement of the mandible will be impossible. Some further reduction in the height of the lower incisors can be achieved by the grinding of their incisal edges. Finally, at operation the lower incisor alveolar process is separated, and a strip removed from below it so that the whole segment can be lowered. The excised strip can be added to the chin, if desired, to increase its prominence. Alternatively, if the overeruption of the lower incisors is not too marked the mandible may be placed so that the lower incisors contact the palatal surfaces of the uppers and the molar occlusal surfaces are in contact. Provided the open bite in the pre-molar region is not too great the teeth will come into contact within a year to 18 months as a result of various tooth movements (Hovell, 1970). Bilateral sagittal splitting procedures of the ramus permit the jaw to be advanced to the new position. Localization and immobilization of the lower incisor segment is by pre-localized and soldered locking plates and intermaxillary fixation by sectioned-tube quick-release locking plates Seward and Foreman (1972) (*Fig.* 27F).

Class II, division 2 patients are less often concerned about the distal position of the mandible since the retroclination of the upper central incisors is an effective disguise. Even so, the deep overbite can result in damage to the periodontal attachment of both upper and lower incisors and surgical rearrangement of the position of the appropriate alveolar segments can be used to overcome the problem.

Extreme Retrognathia.—Provided that the agent which resulted in the extreme retrognathia did not also damage the soft tissues unduly, advancement of the mandible may be successful. Considerable forward movement of the mandible using an Obwegeser sagittal splitting osteotomy results in lateral displacement of the posterior fragments by the anterior one. Moderate advancement, therefore, should be used together with a sliding genioplasty to increase the chin prominence.

The Trauner inverted L osteotomy of the ramus may be used, with a bone-graft, but to gain stable bone-to-bone contact a long additional cut is made forwards just short of the lower border (Seward, 1970) (*Fig.* 27G). In other cases Eiselsberg's and Pichler's Z-shaped body osteotomy is used with bone-grafts at the upper border distal to the 3rd molar and at the lower border below the premolars. To retain sensation in the lower lip the mental nerve is dissected out in continuity with the inferior dental and freed from the bone by cutting the incisive branch. Even so the nerve may be stretched and lip sensation reduced.

If developmental deficiencies are tackled, the chances of relapse must be understood by all concerned. Care must be taken to assess the part played by soft-tissue deficiencies for these may require additional procedures such as epithelial inlays, padding, and onlay grafting to disguise them. Serial grafting in the ramus is the usual procedure, but a Köle operation may be used to reduce the height of the lower incisors and alter the chin shape, combined with an oblique body slice to elongate the mandible. Grafts of growing bone ends are not yet out of the experimental stage.

3. PATIENTS IN WHOM THERE IS A TRUE OR RELATIVE MANDIBULAR PROTRUSION

Mandibular protrusion is one of the most common anomalies of the jaw requiring surgical correction. The symmetrically prognathous patient may have this jaw relationship because the mandible is too long or too far forward in relation to a normal maxilla. In some patients the lower dental arch is too far forward, but the remainder of the mandible, including the point of the chin, is not. Most prognathic patients have some degree of underdevelopment of the maxilla, but in a few the mandible is entirely normal in position and shape, and is opposed by a maxilla which is noticeably too far back.

Of course, the deformity may be familial, as in the case of the Habsburgs, but often no other members of the family are affected. The condition may vary from a simple Class III malocclusion without an obvious external deformity to gross mandibular protrusion which interferes with eating and speaking and results in extreme ugliness. In its pronounced form the patient's facies have the heavy coarse appearance of the acromegalic. Mandibular protrusion, except in its most mild form, is usually disfiguring in females, but so far as men are concerned much depends upon the size of the man. A small man with a protruding jaw tends to look abnormal, but a similar degree of mandibular protrusion in a very tall, heavily-built man appears perfectly natural and there is, therefore, no necessity to operate on such a patient merely because the lower teeth bite in front of the uppers. It is also unjustifiable to advise an operation for a patient who has not experienced any difficulty with eating or speaking and has no worries about his appearance.

The operation of bilateral osteotomy or ostectomy is a sizeable surgical procedure and should not be undertaken lightly, especially since the selected procedure is often for cosmetic improvement rather than function and is not without risk, including even mortality.

Preoperative Assessment

In all cases where there is gross mandibular protrusion the possibility of a diagnosis of acromegaly must be considered. This is a comparatively rare disease in which there is hypersecretion by the anterior lobe of the pituitary due to an eosinophil adenoma, the influence being effective after ossification is complete. The patient may complain of temporal headaches, photophobia, and reduction of the lateral visual fields (bitemporal optic hemianopia), and eventual optic atrophy. The terminal phalanges of the feet and hands become large, the lips become thick, and enlargement of the tongue leads to indentations or crenations on its sides from pressure against the teeth. Overgrowth of the lower jaw together with the thickening of the lips gives rise to a very characteristic facies. The hands eventually become spade-like and a lateral radiograph of the skull shows uniform expansion of the sella turcica. There is also enlargement of the nose, supra-orbital ridges, frontal sinus, and superior nuchal line. Should the adenoma occur before the epiphyses have fused, gigantism will result and this possibility must be considered whenever mandibular protrusion is associated with excessive general growth of the patient.

Many diverse methods of preoperative evaluation of mandibular protrusion have been described, many of which are unnecessarily complex. This is especially true if too much emphasis is given to a purely orthodontic assessment of the case, for a satisfactory profile achieved by operation sometimes bears little relationship to a purely theoretical normal occlusion. In this respect the study of soft-tissue true lateral radiographs of the jaws with the teeth in a closed position is most helpful.

A relatively simple method of selecting the most appropriate type of operation in any particular case of mandibular protrusion is to begin by taking an accurate true lateral radiograph of the jaws with the teeth in occlusion. This is laid on an X-ray viewing screen and a tracing of the outline of the upper and lower jaws is made with tracing paper. The tracing must include the upper and lower teeth in occlusion. Several patterns in thick brown paper are then cut from the tracing of the lower jaw and these should, of course, include the lower teeth. With a pair of scissors it is then possible to section the brown paper patterns through various parts of the ramus, angle, or body. That portion of the paper pattern representing the condyle, coronoid process, and upper end of the ramus is then laid over the appropriate marking on the original tracing paper and the anterior fragment of pattern is positioned so that the lower teeth are in a corrected position in relation to the upper jaw. It will be immediately apparent that certain types of osteotomy or ostectomy would be useless in achieving the required result. For instance, a trial horizontal section through the ramus may be seen to result in lack of bony contact between the severed ends of the ramus after the body of the mandible has been displaced backwards for the appropriate distance. This method also allows the extent of a body ostectomy to be visualized. To do this the paper pattern is sectioned vertically in the lower 1st molar area after which the anterior part of the pattern is moved forwards on the tracing to its original position. The gap between the two parts of the pattern will represent the amount of bone which will have to be removed to correct the mandibular prognathism. By playing with several patterns and observing the probable results of the various operation sections, the most suitable operation can be selected for any particular case. Impressions should then be taken of the upper and lower teeth and plaster-of-Paris casts mounted on an articulator, the bite having been taken with a squash wax bite. The routine after this depends on the operator's experience and the complexity of the case.

If the section is to be made through the ramus or angle, duplicate plaster-of-Paris models are mounted on a backslab of plaster with the teeth in the proposed postoperative occlusion. Sometimes this occlusion is not satisfactory and in order to achieve an acceptable occlusion one or more teeth must be trimmed. Before operation this will, of course, necessitate the grinding or even extraction of these teeth so that a similar postoperative position can be attained. If a section of the body of the mandible is contemplated, duplicate models are again positioned using a backslab of plaster but this time in the preoperative occlusion. The central part of the lower model is cut out with a pad saw, leaving only the plaster teeth and alveolar process in the form of a U. This lower model is positioned at its base with another detachable slab of plaster fixed at right angles to the backslab. The lower model is then sectioned vertically through the lower 1st molar area and the posterior part of the model is correctly positioned in relation to the upper model and secured in position with the back and lower plaster slabs. The anterior part of the lower model is cut back at either end using a saw or an emery wheel until the incisor teeth can be made to occlude with the teeth on the upper model in a satisfactory position, while the distal end of the anterior part of the lower model touches the anterior ends of the posterior portions of the lower model. If the anterior fragment is then brought forwards to its original position on the lower plaster slab, the gap between the two ends of the plaster model will represent the amount to be removed from the body of the mandible in order to complete a satisfactory ostectomy. A template should be made from metal and a German silver wire handle is attached. This is used to measure the exact area to be removed at operation.

Where the case is complex or where the operator is comparatively inexperienced, full stone models of the mandible should be constructed with the aid of impressions, tracing from radiographs, and clinical measurements. This is because what happens in three dimensions cannot always be judged from consideration in two dimensions. If this precaution is not taken, an impasse may be reached at the time of the operation.

Choice of Operation

Shortening of the mandible is by far the most common procedure undertaken to correct facial deformity. A multiplicity of osteotomies (simple section through the bone) and ostectomies (excision of a portion of the bone) have been advocated for the surgical correction of mandibular protrusion since Hullihen (1849) reported the correction of a case of anterior open bite by a partial resection of the alveolar process. Since that time, osteotomies and ostectomies of every part of the ramus and body of the mandible have been described. In other aspects of medicine or surgery, whenever an excessive number of different methods of treatment are advocated, it usually means that there is no absolutely satisfactory form of treatment and this is also the case with the operations for surgical correction of prognathism.

In view of the wide variety of operations which can be used to correct mandibular prognathism, difficulty may be experienced in selecting the ideal operation for any particular patient. Many surgeons may have a personal preference for a particular operation or find that they obtain more satisfactory results from a certain technique. For example, the sub-sigmoid or oblique ramus osteotomy or the Obwegeser sagittal split operation can be adapted for use in most cases of mandibular protrusion. However, certain operations are more suitable for certain types of mandibular prognathism, and in order to ascertain the most suitable operation in any particular case a careful study must be made of the radiographs, tracings, and study models.

In certain cases it will be found after study of the radiographs, tracings, and models that several different types of operation would achieve the desired result, while in other cases only one particular type of section will have any chance of success. Much time and thought should be devoted to this preliminary study of all available data before coming to a decision about the type of operation to be performed. Other important considerations are:—

1. Should the Section be made Blind or under Direct Vision through an Open Wound?—The blind section of the mandible was popularized by

Kostecka (1931). In his technique, a Gigli saw is passed through the skin and around the ramus with a special introducer and a horizontal section is made above the lingula. The operation is rapid and relatively easy to perform, but it is difficult to control the position of the upper fragment which tends to be lifted anteriorly by the pull of the temporalis muscle and the subsequent lack of bony contact between the bone-ends leads in some cases to a prolonged period before union occurs. In some instances union never occurs. Carelessly used, the Gigli saw may damage branches of the facial nerve and there have been instances in which the maxillary artery was severed. As a result of its high relapse rate, this surgical technique has gone out of fashion and has been replaced by section under direct vision through an open operation.

2. If an Open Operation is to be used should an Extra-oral or Intra-oral Surgical Approach be made to the Mandible?—Extra-oral incisions give an excellent view of the mandible, but inevitably leave an external scar no matter how carefully the incision is sited and the wound repaired. In a keloid former the result could be disastrous and it would seem illogical to produce a cosmetic deformity in the performance of an essentially cosmetic operation.

The approach to the ramus is made through a submandibular incision at the angle, after which the masseter muscle is detached from its insertion to the lower end of the ramus which is then exposed in its entirety. The body of the mandible is approached by a submandibular incision of varying length depending upon the nature of the operation, but it is seldom less than 5 cm. long. Both the incisions to expose the ramus and the body must be made a finger's breadth or 2 cm. beneath the lower border of the mandible and the mandibular branch of the facial nerve preserved and retracted if it crosses the field of operation. Inadvertent neurotmesis of this branch leads to an ugly postoperative drooping of the corner of the lower lip. Careful suturing of the incisions by making use of skin creases will help to disguise the resultant scars beneath the jaws. One solution to this problem was suggested by the late Sir Harold Gillies (1955), who approached the mandible surgically through a long 'face lift' type incision sited mainly in the hairline and only coming on to the face immediately anterior to the external ear. This technique provides good surgical access and leaves minimal scarring, but is technically difficult and time-consuming.

The intra-oral approach to the mandible is certainly very simple, as the bone lies immediately beneath the mucoperiosteum. The ramus can be approached by a vertical incision down the anterior aspect of the ramus from just below the tip of the coronoid process across the retromolar fossa into the buccal sulcus. The body of the mandible is exposed through an incision of suitable length along the crest of the ridge in the edentulous jaw and around the buccal and lingual gingival margins when teeth are standing. Such an incision will give excellent exposure of the body of the mandible. A buccal incision around the gingival margin from $\overline{6-1|1-6}$ will enable the entire chin to be exposed. The arguments against this surgical approach are:—

a. Risk of Infection.—However, provided bone fragments are removed from the wound and haematoma formation is avoided, there is little risk of infection, particularly if the mouth is clean and suitable antibiotic cover is given.

b. There is Limited Access.—The access from an intra-oral approach is quite adequate for an experienced oral surgeon, but would be more difficult for a surgeon more familiar with surgery in some other regions. Advantages of the intra-oral route are:—

i. Lack of visible scars. Some patients find such scars as aesthetically embarrassing as the original mandibular protrusion.

ii. The operation is carried out within the periosteal sheath with a reduced risk to certain anatomical structures.

iii. Both the occlusal relationship of the jaws and the bone-ends are visible at the same time and a satisfactory arrangement of both more readily achieved.

It is obvious that the size of the oral cavity and rima oris greatly affect the access by this route and must be taken into account.

3. Should the Bone-ends be wired together following Section?—If the mandible is sectioned by an osteotomy or an ostectomy and the anterior fragment is repositioned, the sectioned bone-ends seldom lie naturally in such a position that rapid bony union is encouraged. Following a horizontal section of the ramus, the anterior aspect of the superior fragment tends to be pulled upwards by the temporalis muscle leaving little contact between the bone-ends. Oblique section or subsigmoid osteotomy tends to leave compact bone in contact with compact bone, and a similar condition occurs with the horizontal osteotomy of the ramus in many instances. Osteotomy through the neck of the mandibular condyle usually results in little bony contact and greatly delayed bony union occurs. For this reason this method has been largely discarded as a treatment for mandibular prognathism.

Vertical ostectomies of the body of the mandible usually result in the anterior portion of the mandible being sited within and below the posterior portions of the body of the mandible. This results in inadequate bony contact between the bone-ends with resulting protracted healing or even fibrous or non-union. Some authorities (Fickling and Fordyce, 1955) advocate grafting with bone chips to accelerate healing in such cases. However, if adequate contact between the bone-ends is obtained, the surgical fracture of the mandible produced by an ostectomy heals just as rapidly and firmly as any other traumatic fracture of the mandible. Satisfactory union should occur in six weeks.

Delayed healing can even occur in the sagittal split type operations if there is separation of the cancellous surfaces by soft tissue. It has been suggested that transosseous wiring carries a risk of infection, but with good operative technique no such trouble is experienced. In all cases of osteotomy or ostectomy, therefore, it is advantageous to achieve and maintain bony contact of the opposing bone ends by transosseous wiring with stainless-steel wire.

4. Sacrifice of Teeth in Body Ostectomy.—It should be remembered that if an operation is performed on the body of the mandible some teeth (usually the 2nd premolars or 1st molars) will have to be sacrificed in order that an ostectomy can be carried out. When working from an intra-oral approach, the teeth to be extracted may be removed at the time the ostectomy is performed, but in most other cases it is preferable to remove the teeth in question and then allow the area to heal before performing the ostectomy.

If a ramus osteotomy or ostectomy is to be performed, any unerupted lower 3rd molars must be removed first, for when the body of the mandible is pushed backwards such teeth would be sited well beneath the ramus and their subsequent extraction would be rendered difficult.

Types and Sites of Operations

Over the years a multiplicity of operations has been described for the surgical correction of mandibular prognathism and few sites in the mandible have escaped the attention of the surgeon. For example, bilateral resection of the condyle was suggested by Berger (1897) and Jaboulay and Berard (1898) and by Dufourmentel (1921). Osteotomy of the condylar neck was used by Kostecka (1931) (*Fig.* 28A), while Smith and Johnson (1940) suggested the removal of a small rectangle of bone from the sigmoid notch (*Fig.* 28B). Bilateral osteotomy of the ramus above the lingula was originally described by Blair (1907) for correction of mandibular retrusion, but was used for the correction of mandibular protrusion by Babcock (1909) (*Fig.* 28C, D). Since this time numerous variations of this operation have been carried out from a 'blind' extra-oral route by Henry (1946) and Clarkson (1955), while Kazanzian (1951) suggested an angulated cut in the anteroposterior direction made obliquely from the medial to the lateral aspect in order to obtain a wider area of bone contact.

Subperiosteal osteotomy via the intra-oral route was advocated originally by Ernst (1927). Skaloud (1951) advocated an extra-oral and intra-oral approach to the section by passing a Gigli saw from the skin behind the jaw into the mouth. He also wired the bone-ends together by passing a wire over the sigmoid notch to a hole drilled through the lower end of the ramus. Obwegeser (1957) has devised an intra-oral subperiosteal operation whereby a sagittal split of the ramus is performed. At the suggestion of Dal Pont he moved the buccal cortical cut from the ramus to the body of the mandible, increasing the area of the part which is split (Obwegeser, 1964; Dal Pont, 1958, 1961). This operation not only enables the body of the mandible to be advanced or retropositioned, but also an anterior open bite can be corrected. In all cases a considerable area of raw bone is in apposition to a similar area on the opposing fragment and healing is therefore expedited. (*Fig.* 29G.)

Body ostectomy is the procedure used to shorten the mandible in the region of the dental arch. (*Fig.* 29B.) The operation, done from an extra-oral approach was described by Angle (1898) and Blair (1907). The latter originally performed the operation as long ago as 1897 and the method has since been adopted by numerous oral surgeons. As this operation inevitably resulted in an intra-oral wound continuous with the extra-oral tissues, Ballin (1908) suggested removing the tooth or teeth at the site of the proposed ostectomy some weeks before section from an extra-oral approach of the remainder of the mandible. In this way contamination of the external wound from the mouth is avoided.

In 1917 Aller suggested an intra-oral approach in order to avoid external scarring. There was the obvious inherent danger of contamination of the wound from the mouth at the time of operation and this may have

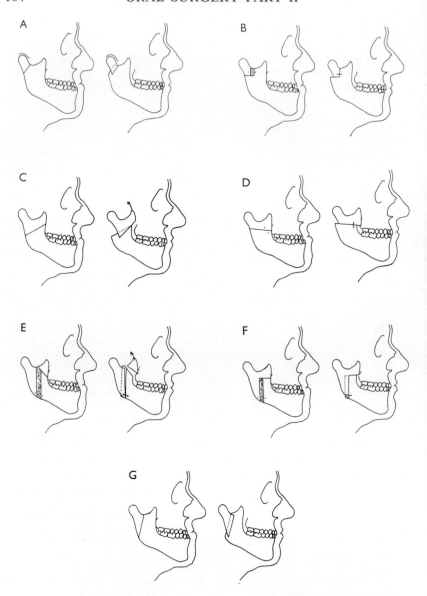

Fig. 28.—Diagrams illustrating some ramus procedures used in the treatment of mandibular prognathism.

A, Section of the condyle neck. B, Section of the condyle neck with removal of bone from below the sigmoid notch (Smith and Johnson). C, Blind section of the ramus (Kostecka). D, Horizontal ramus section. E, The vertical subsigmoid (Caldwell and Lettermann). F, The inverted L (Trauner). G, Oblique osteotomy (Thoma).

led to some lack of popularity of the procedure, but the technique was revived post-war by Thoma (1948), Dingman and Van Alstine (1952), Huebsch (1954), and Converse (1954) in view of the availability of anti-biotic prophylaxis to control any infection. Advantages of the procedure are that it can be safely planned from models of the dental arch only, with or without additional help from cephalometric radiographs. Satis-factory results are achieved, particularly in terms of stability, with few operative risks to the patient. The indications for this type of operation are elongation of the body of the mandible, preferably when the tongue is of normal size and where there is an excess of space to accommodate it. An anterior open bite and low chin may also be corrected by this method, provided that there is a normal articulation as far as the premolar region.

Many operators have found that the healing of the mandible was prolonged following ostectomy and some (Fickling and Fordyce, 1955) have attempted to overcome this problem of delayed or fibrous union of the fragments by chip grafting the operation site. However, it is not always necessary to take iliac crest bone for the graft. Cancellous bone from the excised segment can be used. One way to do this is to remove only the cortex from the unwanted area, permitting the cancellous tissue to crush as the fragments are approximated. However, the main reason for pro-tracted healing of the bone-ends is inadequate bony contact and if the bone-ends are accurately fitted together and united by a transosseous stainless-steel wire, so that maximum bony apposition is obtained, healing occurs as rapidly as with any other mandibular fracture.

A useful variant of the body ostectomy stems from the Y-shaped oste-otomy of Trauner (1929) and Rosenthal (1934). Sowray and Haskell (1968) and then Obwegeser (1969a) have developed this method into a versatile and useful procedure. The mandible is reduced in length by the excision of a tooth socket on either side and reduced in both length and width by the excision of a vertical segment from the midline of the chin. The three ostectomy sites are connected by a horizontal cut below the apices of the anterior teeth. This procedure is of value where the jaw is excessively wide in proportion to its length, where the chin in a woman is square and masculine in shape, or where there are other deformities affecting the anterior part of the jaw. For example, the operation can be combined with the Köle procedure to correct an anterior open bite and a low chin point, so avoiding cuts at several sites in the mandible. The median alveolar segment is raised to close the anterior open bite, and a slice is cut off the lower border of the chin and wedged into the gap below the incisor segment, both to support it and to fashion a new chin prominence at a higher level. (*Fig.* 29.)

Disadvantages of the body procedures are: a marked diminution in tongue space (in some cases a lateral as well as an anteroposterior reduc-tion) and a reduction in the distance between chin and angle producing a dumpy-faced appearance with a tendency to produce a double chin. However, the latter disfigurement tends to regress within nine months to a year after operation. From the foregoing it is obvious that body ostectomy will not be the preferred manœuvre if there is a large Frankfort mandibular plane angle with an obtuse angle to the mandible, or where the patient is plump with a thick subcutaneous layer.

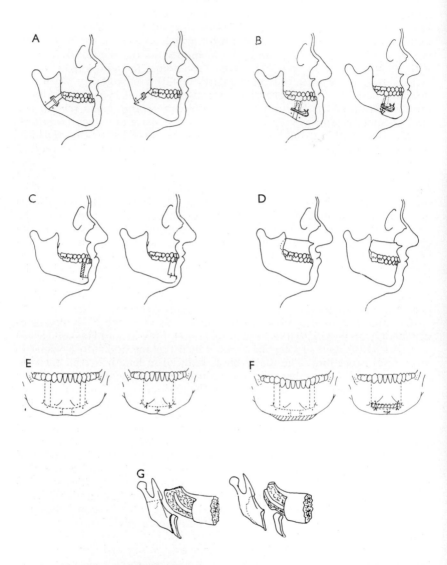

Fig. 29.—Diagrams illustrating some angle, body, and maxillary procedures used in the treatment of mandibular prognathism.

A, The angle ostectomy. B, The body ostectomy. C, Regression of the lower incisor segment. D, Maxillary osteotomy (Wassmund). E, The Y body ostectomy (Sowray and Haskell). F, The Y body ostectomy combined with the Köle procedure whereby the anterior alveolar segment is raised to close on anterior open bite, the height of the chin is reduced, and the point of the chin raised into the chin pad by wedging the chin fragment into the gap (Obwegeser). G, The Obwegeser-Dal Pont operation (left) and the Dal Pont-Hunsuck variant of the sagittal split (right).

Horizontal Osteotomy of the Ramus.—Horizontal osteotomy of the ramus above the level of the inferior dental foramen is one of the oldest and, formerly, must widely used forms of osteotomy for both mandibular protrusion and retrusion. It is the level at which section is carried out in the technique advocated by Kostecka via a blind extra-oral approach, but for reasons already discussed the osteotomy is best effected under direct vision through an open wound and bony healing is expedited by postoperative transosseous wiring of the bone-ends.

Exposure of the site is obtained by an intra-oral incision from the tip of the coronoid process down the anterior border of the ramus across the retromolar fossa and down into the buccal sulcus. The incision is made down to bone and with a Howarth's periosteal elevator the periosteum is raised from the buccal aspect of the ramus. The soft tissues are then retracted by passing the curved end of a Lack's retractor around the posterior border of the mandible. The tissues are raised from the lingual aspect of the ramus to identify the level of the inferior dental foramen so that the cut on the buccal aspect of the ramus can be sited above it. The section of the ramus is best effected with a tapered Meisinger fissure bur used in a straight handpiece. It is a simple matter to gauge the depth of the cut, but as an additional precaution a thin copper strip can be passed on the lingual side of the ramus to act as a guard. Great care must be taken when cutting through the posterior border of the mandible to ensure that the retractor is protecting the soft tissues for the maxillary artery and posterior facial vein are sited just behind the jaw in this area. After the bur cut has been deepened sufficiently the final section can be effected by a light tap with an osteotome on the anterior end of the ramus cut. Alternatively, the cut can be made from the medial to the lateral in the same way as the medial cortical cut of the Obwegeser operation. Various types of saws and drills have been suggested for use in this horizontal section and a Gigli saw can also be passed along the lingual side of the mandible and out behind the jaw to saw the mandible under direct vision. As soon as the section is complete the anterior aspect of the upper fragment will be pulled upwards by the action of the temporalis muscle. It is therefore essential to position the transosseous wire before the section is complete. Holes are drilled through the anterior aspect of the lower fragment about 1 cm. beneath the line of section and a similar hole is drilled in the upper section in a situation appropriate to the position to be taken up by the retroposed mandible. A wire is passed through the holes and the two ends of the wire are left slack. The presence of a wire through the upper fragment enables the operator to maintain control of it after the ramus is sectioned. Skaloud (1951) carried out transosseous wiring by passing the wire through a hole in the lower fragment and then over the sigmoid notch using a Reverdin needle. The wire can also be passed over the notch with a small right-angle aneurysm needle on a handle. Many operators prefer to make their section from the lingual to the buccal aspect of the mandible and this is possibly easier if a Gigli saw or orthopaedic saw is used.

When the ramus is sectioned a similar operation is carried out on the opposite side of the mandible after which the body of the mandible is repositioned and the position of the ramus fragments in relation to the mandible in its new position is checked. If they lie in end-to-end apposition the transosseous wires are tightened, but if there is an overlap on one or both sides either additional bone must be removed from one or the other end of the ramus to obtain end-to-end apposition or an overlap must be accepted. This entails compact bone facing compact bone and healing is much prolonged. When a satisfactory bone apposition is obtained the transosseous wires are tightened and the twisted end is cut short and turned into one of the holes in the ramus. The lower jaw is gently opened and closed to see that the position is maintained with the new occlusion. The wounds are then closed with interrupted black silk sutures.

Mandibular/maxillary fixation has to be maintained for about three months, for the area of bony contact between the fragments of ramus is not very great. It will be obvious that, if the lower fragment is pushed back for about half the total width of the ramus, there will be the equivalent of only half the width of the ramus in contact with half the width of the upper fragment. In fact, of the many jaw sections devised posterior to the dental arch, only the oblique (vertical subsigmoid) and sagittal splitting osteotomies with overlapping of the fragments seem likely to remain in current use. The other techniques practised result in narrow areas of bone contact and slow or unstable bone union unless cancellous bone-grafting of the approximated fragments is practised.

Oblique and Vertical Subsigmoid Osteotomy in Ascending Ramus.—These techniques were described by Thoma in 1948 and Hinds (1958) and Robinson (1958) also reported cases treated by this method in the same year. Strictly speaking, in the oblique osteotomy the lower end of the cut comes to a point on the posterior border of the angle, while in the vertical subsigmoid the cut passes through the lower border of the angle. The differences between the techniques are small however and they will be considered as together in this account. The osteotomy cut is oblique to the posterior border of the mandible and extends from the base of the sigmoid notch to the angle. Thoma regards this operation as useful in cases of mandibular protrusion and retrusion as well as in asymmetry and also valuable in some cases of open bite. It has the advantage that when the mandible is moved posteriorly the gonial angle is improved although such improvement may be temporary. (*Fig.* 28G.)

When a considerable posterior displacement of the anterior fragment has to be effected by this type of osteotomy the coronoid process must be separated or it will impinge on the medial root of the zygoma (*Fig.* 28A). Since complete separation of the coronoid results in gross contraction of the temporalis and elevation of the fragment, the inverted L osteotomy of Trauner seems a more satisfactory approach to this difficulty. (*Fig.* 28F.)

Operative Technique

Thoma (1969) performs the operation from a submandibular approach. A 5 cm. curved incision is made in the skin around and 1·5 cm. below the bony border of the angle on each side. The ramus is exposed by dividing the subcutaneous tissues and raising the masseter from the ramus. A right-angled retractor is used to retract the cheek upwards until the sigmoid notch is in view. The outline of the section is then made with Bonney's blue, and the bone is divided with a bur from the sigmoid notch either to the posterior border of the mandible at the level of the attachment of the stylomandibular ligament (oblique osteotomy), or the section passes vertically downwards to the angle (vertical subsigmoid). The simple vertical cut must be positioned behind the mandibular foramen, but for safety's sake only the buccal cortex is divided over the region of the nerve. The remaining lingual cortex is fractured by wedging the cut open from below. The condylar fragment is freed from its soft-tissue attachments on its inner surface with a Howarth's periosteal elevator and the fragment is allowed to overlap the main mandibular fragment. A sterile swab is then placed over the wound and the operation is repeated on the opposite side. After the bilateral section has been completed the loose mandible is manipulated into its new position and mandibular/maxillary fixation is effected. The external wounds are then inspected and transosseous wiring is carried out between the fragments at the posterior border of the mandible. Thoma regards the transosseous wiring as advantageous but not absolutely essential. Some surgeons advocate decortication of a matching area of the anterior fragment to the overlapping posterior fragment. This ensures a better fit, but it is not essential. If decortication is practised, it is important not to compress the inferior dental bundle for protracted nerve damage can result. If the anterior fragment is not decorticated the upper part of the lingual surface of the posterior fragment may need trimming to ensure that it lies flat against the lateral surface of the anterior fragment.

The masseter muscle is then repositioned and sutured to the lower border of the mandible. For this purpose either a stump of masseter is left at the time of exposing the outer surface of the ramus or the masseter can be sutured to the attachment of the medial pterygoid. The wound is then closed in layers.

This osteotomy can also be carried out through an intra-oral incision as has been described by Winstanley (1968). An incision is made down the anterior border of the ramus from the tip of the coronoid process to the retromolar fossa and is then extended into the buccal sulcus. A Howarth's periosteal elevator is used to separate the soft tissue from the bone on the lateral aspect of the ramus. The sigmoid notch is identified and a Moule retractor is placed around the posterior border of the mandible at the level of the stylomandibular ligament. The ramus is then sectioned obliquely from the sigmoid notch to the posterior border of the mandible using a tapered Meisinger fissure bur in a straight handpiece. Winstanley states that the access is not as good as in the external operation, but the internal operation has the great advantage of avoiding scarring on the face. Following the bilateral osteotomy the mandible is repositioned and the two intra-oral wounds are closed with interrupted black silk sutures.

Mandibular/maxillary fixation is carried out following closure of the wounds at the osteotomy sites, and it should be maintained, according to Thoma, for 6–8 weeks to ensure sound union.

The Sagittal Splitting Technique.—Sagittal splitting of the ramus of the mandible in order to correct mandibular deformity was first described by Obwegeser in 1957, who was the first to appreciate that a halving joint could be constructed by dividing the medial and lateral cortices of the ramus at different levels and then splitting the medullary bone between the cuts. A number of variants of the procedure exist. Two seem to stand out as having particular merit, namely the modification suggested by Dal Pont (1961) and Hunsuck's (1968) operation (*Fig.* 29G). The operation is carried out through an intra-oral surgical approach and so avoids facial scarring and possible damage to anatomical structures such as the mandibular branch of the facial nerve. The full width split permits apposition between a broad surface of cancellous bone in the two fragments and therefore avoids the relapse which occurs following inadequate bony contact.

The sagittal split technique also allows the main fragment to be moved in several directions, but still maintain bony contact over a wide area with the lesser fragment. This enables more than one type of mandibular deformity to be corrected for the technique can be used in cases of mandibular protrusion, mandibular retrusion and in some cases of open bite.

Operative Details

The outer surface of the mandible is exposed through an intra-oral incision from the level of the upper molar occlusal surface down along the external oblique line, across the retromolar fossa, and along the buccal aspect between the gingival margin and the external oblique ridge as far as the 1st molar. The periosteum on the lingual aspect of the mandible is raised between the lingula and the sigmoid notch, and the internal oblique line is drilled away with a large pear-shaped bur to enable the operator to visualize the bone below the sigmoid notch as far back as the posterior border of the mandible. A horizontal cut is made through the inner cortex with a tapered Meisinger bur. The outer cortex of the mandible is then cut vertically in the molar region after which the two cuts are connected by a third linking cut along the anterior border of the ramus. While the cortex is being cut the soft tissues are protected with a retractor which is gutter-shaped in cross-section. A large, thick osteotome is used to start the split and the advancing edge of the instrument must follow the inner surface of the outer cortex. The split is completed by boldly twisting the instrument in the cut in an anticlockwise direction on the right side and with a clockwise motion on the left. Some operators prefer to drive into the line of cut two thick osteotomes which tend to split some mandibles through to the lingual side just short of the angle.

Hunsuck's osteotomy, which Barton (1968) has developed, seeks deliberately to encourage this type of split. When this procedure has been carried out on each side of the mandible, the main fragment can be moved in several directions while the condylar fragment maintains its position. In cases where mandibular protrusion has been corrected, it will be found after mandibular/maxillary reposition that the cortex of the posterior fragment will overlap that of the anterior fragment and this surplus is carefully removed with a surgical bur or bone-cutting forceps. The anterior border of the ramus and the alveolar border of the posterior fragment are also trimmed. Close adaptation of the cortical surfaces of the two fragments is achieved by transosseous wiring in the retromolar area or by looping a circumferential wire around the apposed parts. Bony union should be satisfactory in six weeks.

A problem with almost all mandibular osteotomies is the avoidance of damage to the inferior dental nerve. In the sagittal splitting procedure it is necessary to avoid damage to the nerve at three stages —

a. When the soft tissues are elevated from the medial side of the ramus, particularly if an attempt is made to elevate the attachment of the medial pterygoid.

b. When the vertical cut is made on the lateral side, since it must be made clean through into the medulla.

c. When the final split is executed.

With regard to the last of the specified risk situations, the nerve is particularly in jeopardy in those patients in whom the canal lies laterally and is just beneath the buccal cortex.

One prerequisite for the sagittal split is that there should be cancellous bone between the two cortical plates. Some surgeons for preference use the submento-vertical projection for the radiographic assessment of the thickness of the cancellous tissue, but others rely on the study of good quality oblique lateral radiographs of the mandible. With reference to the latter, if a cancellous bone tracery can be seen then a medullary space exists. If the image is featureless, then it is likely that the two cortices are fused. Fortunately, most mandibles have a medullary cavity in the requisite parts, but the medial cut should be placed low down by the lingula, to be certain that it is entered.

The full width split with the Obwegeser manœuvre provides a large area of bone contact. It is appropriate for moderate degrees of prognathism and anterior open bite, and for forward slides unless the advancement is extreme. (*Figs.* 30, 31.)

Ramus procedures appear to have a number of advantages. The area of bone contact is greater than in body operations and union of the fragments faster and more certain. The attachment of the mylohyoid as well as the genial muscles is moved backwards, so that the tongue is displaced further posteriorly than is the case with body procedures. Furthermore, the size of the lower dental arch is not altered. Thus, size of tongue is less critical than with the body osteotomy.

The length of the body of the mandible is retained and the shape of the angle is initially improved. Unfortunately, the improvement of the angle is not permanent since the bone behind the new insertions of the masseters and medial pterygoids is resorbed during the first two years after the operation.

One of the disadvantages of ramus procedures is the tendency to post-operative swelling of the lateral wall of the pharynx and pillars of the fauces. This is due to oedema of the tissues and/or haematoma at the operation site, but the latter complication can be mitigated by the use of vacuum drains and careful haemostasis. The lips and cheeks should be protected from rubbing by instruments and this measure, coupled with a gentle surgical technique, should reduce the amount of postoperative oedema. The combined use of hypotensive anaesthesia and local vaso-constriction should be avoided since this results in excessive local tissue cyanosis and predisposes to excessive postoperative oedema.

Body Ostectomy.—Ostectomy of the body of the mandible is usually carried out in the $\overline{65|56}$ area and it can be performed through either a submandibular or an intra-oral incision, but for the reasons already emphasized the intra-oral operation is preferable in most cases. If a submandibular approach is adopted, it is essential to remove the specified tooth or teeth prior to performing the ostectomy. In the case of the intra-oral procedure extraction of the selected tooth or teeth prior to

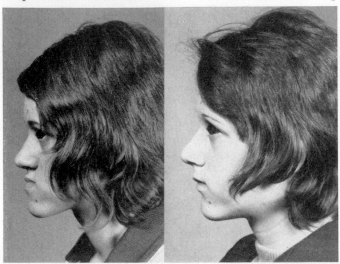

Fig. 30.—Marked prognathism treated by Hunsuck's modification of the sagittal splitting procedure: pre- and postoperative photographs.

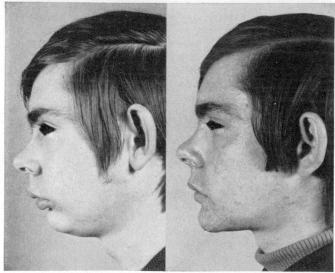

Fig. 31.—A marked degree of retrognathism (Angle's Class II, division 1) treated by the advancement of the mandible using bilateral Obwegeser-Dal Pont procedures concurrently with a lowering of the lower anterior alveolar segment: pre- and postoperative photographs.

operation is helpful, but this measure can be deferred till the time of the ostectomy without much added inconvenience. Preoperative extractions should be carried out at least six weeks prior to the ostectomy in order to allow the extraction site to heal fully and eliminate the possibility of residual infection.

Intra-oral Operation.—A local analgesic solution containing a vaso-constrictor (Xylocaine and 1 : 80,000 adrenaline) is injected buccally and lingually in the operation area to control local bleeding, and then an incision is made around the gingival margins buccally and lingually from the retromolar area to the lower canine and on the buccal side, anteriorly, taken into the sulcus for a distance of half an inch. Buccal and lingual flaps are raised with a Howarth's periosteal elevator to expose the body of the mandible down as far as the lower border of the mandible at the operation site. Retraction is obtained either with 2·5-cm. copper strips bent at one end to pass underneath the lower border of the mandible or preferably by the use of two Lack's retractors. The retractor's handle is bent in the opposite direction so that the blade with the slight curve on the end can be passed under the lower border of the mandible on each side.

When adequate exposure of the operative site is obtained the template pattern of the area to be removed is laid on the buccal aspect of the mandible, care being taken to see that the edges are well clear of the roots of adjacent teeth. Two parallel vertical cuts are then marked out either side of the marker plate using the point of a Meisinger tapered fissure bur. The template pattern is then removed and the cuts are deepened with the tapered fissure bur to penetrate the buccal cortex. Study of the oblique lateral radiographs will show the approximate level of the neurovascular canal and the cuts can be deepened at the lower border so that they penetrate through to the lingual side for a distance of about 0·5–1 cm. and still avoid the neurovascular bundle. Care must be taken to ensure that the lingual retractor is in its correct place while these cuts are made. At the upper end of the body of the mandible the two cuts are also deepened through to the lingual side until the approximate site of the neurovascular bundle is reached. A gentle tap with a chisel on the buccal plate between the bur cuts first at the lower border and then at the upper end of the mandible will remove the lower border of the mandible and upper bone almost to the site of the mandibular canal. The buccal plate covering the neurovascular canal is then knocked off by positioning a chisel on its lingual side and tapping it buccally. This manœuvre exposes the neurovascular canal.

While the mandible is still intact, holes are drilled diagonally through the buccal plate of the mandible on each side of the defect and just above the neurovascular bundle. A 0·5-mm. soft stainless-steel wire is threaded loosely between the bone-ends. It is easier to put the transosseous wire in place before finally sectioning the mandible because difficulty may be experienced when working on two mobile bone-ends. The neurovascular bundle is then exposed and identified and a Howarth's periosteal elevator is placed first above and then below the bundle to act as a guard while the Meisinger bur is used to deepen the parallel cuts through to the lingual side of the mandible. The lingual plate is knocked off with a chisel and the section is complete.

The neurovascular bundle is allowed to take up a position between the bone-ends and the transosseous wire is loosely tightened across the fracture line. The opposite side of the mandible is sectioned in a similar manner and the predetermined amount of bone removed, after which both transosseous wires are adjusted until the bone-ends are seen to be in apposition. The transosseous wires should not be too tight or they will damage the neurovascular bundle which has been allowed to curl up between the bony interfaces. It is not necessary to cut out a special recess in one of the two bone-ends to receive the slightly coiled nerve and vessels, for if the bundle is permitted to take up its own place between the sliced bone-ends and the transosseous wires are fairly slack, nerve damage will be negligible and mental anaesthesia avoided. Indeed, transosseous wires are used merely to hold the alined bone-ends in apposition to facilitate healing, and they do not need to be twisted tightly. The ends of the twisted transosseous wires are cut short and the free end is turned neatly into one of the holes.

With the fragments fixed, the soft-tissue wounds are then closed with interrupted silk sutures. When teeth are present in the lower jaw, on the anterior and posterior fragments, fixation is best effected in the following manner: a silver copper alloy cap splint which has a locking plate on each side in the lower premolar area is cemented to the lower anterior teeth, and soldered to the locking plate is a perforated arch bar which can be wired to the adjacent molar tooth or teeth on the posterior fragments. The centre part of an 20-cm. length of wire is placed over individual teeth, (8 and/or 7|7 and/or 8) on the posterior fragment in the form of a clove-hitch knot and secured to each tooth with a couple of twists on the free ends. These free ends are then threaded through the holes in the arch bars, crossed and tightened. This method provides a very effective and rigid fixation between the anterior and posterior fragments. The use of the arch bar in conjunction with a cap splint allows some flexibility when immobilizing the parts, for it is difficult to calculate exactly the final correct position of the stabilized fragments and their relation to any oral fixation. If posterior teeth are also splinted and pre-arranged localizing bars are constructed, there is the possibility that when the prefabricated connecting bars are fitted there will be a gap between the bone-ends. The other problem with silver copper alloy cap splints fitted to single teeth is that they have a tendency to become detached no matter how well the splint is constructed or how carefully it is cemented in position.

After the surgical fractures in the mandible have been immobilized, mandibular/maxillary fixation is effected with elastic bands between the hooks on the upper and lower teeth. Postoperatively a suitable antibiotic should be administered to the patient for seven days. The sutures are removed at the end of the first week and clinical union should have occurred after a six-week period of immobilization. If so, the fixation is dismantled and it is then important to balance the occlusion by the provision of a suitable partial denture to fill any gaps in the dentition. This prevents the patient from adopting a bite of convenience which might place a strain on the newly healed fracture sites. Sensory function in the mental region should be unaffected.

Symphysial Alveolar Osteotomy.—With patients in whom the dental arch only is too far forward, a backwards movement of the jaw as a whole will produce a 'weak chin'. Extraction of a first premolar tooth on each side followed by movement of the sectioned lower anterior alveolar segment to a more posterior position should produce the desired result. (*Fig.* 29C.)

Patients with a Retrusion of the Upper Jaw

A mild degree of retrusion of the upper jaw can be corrected cosmetically by fitting an upper denture which comes into correct occlusal relationship with the lower incisors and pushes the upper lip into an aesthetically satisfactory position. When the patient is edentulous the procedure is simple, but if maxillary anterior teeth are present these should be extracted if they are decayed or unsightly. If the upper teeth are sound the denture can be designed to cover them, or, alternatively, the natural teeth are allowed to protrude through the denture behind the artificial incisors. If the maxillary retrusion is more pronounced, such a solution is impossible, for if the incisor teeth of the denture are pushed forwards too far off the ridge the denture will, of course, become unstable. In such an eventuality there are three possible alternative procedures: (1) A buccal inlay and prosthesis, (2) Alveolar osteotomy, (3) Maxillary osteotomy.

1. Buccal Inlay and Prosthesis.—In cases of extreme retrusion of the upper jaw the buccal inlay and prosthesis achieves an excellent cosmetic result.

Preliminary Treatment.—Before operation a silver copper alloy cap splint is cemented to the upper teeth with Ames black copper cement. To the anterior aspect of the splint a square post is soldered and over this post a square tube is fitted to which is attached a small perforated German silver tray which projects out horizontally over the upper buccal sulcus. The square tube can be attached to the square post by a grub screw so that when the screw is undone the German silver plate can be removed.

Operation.—An incision is made around the upper buccal sulcus from approximately 6|6. The incision is taken through the mucous membrane and is then deepened vertically upwards, the cut lying just superficial to the periosteum. In this manner a large surgical pocket is made in the upper buccal sulcus and the periosteum covering the bone on the anterior aspect of the premaxillary area is exposed over a wide area. A large gutta-percha mould is then constructed to fill this pocket and correct the maxillary retrusion and the mould is held in position by the German silver tray. After the mould and tray are satisfactorily adjusted, a split skin-graft is taken from some non-hair-bearing area of the patient (inner aspect of the arm or thigh) and this graft is draped over the mould with its raw surface outwards so that when the mould is in position the skin-graft will cover the raw area of the periosteum. Complete haemostasis of the wound must be achieved before positioning the graft because haematoma formation beneath the graft may lead to its destruction. The mould is secured in place by screwing the German silver plate to the square post on the splint.

The skin-graft will take in about seven days, but the mould can be left in position for about fourteen days in the upper jaw. After this time the mould should be removed by unscrewing the grub screw and lifting out the plate and mould. The graft is inspected and the gutta-percha washed, after which the mould is replaced quickly to prevent contracture of the skin-graft. The mould should be changed daily and the patient can be trained to perform this task.

After a few weeks, the actual time depending on the area covered by graft, the gutta-percha mould can be replaced by an upper prosthesis which corrects the profile of the upper part of the patient's face. The gutta-percha mould should overcorrect the maxillary retrusion to allow for any subsequent contracture of the graft before the prosthesis is fitted.

2. **Alveolar Osteotomy.**—The upper incisors and canines can be advanced by carrying out an alveolar osteotomy as described for cases of maxillary protrusion, after which the anterior fragment is brought forward. To prevent the fragment relapsing, a bone-graft is placed on each side in the osteotomy gap created in the bone in the bucccal culcus. This is an extensive surgical procedure and owing to the limitations imposed by the palatal mucoperiosteum and its attendant blood-supply from the greater palatine arteries, any advance of the anterior fragment is of necessity limited in extent, unless the palatal mucosa is divided behind the greater palatine vessels and advanced as an island flap. Bilateral bridges may be placed to help to prevent relapse.

3. **Maxillary Osteotomy.**—A maxillary osteotomy is an extensive surgical procedure in which a Guerin- or Le-Fort-I-type fracture is created surgically and the entire tooth-bearing portion of the upper jaw is advanced. This procedure is usually undertaken when the upper occlusion has not only to be advanced, but also brought down to correct a gross open bite. The techniques employed stem from the work of Wassmund, Axhausen, and Gillies. Unfortunately, even though maxillary osteotomy has been practised for over 40 years it has not been used by so many operators as the mandibular procedures and the number of cases in which it is indicated are far fewer. Hence, there is not the same solid body of experience to help in planning and management. (*Fig.* 29D.)

Wassmund effects an osteotomy at a Le Fort I level. Through an incision in the upper buccal sulcus from the 1st molar region around to 1st molar region, the nasal septum and the medial and lateral walls of the maxillary sinuses are sectioned. A curved osteotome is directed behind the tuberosities to separate the maxilla from the pterygoid plates. Any nasal mucoperiosteum which resists movement of the fragments into the desired position with dissecting forceps is also divided (Obwegeser, 1969b). Thus, the maxilla is pedicled on the soft palate, the greater palatine vessels, and the molar sulcus mucosa.

Some operators feel this bold approach puts the blood-supply to the fragment in jeopardy since the greater palatine vessels can be damaged in the palatine canal when the maxilla is separated from the pterygoid plates. These operators prefer to keep a second strip of sulcus mucosa intact in the premolar-canine-incisor region.

Obwegeser maintains that the insertion of a block of bone between the maxilla and the pterygoid plates and flakes of bone over the lateral bony cuts are essential to the achievement of a stable bony union. Even so, there seems to be a greater tendency to relapse than with certain mandibular procedures.

More recently adventurous attempts have been made to deal with retrusion of the mid-face and even malposition of the orbits and hyper-teliorism have been tackled (Tessier and others, 1967; Obwegeser, 1969b).

Henderson and Jackson (1973) have used oblique incisions below the medial corners of the orbits to effect a Le Fort II level osteotomy. Where the nasal complex also needs advancement or lengthening the incisions are joined into an inverted 'V' over the bridge of the nose.

A Le Fort II osteotomy may be carried out in the following fashion (Seward, 1973). Bilateral incisions are made over the infra-orbital margins opposite the medial two-thirds of the margin. Through these the perios-teum is stripped from the orbital floor back to the inferior orbital fissure, laterally to the lateral side of the orbital floor and medially as far as the lacrimal duct. The nasal soft tissues are elevated subperiosteally over the frontal processes of the maxilla and nasal bones until the undermining from one side reaches that on the other. The anterior margins of the frontal processes and nasal bones can be visualized at this stage through the wounds by careful retraction.

By tunnelling upwards along the orbital rim the periosteum is raised between the medial canthal ligament and the lacrimal sac and a bur cut made from the point at which the anterior end of the nasal bone joins the frontal process of the maxilla back to the orbital rim between the ligament and the lacrimal sac (above the inferior concha). The cut is carried back-wards medial to the sac and then with small osteotomes laterally behind the sac.

The orbital contents are retracted upwards and the cut carried laterally through the thin roof of the orbit with a rose head bur. When the infra-orbital nerve is reached it is mobilized and the bone cut carried above and below it. At the lateral end of the orbital floor the bone is divided in a forward direction in a line which diverges laterally until the orbital rim is reached. The periosteum may be raised from the lateral rim of the orbit to permit onlay grafting if this is desired. The tissues are next raised from the bone vertically down the body of the zygomatic bone until the zygo-matico-alveolar crest is reached. With a long-shank taper-fissure bur the bone is sectioned from the zygomatico-alveolar crest upwards, into the zygomatic extension of the antrum and to join the lateral cut in the orbital rim.

The mouth is entered and incisions made in the sulcus from the zygo-matico-alveolar crest backwards. The lower ends of the bone cuts are identified and continued horizontally backwards above the apices of the teeth with a No. 8 rose head bur. Through this cut and using a smaller long-shank rose head bur the cut is carried along the posterior and medial wall of the antrum. On the medial wall the cut slopes upwards, above the inferior concha, to the region of the hiatus semilunaris. With a rose head bur there is less risk of damage to the anterior palatine artery than with an osteotome.

Separation of the tuberosity from the pterygoid plates is with a curved Obwegeser chisel. The nasal septum must be divided with care right to the back, or the maxilla will not move. This is best done through short vertical incisions just behind the columella. Where the nose needs to be advanced Henderson and Jackson's (1973) method is advocated.

If a mandibular osteotomy is to be combined with the maxillary one the mandibular sites are prepared short of final section before the maxilla is mobilized. Then the maxilla is mobilized with Rowe forceps and advanced, using the mandibular arch as a reference point, and fixed to a halo frame. The mandibular cuts are completed and the jaws fixed together.

A block of iliac crest bone-graft is wedged between the pterygoid plates and the back of the tuberosity on both sides. Thin curved flakes are used to cover the defects in the oribital floors and blocks and chips used to fill all other defects. Onlay grafts may be inserted over the lateral orbital rims to smooth their contour into the displaced infra-orbital rims.

Provided Barton and Harris's (1970) method of fixation with the jaws apart is used, Le Fort II osteotomies can be completed using nasal intubation and bilateral nasopharyngeal airways postoperatively. If both mandibular and maxillary osteotomies are performed, or Henderson and Jackson's (1973) nasal procedures, a tracheostomy will be required.

4. ASYMMETRICAL MANDIBULAR DEFORMITY

In broad terms, mandibular asymmetry can be the result of overgrowth or undergrowth of one side. Condylar hyperplasia is the most common cause of mandibular overgrowth. Two main types seem to occur and have been given a variety of names. In one type the condyle head is not greatly enlarged and often moves normally in the fossa. The condyle neck is elongated and angulated downwards and forwards, displacing that side of the mandible forwards. The angle of the mandible comes to lie more anteriorly than on the other side. There is no open bite, no tilting of the occlusal plane, or increase in depth of the mandible. The condition, therefore, produces asymmetrical prognathism.

In the other type the condyle head is greatly enlarged and may simply rotate when the mouth is opened. The condyle neck is considerably elongated and leaves the condyle either vertically or even in a downwards and backwards direction. The midline of the mandible is usually centrally placed in the face, but the lower border may be tilted towards the opposite side and the lower incisors tilted towards the same side as the deformity. There is a marked downward and inward bowing of the mandible and separation of the posterior teeth. A compensatory downgrowth of the maxillary alveolar process attempts to close the gap. This increases the vertical height of the maxilla on this side. However, it seems probable that some patients have a degree of unilateral gigantism since the appropriate nostril may be enlarged and the ipsilateral supra-orbital ridge may slope upwards. The degree of orbital asymmetry may even be sufficient to require the patient to tilt the head to bring the visual axes horizontal. At operation an enlarged parotid gland and a complex of facial nerve branches may be encountered. The opposite side of the mandible may be either of normal size, or smaller than average.

Minor degrees of this deformity which do not require treatment are not uncommon, but gross examples are far less frequent than in the case of the first type. Asymmetrical prognathism can be managed by the procedures for shortening the mandible outlined previously. In some cases one side only needs to be sectioned, but in many both sides will have to be sectioned to permit a proper interdigitation of the teeth. Since the patient has a near normal joint movement condylectomy should *never* be performed in these cases.

The second type is more difficult. Hovell (1956) has shown dramatically that a condylectomy at the right age will produce a normal facial appearance. However, it seems a pity to sacrifice a joint even if the function is imperfect and a subcondylar procedure to shorten the ramus should be considered, particularly in the adult. More recently Hovell (1970) has used a condyle shave only.

An intra-oral approach to the condyle is described by Sear (1972) who showed that provided a subperiosteal resection of the condyle was effected a new condyle of more reasonable proportions developed. A satisfactory correction of the occlusion and appearance was achieved by this technique. It should be emphasized that this method is for the experienced oral surgeon as potentially marked haemorrhage in a confined wound could be produced by incautious surgery.

Some of the deformity in the lower border of the mandible appears to be secondary to the condylar deformity and condylectomy results in its resorption. Where the mental tubercle is involved, however, this part does not remodel.

A vertical movement of the ramus can only be achieved if an open bite exists or can be created on that side. Trimming of the lower border and onlay grafting of the other side if it is underdeveloped may also be needed.

As in the case of severe degrees of retrognathism, unilateral underdevelopment of the mandible may be the result of a congenital or developmental defect or the result of damage to the condylar growth centre.

The major problem in these patients is that the normal side of the mandible is bent round to meet the abnormal, producing a jaw which is shorter than average, flattened on the abnormal side, and with the central incisor region bent round to the abnormal side. The upper arch adjusts itself to fit the lower. Thus, correction requires expansion of the upper arch and remodelling of the lower incisor region. In many cases a choice lies between serial bone-grafts, which attempt to prevent some of the compensatory changes, and a disguising procedure. Neither are entirely satisfactory. Serial grafting means multiple operations during the patient's childhood and schooldays. Disguising procedures tend to relapse.

In recent years experiments have been tried with the grafting of growing epiphysial bone-ends. The results of these operations are not yet certain. A further complication where the deficiency is due to a congenital malformation is that there is often hypoplasia of the skin, muscle, and other soft tissues and delayed tooth eruption or absent teeth. The soft-tissue defects materially increase the asymmetry and accentuate it in function.

5. PATIENTS WITH MALOCCLUSION NOT ASSOCIATED WITH A GROSS SKELETAL ANOMALY OF THE UPPER OR LOWER JAW

The correction of gross malocclusion is achieved to a greater or lesser extent following all the osteotomy and ostectomy operations performed upon the upper and lower jaws. In the mandible these operations involve, of course, a complete section of the jaw. Surgical correction of occlusal anomalies can also be achieved by alveolar surgery whereby a portion of the upper or lower alveolar process is detached from the underlying bone and repositioned *en bloc*.

One such procedure (alveolar ostectomy and osteotomy) has already been described for the correction of maxillary protrusion and retrusion. This type of alveolar surgery has also been termed 'subapical osteotomy', dento-alveolar surgery, and surgery of the labial segments. The technique can also be used in the lower jaw to reposition the lower incisor segment in an Angle's Class II, division 1 type of malocclusion to correct a deep overbite. This is achieved surgically by detaching the $\overline{321\mid123}$ by an osteotomy in which both the teeth and their investing bone are separated from the body of the mandible. A section of the body of the mandible is then removed from below these teeth so that the segment containing the teeth can be lowered, so restoring a normal occlusal plane to the mandible. Following a similar mobilization of the lower anterior segment the fragment can be raised to close an anterior open bite (Köle procedure). A slice of chin is removed and wedged into the gap below the fragment to bring the chin eminence up behind the chin pad. The blood-supply to the lower teeth is maintained through the soft tissue attached to its lingual aspect.

Maxillary ostectomy for the correction of protruding upper teeth has already been described (p. 155). A similar technique for repositioning upper buccal segments can also be carried out and was described by Schuchardt (1954) for the correction of anterior open bite. The procedure was carried out in two stages in order to preserve an adequate blood-supply to the segments. The palatal cuts are completed at the first operation and the buccal cuts are made four weeks later when an adequate blood-supply has been established through the reattached palatal mucoperiosteal flap. By means of an ostectomy on the buccal aspect, the vertical depth in the molar region can be reduced. In all alveolar osteotomy and ostectomy procedures a very exact diagnostic plan must be made preoperatively with a full evaluation of the soft-tissue morphology. Careful sectioning of plaster-of-Paris models will enable the operator to calculate the exact site of the osteotomy cuts and the amount of bone to be removed in the case of an ostectomy.

Alveolar osteotomy and ostectomy procedures can, of course, be carried out in conjunction with osteotomy and ostectomy procedures which involve a complete section of the mandible. It should be remembered that alveolar osteotomy and ostectomy operations must be time-consuming otherwise there is the possibility of postoperative loss of teeth or alveolar process through inadequate blood-supply to the fragment. This should not occur in an adequately planned and skilfully performed operation, but there is always a risk.

Immobilization of Fragments following Osteotomy or Ostectomy.—Immobilization of the fragments following osteotomy or ostectomy can be effected by any of the methods used in the immobilization of jaw fractures. The fixation of choice must vary from case to case and much depends upon whether teeth are present in the fragments.

Patients with Teeth on all Fragments.—

*Cap Splints.—*When teeth are present the method of choice in Great Britain is the provision of silver-copper alloy cap splints on all fragments, with either prearranged localizing bars or with localization carried out postoperatively. In the case of mandibular operations when only one tooth is present on the posterior fragment, some difficulty may be experienced in cementing securely the cap splint on a single tooth and a safer fixation is to have an arch bar attached to each side of the anterior splint and secured to the tooth on the posterior fragment by means of direct wiring. If there is an edentulous posterior fragment in the lower jaw, upper border transosseous wiring (above the mandibular canal) forms a secure fixation.

*Arch Bar.—*Some operators prefer to use arch bars in place of cap splints and this is, of course, the method of choice when facilities for the construction of cap splints are not available.

*Orthodontic Bands.—*Orthodontic banding of the teeth tends to be a time-consuming procedure and requires the expert co-operation of a skilled orthodontist.

The Edentulous Patient.—

*Transosseous Wires.—*Transosseous wires above the mandibular canal may be used following mandibular operations and the fixation can be reinforced with Gunning-type splints fixed with peralveolar and circumferential wiring.

*Bone Plating.—*Bone plates may be used following mandibular operations and they provide a more rigid fixation, although more difficult to fit during the intra-oral type of operations.

*The Edentulous Upper Jaw.—*Alveolar osteotomy and ostectomy would not be considered in the edentulous upper jaw, for adequate adjustments to the ridge and occlusion can be effected by suitable alveolectomies and the provision of dentures.

REFERENCES

ALLER, T. G. (1917), 'Operative Treatment for Prognathism', *Dent. Cosmos*, **59**, 394.

ANGLE, E. H. (1898), 'Double Resection of the Lower Maxilla', *Ibid.*, **40**, 635.

AXHAUSEN, E. (1939), *'Die operative orthopädie bei den fehlbildungen der kiefer'*, *Dt. Zahn- Mund- u. Kieferheilk.*, **6**, 582.

BABCOCK, W. W. (1909), 'The Surgical Treatment of Certain Deformities of the Jaw associated with Malocclusion of the Teeth', *J. Am. med. Ass.*, **53**, 833.

BALLIN, M. (1908), 'Double Resection for Treatment of Mandibular Protrusion', *Dent. Items*, **30**, 422.

BARTON, P. (1968), Paper read to the Autumn Meeting of the British Association of Oral Surgeons. Royal College of Surgeons, England, London, 26th Oct.

— — and HARRIS, A. N. (1970), 'An Investigation into the Efficiency of the Oral Airway and a Technique for improving the Airway in the Early Post-operative Period following Mandibular Osteotomy', *Br. J. oral Surg.*, **8**, 16–20.

— — and RAYNE, J. (1969), 'The Role of Alveolar Surgery in the Treatment of Malocclusion', *Br. dent. J.*, **126**, 11.

BERGER, P. (1897), *Du traitement chirurgical du prognathisme*. Thesis, Lyons University.

BLAIR, V. P. (1907), 'Operations on the Jaw Bone and Face', *Surgery Gynec. Obstet.*, **4**, 67.

CALDWELL, J. B., and AMARAL, W. J. (1960), 'Mandibular Micrognathia corrected by Vertical Osteotomy in the Ramu and Iliac Bone Graft', *J. oral Surg.*, **18**, 3.

CLARKSON, P. (1955), 'Late Result of Kostecka's Operation for Prognathism', *Proc. R. Soc. Med.*, **48**, 984.

CONVERSE, J. M. (1954), 'Bone Grafting Malformations of the Jaws', *Am. J. Surg.*, **88**, 858.

CRADOCK-HENRY, T. (1966), in *Oral Surgery* (ed. W. H. ARCHER), 4th ed., p. 984. Philadelphia: Saunders.

DAL PONT, G. (1958), 'Die retromolare osteotomie zur korrection der retrogenic und der morden apertus', *Osterr. z. stomat.*, **58**, 8.

— — (1961), 'Retromolar Osteotomy for the Correction of Prognathism', *J. oral Surg.*, **19**, 42.

DINGMAN, R. O. (1948), 'Surgical Correction of Developmental Deformities of the Mandible', *Plastic reconstr. Surg.*, **3**, 124.

— — and VAN ALSTINE, R. S. (1952), 'Correction of Mandibular Protrusion in the Edentulous Patient', *J. oral Surg.*, **11**, 273.

DUFOURMENTEL, L. (1921), 'Surgical Treatment of Prognathism', *Presse méd.*, **29**, 235.

EISELSBERG, A. (1906), 'Plastik bei ektopium der unterkiefers', *Wien. klin. Wschr.*, **51**, 1505.

— — (1907), 'Über plastik bei ektopium der unterkiefers', *Munch. med. Wschr.*, **54**, 36.

ERNST, F. (1927), 'Progenie', in *Die Chirurgie* (ed. KIRSCHNER, M., and MORDMANN), vol. 4, part 1, p. 802. Munich: Urban.

FICKLING, B. W., and FORDYCE, G. L. (1955), 'Mandibular Osteotomy for Facial Asymmetry', *Proc. R. Soc. Med.*, **48**, 989.

GILLIES, H. (1955), personal communication.

HENDERSON, D., and JACKSON, I. T. (1973), 'Nasomaxillary Hypoplasia: The Le Fort II Osteotomy', *Br. J. oral Surg.*, **11**, 77–93.

HENRY, C. B. (1946), 'Case of Kostecka's Operation of Prognathous Mandible', *Proc. R. Soc. Med.*, **39**, 646.

HINDS, E. C. (1958), 'Correction of Prognathism by Subcondylar Osteotomy', *J. oral Surg.*, **16**, 209.

HOVELL, J. H. (1956), 'The Surgical Correction of Variations in the Facial Skeletal Pattern', *Proc. R. Soc. Med.*, **49**, 546.

— — (1970), 'Surgical Correction of Facial Deformity', *Ann. R. Coll. Surg.*, **46**, 92.

HUEBSCH, R. F. (1954), 'Correction of Mandibular Prognathism by Intra-oral Ostectomy', *J. oral Surg.*, **12**, 214.

HULLIHEN, S. P. (1849), quoted by HOGEMAN, K. E. (1951), *Acta chir. scand.*, Suppl. 159, *Am. J. dent. Sci.*, **9**, 157.

HUMPHREY, A. (1856), quoted by RUSHTON, M. A. (1946), *Proc. R. Soc. Med.*, **39**, 431.

HUNSUCK, E. E. (1968), 'A Modified Intra-oral Sagittal Splitting Technique for Correction of Mandibular Prognathism', *J. oral Surg.*, **26**, 249.

JABOULAY, M., and BERARD, L. (1898), 'Traitement chirurgical de prognathisme', *Presse méd.*, **6**, 173.

KAZANZIAN, V. H. (1951), 'The Treatment of Mandibular Prognathism', *Oral Surg.*, **4**, 680.

KOSTECKA, F. (1931), 'Die chirurgische therapie der progenie', *Zahnärztl. Rdsch.*, **40**, 780.

LIMBERG, A. A. (1928), 'A New Method of Plastic Lengthening of the Mandible in Unilateral Micrognathia and Asymmetry of the Face', *J. Am. dent. Ass.*, **15**, 851.

MARKWELL, B. D. (1967), 'The Correction of Maxillary Prognathism by One Stage Ostectomy', *Br. J. plast. Surg.*, **20**, 179.

MATRAS, H. (1967), 'Observations in Connection with the Maxillary Protrusion by Method of the Frontal Pedicle Maxillary Fragment', *Trans. int. Ass. oral Surg.*, p. 103.

MOHNAC, A. M. (1966), 'Maxillary Osteotomy in the Management of Oral Deformities', *J. oral Surg.*, **24**, 305.

MURPHY, P. J., and WALKER, R. V. (1963), 'Correction of Maxillary Protrusion by Ostectomy and Orthodontic Therapy, *Ibid.*, **21**, 275.

NICOLSKY and PEHRGADD. Quoted by REICHERBAD, E., KOLE, H., and BRUCHL, H. (1965), *Chirurgische kieferorthopädie*, p. 208. Leipzig: Barth.

OBWEGESER, H. (1957), 'The Surgical Correction of Mandibular Prognathism and Retrognathia with Consideration of Genioplasty', *Oral Surg.*, **10**, 677.

— — (1964), 'The Indications for Surgical Correction of Mandibular Deformity by the Sagittal Splitting Technique', *Br. J. oral Surg.*, **1**, 157.

— — (1969a), 'Die bewegung des unteren alveolarfortsatzes zur korrektur von kieferstellungsanomallen', *Dt. zahnärztl. Z.*, **24**, 5.

— — (1969b), 'The Surgical Correction of Small or Retrodisplaced Maxillae—Dishfaced Deformity', *Plastic reconstr. Surg.*, **43**, 351.

CORRECTION OF JAWS IN FACIAL DEFORMITY   183

PICHLER, H. (1912), 'Über progenie-operationen', *Wien. klin. Wschr.*, **41**, 1333.
— — (1948), in *Mund-und Kieferchirurgie* (PICHLER, H., and TRAUNER, R.), vol. 2, part 2, p. 621. Munich: Urban.
ROBINSON, M. (1958), 'Prognathism Corrected by Open Vertical Sub-Condylar omy', *J. oral Surg.*, **16**, 215.
— — and SHUKEN, R. (1969), 'Bone Resorption under Plastic Surgery Implants', *Ibid.*, **27**, 116.
ROSENTHAL, W. (1931), 'Chirurgische Fragen in der Zahnheilkunde', *Dt. Zahnärztl. Wscht.*, **34**, 655.
RUSHTON, M. A. (1946), 'Unilateral Hyperplasia of the Mandibular Condyle', *Proc. R. Soc. Med.*, **39**, 430.
SCHUCHARDT, K. (1954), 'Die chirurgie als helferin der kieferorthopädie', *Fortschr. Kieferorthop.*, **15**, 1.
SEAR, A. J. (1972), 'Intra-oral Condylectomy applied to Unilateral Condylar Hyperplasia', *Br. J. oral Surg.*, **10**, 143–153.
SEWARD, G. R. (1970), personal communication.
— — (1973), personal communication.
— — and FOREMAN, B. C. (1972), 'Quick-release Locking Plates', *Br. Dent. J.*, **132**, 366–368.
SKALOUD, F. (1951), 'A New Surgical Method for Correcting Prognathism of the Mandible', *Oral Surg.*, **4**, 689.
SMITH, A. E., and JOHNSON, J. B. (1940), 'Surgical Treatment of Mandibular Deformities', *J. Am. dent. Ass. dent. Cosmos*, **27**, 689.
SOWRAY, J. H., and HASKELL, R. (1968), 'Ostectomy at the Mandibular Symphysis', *Br. J. oral Surg.*, **6**, 97.
STRAITH, R. E., and LAWSON, J. M. (1967), 'Surgical Orthodontia: A New Horizon for Plastic Surgery', *Plastic reconstr. Surg.*, **39**, 366.
TAYLOR, R. S., and COOK, H. P. (1958), 'The Surgical Correction of Skeletal Deformities of the Mandible', *Br. dent. J.*, **105**, 349.
TESSIER, P., and others (1967), 'Osteotomies Cranio-naso-orbito-faciales. Hypertelorisme', *Annls Chir. plastic.*, **12**, 103.
THOMA, K. H. (1948), *Oral Surgery*, vol. 2. St Louis: Mosby.
— — (1969), *Ibid.*, 5th ed.
TRAUNER, F. (1929), 'Unterkieferplastik nach Verlast beider Gelenkköpfchen', *Zbl. Chir.*, **56**, 1986.
TRAUNER, R., and OBWEGESER, H. (1957), 'The Surgical Correction of Mandibular Prognathism and Retrognathia with Consideration of Genioplasty', *Oral Surg.*, **10**, 787.
WASSMUND, M. (1935), *Lehrbuch der praktischen chirurgie des mundes und der kiefer*, vol. 1. Leipzig: Meuser.
WINSTANLEY, R. P. (1968), 'One Stage Maxillary Ostectomy for Correction of Class II, Division I Malocclusion', *Br. J. oral Surg.*, **2**, 173.
WUNDERER, S. (1962), 'Die prognathie operation mittels frontal gestieltem maxilla fragment', *Öst. Z. Stomat.*, **59**, 98.

CHAPTER XVI

THE REPLACEMENT OF BONE

BONE which has been destroyed by accident, disease, or surgery in any quantity must be replaced, for there are limits to the degree to which such bone will regenerate. Bone can be replaced by bone-grafts or by allelografts. Bone-grafts can be taken from the host himself (autograft), from a donor of the same species (homograft), or from a donor of another species (heterograft). Cortical bone, cancellous bone, or mixed cortical cancellous slabs may be used. Such grafts can be applied as chips, flakes, or shaped blocks. The bone can be used when freshly cut or after storage. Heterogenous material is usually prepared for use in ways which remove the soft tissues, or attempt to destroy their antigenicity. Allelografts can be of metal, plastic, or silastic.

It is, perhaps, worth while considering the circumstances in which new bone will successfully regenerate before considering the indications for grafts. For example, new bone will be produced to unite the fragments of a fractured bone. Ideally the bone-ends should be held firmly together without movement until union occurs, the tissues, of course, being free from infection, healthy, and vascular. However, fractures will unite in spite of movement, though the time required may be considerable. Movement, of course, implies movement of one fragment relative to the other. Considerable movement will have little effect if the fragments move together with little relative movement of the bone-ends. Thus, one should not be too dogmatic about the prognosis for an un-united fracture of the mandible with rounded and eburnated bone-ends. Even without fixation, freshening of the bone-ends, or grafting it will be found that some such fractures are united if the patient is seen 2–3 years later.

A gap between the bone-ends will delay union, but again a significant gap can be bridged. Provided the gap width is less than the cross-section of the bone-ends, there can be reasonable hope of success if immobilization is continued for an adequate time.

Even following full-thickness resection of part of the mandible, there can be a surprising amount of new bone deposited, particularly if the periosteum has been retained and especially during childhood and adolescence. Indeed, where a metallic implant has been placed within the periosteum in a child to replace part of the mandible which has been resected, a layer of bone will often be deposited over the surface. A surprising regeneration of bone can occur after a marginal or partial-thickness resection of the mandible. In fact, restitution of the full width of the basal bone can be hoped for. In the maxilla a similar state of affairs exists. Quite sizeable bony perforations penetrating into the nose or maxillary sinus will be repaired if the soft-tissue covering is lined by periosteum.

Because of the difficulty which was experienced in the past with the reduction and fixation of maxillary fractures, the story grew up that bony union did not occur in this bone and that bone regeneration was poor. In fact, fractured maxillae do unite; indeed impacted fractures become solid with considerable speed, and full-thickness defects in the flat bones heal provided that periosteum covers them. On the other hand, there seems a greater likelihood of cyst cavities in the maxilla filling slowly, or incompletely, after marsupialization than in the mandible, particularly where the lining has reached the palatal, nasal, or maxillary sinus mucoperiosteum.

Bone-grafts are used in oral surgery in the following situations:—

1. In the treatment of un-united fractures.

2. To speed the union of the fragments after certain osteotomies.

3. To replace excised segments of mandible or to repair large defects in the maxilla.

4. To restore continuity in the bone where osteotomies have been performed to lengthen the mandible or radically displace the maxilla.

5. As onlay grafts to improve the contour of a bone.

6. To increase the height of the alveolar process so as to improve the foundation for a denture.

7. To fill bony cavities left after the enucleation of cysts or benign neoplasms and hasten healing, or to maintain the normal contour of the bone.

The Fate of Fresh Bone-grafts

If all the cells of a bone-graft were to die and osteogenetic activity spread into the mass only from the site of contact with the adjacent bone, then the process of incorporation would take a considerable time, far longer than is found in practice. That, at best, the vast majority of the original cells within the graft die, even with autografts, can be confirmed by histological section. However, shortly after the invasion of the cancellous spaces by granulation tissue, both osteoclastic resorption of the graft trabeculae and deposition of new bone upon the graft trabeculae is evident throughout the mass. While there is considerable circumstantial evidence that a few of the superficial osteoblasts survive in autografts, much of this activity must result from inductive changes brought about by the bony mass on the cells of the invading granulation tissue. Some believe that a chemical substance, which Lacroix (1951) terms 'osteogenin', is present in the graft and brings about this inductive change.

It is obvious that porous cancellous bone is more easily invaded and incorporated than cortical bone; thus within six weeks most cancellous bone-grafts will be firmly united to the recipient bone.

The Fate of Stored Bone

If grafting between twins and between individuals of an inbred population is excluded, then whenever tissue is transferred from one individual to another an immunological reaction is induced, unless, of course, immunosuppression has been used, as when organ transplantation is attempted. Following a first transfer of tissue there is initial acceptance of the transplant, followed by rejection after about 10–14 days. If tissue is transferred between the same two individuals a second time, the rejection process starts immediately and is more severe. In the process of homografting of bone, there is no practical reason for transferring tissue a second time, so that only the first type of reaction is relevant.

Homografts are invaded by granulation tissue in the same way as autografts, and necrotic soft tissue is removed. Because an immune response must be elicited by the graft, almost certainly no donor cells survive. Unlike the situation with other tissues, with bone homografts there is a calcified matrix which is not destroyed by the host's response. Furthermore, this calcified matrix seems to be capable of exerting an inductive influence on the invading granulation tissue resulting in osteogenesis. Thus, by twelve weeks there is little difference between an autograft and a homograft. However, clinically, there is a somewhat smaller chance of a successful 'take' with homograft bone compared with autograft bone.

The attraction of homo- and heterograft bone is that a second and often debilitating surgical procedure is not necessary in order to obtain the bone. It is rare that suitable homograft bone is available in the fresh state at the right time for a grafting procedure. The bone has therefore to be stored. Healthy sterile bone may be obtained when ribs are resected during thoracotomy or nephrectomy operations. In some countries it is possible to obtain suitable bone from cadavers. Any flesh is carefully removed and the bone freeze-dried.

There is a considerable attraction in the concept of having available for use regular supplies of bone suitable for grafting and of a convenient size. A number of attempts have been made to satisfy this need. One of the earliest was to take the excised diseased segment of bone and to boil it. This destroyed any neoplastic cells or infection. The boiled and defleshed bone was replaced in its original site. As such a graft is composed of cortical bone on the outside so invasion by granulation tissue is difficult and slow and success proportionately low. Os purum, or bone from which some of the organic elements had been removed, was advocated by Orell in 1937. More recently a number of other materials have become available: anorganic bone, Kiel bone, and Boplant bone.

Anorganic bone is prepared by boiling the bone in ethylenediamine for several days. At the end of this time the ethylenediamine is washed out. The anorganic bone can be stored indefinitely without refrigeration. Although brittle it can be trimmed with a scalpel and cut up into chips.

Kiel bone is bovine bone treated with hydrogen peroxide and a de-fatting agent. Boplant is similar save that the bovine bone is treated with β-propiolactone to sterilize it and detergents and organic solvents to remove the fat. They are freeze-dried for storage. Killey, Kramer, and Wright have investigated these substances with the object of determining their possible usefulness for grafting procedures in oral surgery (Killey, Kramer, and Wright, 1966, 1970; Kramer, Killey and Wright, 1968 a, b, c.

Unfortunately these materials appear to be of limited usefulness in this field. Anorganic bone is largely inert. It is neither subject to osteoclastic resorption, except very slowly, nor does it induce osteoblastic activity. Indeed, it impedes the normal repair of a bony defect. Once incorporated in the part, it remains virtually unchanged for many months. Its only place would appear to be as a cavity filler where contour of the bone is of more importance than strength, or as a subperiosteal onlay graft, when it can be placed reasonably deep in the tissues, and where its inertness might prove an advantage. Other forms of onlay graft tend eventually to be resorbed.

Both Kiel bone and Boplant are treated by the host in a similar manner. Initially the graft is invaded rapidly by granulation tissue and trabeculae adjacent to the host bone are covered by new bone. Then giant cells appear on the surface of the uncoated graft bone trabeculae and they are surrounded by lymphocytes, plasma cells, macrophages, and even a few polymorphs. This reaction appears to be immunological in type and induced by the considerable amount of bone matrix and dead osteocytes which remain after the chemical preparation. Fragmentation and destruction of all the uncovered trabeculae follows, but the activity of the giant cells differs from that seen in normal osteoclasis. The inflammatory cell infiltration does not disappear until all the exposed graft bone has been destroyed.

It would appear that these products can only be used with success where rapid coating of the graft bone with new host bone can occur. That is, where the graft can be protected from the immunological response.

The Conditions for Success in Bone-grafting

In the rest of this chapter only autogenous bone-grafting will be described, since this is in general the most successful type of procedure. The conditions for success in bone-grafting are as follows:—

1. Absence of Infection.—It is obviously desirable that there should be an absence of infection, for should the graft become infected before it has been revascularized it will constitute a sequestrum. Even if the infection should not become established until after the graft has been revascularized, then the situation would be the same as an infected fracture.

Ideally, therefore, bone-grafts are inserted through skin incisions since the skin can be more thoroughly cleaned and disinfected on the surface than the more delicate mucous membranes of the mouth. Further, the wound edges can be covered with adhesive drapes or wound towels. Nevertheless, after careful preparation of the oral cavity bone-grafts can be successfully placed through oral incisions (Obwegeser, 1966 and 1968), even where a sizeable opening into the mouth exists. Meticulous multilayer closure and the postoperative use of antibiotics are necessary aids to a good result.

It is even possible to replace parts of the mandible affected by chronic osteomyelitis by an immediate bone-graft, but it is important to ensure that wound contamination is reduced to a minimum by the technique of excision. Thorough irrigation of the wound, the local instillation of an antibiotic to which the organisms are sensitive, and the postoperative administration of systemic antibiotics increase the chances of success.

The reason for attempting immediate grafting in these circumstances is that once the space for the segment of jaw has been allowed to collapse it is difficult to re-open it since the area becomes considerably scarred. Should the attempt fail, however, the graft will have to be removed and the infection cleared up before a further attempt can be made. Also the first donor site will have been operated on in vain.

Chip grafts are in general more rapidly vascularized and therefore more resistant to infection than block grafts. In fact, if infection does supervene only some of the chips may be lost. Curiously, there is a minimum size below which cancellous bone chips cease to act as grafts and are treated as foreign bodies (Hey Groves, 1917; Anderson, 1961).

2. A Vascular, Unscarred Bed.—Unless the recipient site has an adequate blood-supply to ensure rapid invasion of the graft by granulation tissue and its adequate nourishment, the graft will fail. The greater the proportion of cortical to cancellous bone, the more vascular must be the graft bed to ensure success. In general, rib grafts require a more vascular bed than iliac crest grafts (Gillies and Millard, 1957).

3. An Adequate Area of Contact between Graft and the Bone-end.—A good broad contact between the graft and the medullary bone of the recipient bone is essential for union of the graft.

4. Immobilization.—As in the case of union of a fracture, firm contact of the parts with complete immobility produces the best environment for the early stages of union of the graft to the recipient site. Even when chips are used, the fragments should be packed tightly together so that the necessary degree of contact and lack of movement is obtained.

Once new bone unites the graft to the host bone, a degree of functional stress leads to the most rapid consolidation of the graft (Steinhäuser, 1967). Radiographic density increases as new bone is deposited throughout the graft. A layer of bone appears over the whole surface of the mass to form a new cortex, but while there is some remodelling of the inner architecture, only in the young does the graft completely loose the trabecular characteristics of the donor bone.

It is important that all parts of the graft function. For example, a nicely shaped angle on a graft replacing part of the mandible will not be retained unless the masseter and medial pterygoid can be reattached to it. Indeed, in the long term, that is over twenty to thirty years, there seems to be a tendency for all mandibular grafts to be reduced in bulk. Particularly is it true of those replacing the ramus and condyle. Indeed, if it is possible without prejudice to the procedure, the condyle and condyle neck should be conserved and attached to the graft.

Chip and Flake Grafts

In the adult, bone for grafting is usually taken from the iliac crest. Iliac crest bone has a large bulk of cancellous tissue compared with cortex and grafts of a uniform porous texture can be cut from it.

The assistant places his hand on the skin above the iliac crest and depresses it towards the abdomen. This draws the skin upwards so that the scar will lie in the 'bikini' line and not over the crest where it will be subject to friction. The incision follows the line of the outer lip of the crest and is deepened to the muscles. The periosteum is incised between the external oblique origin and the gluteus medius. About 2·5 cm. of the gluteus medius origin is elevated from the bone and a strip of cortex of adequate length and about 2 cm. in width removed from just below the crest. Flakes of cancellous bone can now be removed with a chisel, or blocks separated through as far as the inner cortex. The blocks can be cut up into chips of a size suitable for the procedure.

Where larger amounts of cancellous bone are required, the crest is divided across through the muscle with an osteotome and then separated by a cut parallel with the crest, so that it hinges upwards on the oblique muscles and periosteum. Osteotomes are then driven in to separate a length of ilium about 2 cm. shorter than the crest 'lid'. The crest can be reattached either with braided wire suture or No. 1 chromic cat gut. A disadvantage of this approach is that comfortable walking is delayed until the crest has united to the rest of the bone—about 3–4 weeks. Where it is necessary to take grafts in children or young adolescents, however, it is necessary to conserve the crestal epiphysis and this approach may be required.

Ooze from the bone is controlled by crushing bleeding points and by the use of bone wax and Surgicel. The wound is closed in layers with vacuum drainage.

If a small amount of chips is required, as in the grafting of an un-united fracture or an osteotomy site, a 5-cm. incision only is made. A 1–2-cm. square of cortex is lifted off from just below the crest and a straight curette used to remove the cancellous bone. It can be swept laterally between the cortical plates and surprising amounts removed. The technique was described by Scott, Petersen, and Grant (1949) and by Flint (1964).

BLOCK GRAFTS

Block grafts are used to replace full thickness segments of a bone, since they are mechanically stronger and easier to handle for this purpose than chips. Chips can be packed into a relatively short gap between bone-ends, but some form of strut must be used to give the mass cohesiveness over a long stretch. In addition, block grafts can be contoured more accurately than an aggregate of chips and are used where this aspect is important.

The end or ends of the bone to which the graft is to be fixed are recessed by removing the cortex. This not only forms a lap joint, but exposes medullary bone against which the graft can be fixed.

After applying an adhesive skin drape the iliac crest is exposed as before. The periosteum and muscles are elevated from the crest of the ridge and the medial surface of the ilium is exposed. The iliacus is not as tightly attached to the medial surface of the ilium as the gluteus medius to the lateral and its elevation causes less disturbance to the gait.

A template cut from a thin sheet of malleable metal, such as relief chamber metal, is applied to the bone. Where a replacement for one-half of the mandible is to be cut, the ilium on the same side is exposed and the template inverted. The lower border follows the crest, the angle lies just posterior to the anterior superior spine and the anterior end lies towards the sacro-iliac joint.

An outline of the proposed graft is traced on the bone either with the corner of a narrow osteotome or a No. 10 rose head bur. The outline should be somewhat oversize to allow for trimming. It is particularly important to have some excess in length to ensure an accurate joint with the bone-end. The outline is deepened either with osteotomes or drill up to the outer cortex. This cortex should be penetrated in the region of the condyle but not elsewhere. Only in some thin male pelves is it necessary to take the full thickness of the bone.

With a thin-bladed osteotome the graft is separated from the outer cortex. This should be done with patience, deepening the cut a little at a time, or either the graft or the osteotome will be fractured. Haemostasis is achieved and the wound is closed as before. To avoid a haematoma a tube drain connected via a bottle to a pump is used.

Careful contouring with sharp osteotomes, bone nibblers, and vulcanite burs will produce a suitable replica of the missing part. The graft is fitted into place and wired securely to the bone-end. The inner cortex of the

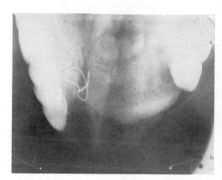

Fig. 33.

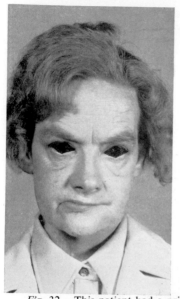

Fig. 32.

Fig. 32.—This patient had a primary carcinoma of the right side of the tongue treated by radiotherapy and a block dissection of neck. There has been no recurrence. A fresh primary has arisen in the left lingual sulcus and the new neoplasm has been excised together with the left mandible, left half of tongue, and contents of the left submandibular region. An immediate bone-graft was placed giving good function and a good aesthetic result.

Fig. 33.—A 0·5 cm. squamous carcinoma of the palate has been excised with a block of maxillary bone. An immediate iliac crest bone-graft has been inserted to replace ridge and palate and chips packed in to restore the contour of the floor of the nose. Bilateral sulcus and cheek flaps were used to cover the graft. The X-ray shows good union and acceptance of the graft.

ilium gives the graft reasonable strength and the cancellous surface aids early vascularization.

There has been considerable improvement in the aesthetics of bone-grafts to the mandible. (*Fig.* 32.) Manchester emphasizes how it is possible to provide a graft which closely mimics the original in appearance and function (Manchester, 1965), and Obwegeser (1966) has encouraged the intra-oral excision of the part and its immediate replacement through the same incision. (*Fig.* 33.) Provided an adequate margin of tissue can be removed without trespassing on the lesion, this approach has advantages. Great care must be taken to avoid a haematoma forming, as this will put tension on the suture line. Vacuum drains, circumferential sutures, and careful closure in layers are all aids to this end.

CURVED BONE-GRAFTS

From time to time it will be necessary to replace segments of bone of such a curvature that part of the iliac crest will not do, for example, in the replacement of the anterior part of the mandible. (*Fig.* 34.) Several approaches can be made to this problem. Sizeable chips of ilium can be threaded on a stout wire (Kirschner wire) which has been bent to the

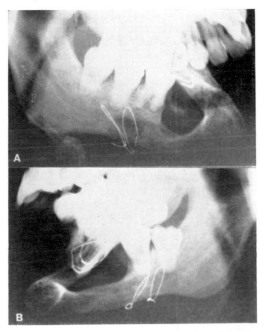

Fig. 34.—Right and left oblique lateral jaw radiographs showing replacement of the anterior part of the mandible by a single horseshoe-shaped piece of bone. A, A radiograph of the left side at three months postoperative and, B, a radiograph of the right side at one year.

desired shape. The ends of the wire are thrust into the medullary cavities of the bone-ends and more chips built up around the strut as the wound is closed.

Another technique (Albee, 1919; Dingman, 1950; Seward, 1967) utilizes a 'U' of bone cut from the surface of the ilium. A graft from molar region to molar region can be managed in this manner. A further alternative uses a length of rib which is notched with a saw so that it can be bent with a series of green-stick fractures (Steiss, 1949; Gillies and Millard, 1957). Finally, where all or almost all of the mandible has been removed the two sides are replaced by cortico-cancellous blocks cut as already described. The front ends of the blocks are cut to form a step. A third piece cut to include the tubercle from one iliac crest is fixed across between the bone-ends. It is shaped at each end to complement the steps cut in the lateral pieces and fixed to them with two wires on each side.

Rib Grafts

Because it is denser bone and not of a size that favours contouring, rib is not generally used to replace parts of the jaws, though there are special circumstances where it is used.

Ribs removed by subperiosteal dissection are replaced. Indeed, in a child the replacement may defy detection in a radiograph. Thus, rib is used in infants for grafting alveolar clefts and in young children in preference to iliac bone. An incision is made over the 7th rib and deepened to its surface. The periosteum is raised and divided at right angles to the line of the rib at each end. A Doyen periosteal elevator is used to separate the periosteum on the inner surface. This must be done with care, since the parietal pleura is close below and a tear in the rib bed will almost certainly open the chest cavity. A cuffed tube should be used by the anaesthetist so that if necessary the lungs can be inflated and, if the chest is accidentally opened, an underwater drain must be inserted.

The required length of rib is resected and the wound closed in layers. It is common practice to split the rib lengthwise so that medullary bone is exposed in the graft.

Cartilage Grafts

These may be cut for onlay grafting from the costo-chondral junction region of the 8th, 9th, and 10th ribs. Full-thickness removal of cartilage should be avoided. Where sizeable quantities are required freeze-dried, bank cartilage should be used if it is available.

Allelografts

The concept of tailor-made or ready-made allelografts which can be screwed, or bolted into place is one which holds great attractions for those doing radical surgery for malignant neoplasms. Acrylic resin, silastic, teflon, tantalum, stainless steel, and various chrome-cobalt alloys have been used in this way.

Such appliances can be used in several ways: one way in which allelografts are used is as a temporary replacement for a segment of jaw until bone-grafting can be undertaken at a second operation. Such a use prevents the collapse and scar contracture which otherwise occurs and impedes the establishment of a bed for the graft at the next procedure. The simplest appliance of this type is a Kirschner wire which has been threaded at each end to take a nut. Henny and McClelland (1959) have used such an appliance by impacting the wire into the bone-ends so that the nuts prevent the wire from working farther into the bone-ends. Provided that full intermaxillary fixation is used, such appliances do not become displaced and work well.

Others (see Henny and McClelland, 1959) use the appliance as an aid to immobilization during the actual grafting. A stout wire or a tray screwed to the lower borders of the bone-ends may be used in this manner.

Finally, permanent implants may be used. These may be either made for the individual occasion or system-built commercial appliances assembled to meet the operator's requirements. They are usually bolted to the remaining bone fragment. Dewey and Moore (1962), Mallet (1963),

Cooke (1969), and Bowerman and Conroy (1969) have described examples of these systems.

It is perhaps unfortunate that the long-term success of these prostheses is poor. Even in the hands of experts the soft tissues seem ultimately to break down over some prominence. Perhaps the depth to which it is possible to bury them in these regions is too little. Alternatively, the fixation of the implant to the jaw works loose. Initially, all are agreed, the fixation must be very strong indeed but, even so, should the slightest movement start to occur, osteoclastic resorption will result in rapid loosening. Neither does it seem easier to get the wound to heal over these materials. Indeed, bone-grafts are far less demanding in terms of environment. For example, if the flaps are thin, or the tissues have been irradiated, an allelograft will not be a success.

In the authors' opinion, in spite of the additional operative trauma, an immediate, but not elaborate, iliac crest bone-graft is preferable in many cases where an implant would be used.

ELECTIVE TRACHEOSTOMY

After resection of large segments of the mandible and adjacent tissues, and the insertion of bone-grafts, the patency of the airway is of concern. In certain patients a tracheostomy is necessary to safeguard the airway during the early postoperative days.

The head is extended on the neck by means of a small sandbag between the shoulders. A collar incision about 5 cm. long is made a finger's breadth above the medial ends of the clavicles. It is deepened through the platysma and flaps raised mainly upwards, but also downwards.

The midline is carefully identified and the strap muscles separated to expose the thyroid gland. The upper edge of the thyroid isthmus is separated from the front of the trachea. Blunt dissection with an artery forceps releases the rest of the isthmus and the forceps emerge below its lower border. Any adjacent inferior thyroid veins are gently picked up and a retractor inserted under the lower border of the isthmus. This both exposes the second, third, and fourth rings of the trachea and lifts the trachea up into the wound. Cautiously the trachea is incised, so that neither the anaesthetist's tube nor the vulnerable posterior wall of the trachea are damaged. With cartilage shears an oval window, of suitable size and with its long axis vertical, is cut in the front of the second and third rings. The fragment is grasped before it is finally cut off so that it is not dropped into the lumen of the trachea. Tracheal dilators are inserted and a cuffed, plastic tracheostomy tube is inserted as the anaesthetist withdraws the endotracheal tube.

The strap muscles, platysma, and the skin are closed in layers about the tube, but not too tightly. The wound is sprayed with a plastic dressing, a dry dressing applied, and the tapes of the tube tied behind the neck.

REFERENCES

ALBEE, F. H. (1915), *Bone Graft Surgery*, p.35. Philadelphia: Saunders.
—— (1919), *Orthopedic and Reconstructive Surgery*, p. 1062. Philadelphia: Saunders.
ANDERSON, K. (1961), 'A Histological Study of the Effect of Size of the Implant', *J. Bone Jt Surg.*, **43A**, 980.

BOWERMAN, J. E., and CONROY, B. (1969), 'A Universal Kit in Titanium for Immediate Replacement of the Resected Mandible', *Br. J. oral Surg.*, **6**, 223.

COOK, H. P. (1969), 'Titanium in Mandibular Replacement', *Ibid.*, **7**, 108.

DEWEY, A. R., and MOORE, J. W. (1962), 'Mandibular Repair after Radical Resection', *J. oral Surg.*, **20**, 34.

DINGMAN, R. O. (1950), The Use of Iliac Bone in the Repair of Facial and Cranial Defects', *Plastic reconstr. Surg.*, **6**, 174.

FLINT, M. (1964), 'Chip Bone Grafting of the Mandible', *Br. J. plast. Surg.*, **17**, 184.

GILLIES, Sir H., and MILLARD, D. R. (1957), *The Principles and Art of Plastic Surgery*, vol. 2, p. 527. London: Butterworths.

GROVES, E. HEY (1917), 'Methods and Results of Transplantation of Bone in the Repair of Defects caused by Injury or Disease'. *Br. J. Surg.*, **5**, 185.

HENNY, F. A., and MCCLELLAND, W. D. (1959), 'Methods of Fixation in Mandibular Bone Grafts', *J. oral Surg.*, **17**, 34.

KILLEY, H. C., KRAMER, I. R. H., and WRIGHT, H. C. (1966), 'The Effects of Implanting Heterogenous Compact and Cancellous Anorganic Bone into Long Bones of Rabbits', *Archs oral Biol.*, **11**, 1117.

— — — — — (1970), 'The Response of the Rabbit to Implants of Processed Bovine (Kiel Bone) and the Effects of Varying the Relationship between Implant and Host Bone', *Ibid.*, **15**, 33.

KRAMER, I. R. H., KILLEY, H. C., and WRIGHT, H. C. (1968a), 'The Replacement of Bone', *Aust. dent. J.*, **13**, 17.

— — — — — (1968b), 'A Histological and Radiological Comparison of the Healing of Defects in the Rabbit Calvarium with and without Implanted Heterogenous Anorganic Bone', *Archs oral Biol.*, **13**, 1095.

— — — — — (1968c), 'The Response of the Rabbit to Implants of Processed Calf Bone (Boplant)', *Ibid.*, **13**, 1263.

LACROIX, P. (1951), *The Organisation of Bones*. London: Churchill. Translation of 1949 French edition.

MALLET, S. P. (1963), 'A Method of Preparing and Using Stainless Steel in Oral Surgery', *Oral Surg.*, **16**, 1160.

MANCHESTER, W. M. (1965), 'Immediate Reconstruction of the Mandible and Temporomandibular Joint', *Br. J. plast. Surg.*, **8**, 291.

OBWEGESER, H. L. (1966), 'Simultaneous Resection and Reconstruction of Parts of the Mandible via the Intra-oral Route in Patients with and without Gross Infections', *Oral Surg.*, **21**, 693.

— — (1968), 'Primary Repair of the Mandible by the Intra-oral Route after Partial Resection in Cases with and without Preoperative Infection', *Br. J. plastic Surg.*, **21**, 282.

ORELL, S. (1937), 'Surgical Bone Grafting with Os Purium, Os Novum and Boiled Bone', *J. Bone Jt Surg.*, **19**, 873.

SCOTT, W., PETERSEN, R. C., and GRANT, S. (1949), 'A Method of procuring Iliac Bone by Trephine Curettage', *J. Bone Jt Surg.*, **31A**, 860.

SEWARD, G. R. (1967), 'A Method of Replacing the Anterior Part of the Mandible by Bone Graft', *Br. J. oral Surg.*, **5**, 99.

STEINHÄUSER, E. (1967), 'Influence of Function on Bone Grafts reconstructing the Mandible—An Experimental Study', *Excerpta Medica*, **174**, 137. 4th International Congress of Plastic and Reconstructive Surgery, Rome, 1967.

STEISS, C. F. (1949), 'Utilization of the Tube Pedicle in the Reconstruction of Facial Defects', *Plastic reconstr. Surg.*, **4**, 545.

CHAPTER XVII

SOME SKELETAL DISEASES OF INTEREST TO THE ORAL SURGEON

FIBROUS DYSPLASIA OF BONE

MUCH of the confusion in the literature surrounding fibrous dysplasia stems from the multiplicity of titles under which cases have been described, for Lichtenstein and Jaffe (1942) reported no fewer than 37 such synonyms. In order to understand this aspect of the problem more clearly, it is necessary to consider a chronological history of the condition.

In 1891 Von Recklinghausen published a monograph in which he described several cases of bony dysplasia which appeared to fall into one group but which, in fact, represented several different conditions. Two of the cases in this series were generalized osteitis fibrosa and his name is still attached to this condition.

In 1904 Askanazy reported a case of osteitis fibrosa in which a parathyroid tumour was discovered after death, and in 1926 Mandl successfully performed a parathyroidectomy for a case with the characteristic bone changes. Hunter and Turnbull (1931) pointed out that there was a large group of dysplasias which were obviously not due to hyperparathyoidism and called them 'diffuse osteitis fibrosa' in contradistinction to the lesions associated with hyperparathyroidism, which were known as 'osteitis fibrosa cystica generalisata'. The non-hormonal group continued to be classified as varieties of osteitis fibrosa until it was observed that some of the lesions were associated with extraneous pigmentation and other extra-skeletal manifestations. The first of these cases was described by Weil in 1922, but subsequently cases were reviewed by McCune and Bruch (1937) and by Albright, Butler, Hampton, and Smith (1937). The condition is now referred to as Albright's syndrome. The subjects are usually children and the classic triad consists of:—

1. Polyostotic fibrous dysplasia with a tendency to a unilateral distribution.

2. Abnormal pigmentation of the skin and occasionally of the mucous membrane.

3. Sexual precocity especially in females due to endocrine dysfunction.

Skin Pigmentation.—The pigmentation is of the *café-au-lait* type and is usually scattered over the back, thighs, and buttocks. Cases have been reported with oral pigmentation.

Endocrine System.—The most common feature is precocious puberty with the menarche at from 1 to 5 years of age in 50 per cent of cases and from 6 to 10 years in another 33 per cent. Breast development and pubic and axillary hair appear after the menarche. Occasionally precocious puberty occurs in males and it may be accompanied by gynaecomastia.

In 1938 Lichtenstein observed that the bone lesions which were the essential feature of the disease could occur in the absence of the extra-skeletal manifestations and suggested the term 'polyostotic fibrous dysplasia'. In 1942 Lichtenstein and Jaffe made the further observation that the condition could be confined to a single bone and, therefore, suggested the term 'fibrous dysplasia' to describe the entire group, but stipulated that monostotic or polyostotic varieties could occur.

Aetiology.—The aetiology of fibrous dysplasia is unknown, but most workers now regard it as a developmental defect. The disease is neither familial nor hereditary, and where an identical twin is affected it is usual for the other to be entirely normal.

Jaffe (1958a) suggested that it may have its basis in some deep-rooted defect. Caffey (1956) considered that the dystrophy was of neurogenic origin. Tannhauser (1944) related it to neurofibromatosis. Snapper (1949) considered fibrous dysplasia should be linked with lipoid histiocytosis, a view discarded by Falconer, Cope, and Robb Smith (1942) and Fairbank (1950). Schlumberger (1946) attributed the lesion to injury.

Incidence.—The Memorial Sloan-Kettering Cancer Centre found 47 cases of craniofacial fibrous dysplasias in the period 1930–65. The classic Albright's syndrome is rare and only occurs once for every 20 to 30 cases of monostotic or polyostotic fibrous dysplasia without extra-skeletal manifestations. In a series reported by Zimmerman, Stafne, and Dahlin (1958) from the Mayo Clinic, only 1 out of 69 patients with jaw lesions had polyostotic fibrous dysplasia and of 13 patients with polyostotic fibrous dysplasia only 2 had jaw involvement.

Stewart, Gilmer, and Edmonson (1962), at the Campbell Clinic, Memphis, Tennessee, found 20 cases of fibrous dysplasia in a 30-year period. Reviewing the world literature in 1951, Pritchard found 256 cases. He found an equal distribution between male and female. However, Stewart and others (1962) who reviewed 20 cases found 15 males and 5 females.

Sex and Race.—Ramsey, Strong, and Frazell (1968), in their series of 47 patients, found 26 female and 21 male. Most authorities consider the condition more common in females.

Age.—Age of onset of symptoms in Ramsey and others' (1968) series varied from one and a half years to 73 years of age and 83 per cent noted symptoms within the first two decades of life.

Bones Involved.—Any bone may be involved, but the long bones are most frequently affected, especially the upper end of the femur, and this may result in bowing of the leg.

The condition may be asymptomatic, but pain and even fracture may occur, the fractures being multiple and recurrent. Facial asymmetry may develop due to involvement of one or more facial bones, and occasionally there may be proptosis of the eye with associated visual disturbance. The calvarium may be involved and thickened with frontal bulging. The bossing may be asymmetrical and sometimes there is unilateral or bilateral obliteration of the sinuses. The facial bones are involved in about half of the cases. Lesions of the skull are found in about one-half of the cases with a moderate degree of skeletal involvement, and in severe cases the skull is almost always affected (Lucas, 1962).

Oral Manifestations.—The jaws may be enlarged, expanded, and distorted. Radiographs show a dense mass often 'ground glass' in appearance which in the upper jaw expands into and can obliterate the sinuses. In the mandible the jaw may be expanded and distorted and occasionally radiographs reveal a radiolucent area similar to that seen in the long bones. In a few instances there is oral pigmentation. The mandible was the bone most frequently involved in Ramsey's series of 47 cases (Ramsey and others, 1968), but Lucas (1962) states that the lesion is more commonly found in the maxilla. The lesions tend to become inactive after the normal period of bodily growth has terminated, but cases have been reported where the lesion continued to enlarge after this time (Seward, 1970).

The monostotic type of fibrous dysplasia of the craniofacial bones is rarely accompanied by extra-skeletal manifestations, although it is identical histologically to the polyostotic form. The cranial bones are often involved, particularly the base of the skull.

Signs and Symptoms.—The presenting symptom in most instances is swelling and this occurred in 80 per cent of Ramsey's series.

Pain is a less common symptom in jaw cases (Lucas, 1962). Pathological fracture of long bones may occur, but there is no reported case of fracture of the mandible. Harris, Dudley, and Barry (1962), in a series of 50 cases, reported that 85 per cent sustained a fracture of a long bone.

There is little disturbance of function, though teeth may be displaced and occlusion upset. In children, teeth in the affected part may fail to erupt (Lucas, 1962).

Radiology.—The radiological picture of fibrous dysplasia depends on the proportions of fibrous and osseous tissue in the lesion. When the bone in the affected area is predominantly replaced by fibrous tissue an area of radiolucency results and the cortex is thinned and expanded. As ossification occurs in the fibrous tissue, the radiograph becomes more opaque.

With regard to the facial bones the area affected by fibrous dysplasia may vary from a minimal lesion in a single bone, often the maxilla, to the most extensive involvement of both mandible and maxillae with further lesions in the skull. Often the fibrous dysplasia is confined to one side of the face and the deformity may assume bizarre shapes. In the mandible the lesion is usually confined to one side and results in considerable bony expansion. Not infrequently in young patients there is a cyst-like area in the involved bone (Stafne, 1964). In the upper jaw the lesion is usually confined to one maxilla and its neighbouring bones and the maxillary sinus is reduced in size by the dysplasia.

Fibrous dysplasia can be demonstrated on radiographs from a very early age, but in the very young patient the affected area appears almost translucent. As the patient grows the area affected increases in size and becomes more opaque as the fibrous tissue becomes more calcified. At this stage the area involved has a uniform density and assumes the radiographic appearance of ground glass. (*Fig.* 35.) Sometimes the affected bone has the appearance of orange peel. If the lesion involves the teeth the lamina dura may sometimes be lost (Worth, 1963).

When the skull is involved, unusual radiographic appearances may result and often there is an irregular radiolucent area similar to that seen in osteoporosis circumscripta of Paget's disease. There is often an increased density and thickening of the base of the skull.

With the passage of time there is a change in structure of the lesion (Worth, 1963). Serial radiographs have shown that in some cases the lesion becomes more calcified with increasing age of the patient, but exceptions to this are not uncommon (Stafne, 1964).

When such changes occur, the uniform ground-glass appearance of the radiograph gives way to patchy areas of sclerosis until eventually the radiographic appearance is similar to the cotton-wool effects seen in Paget's disease. (*Fig.* 36.) At operation such bone is found to be extremely hard and avascular.

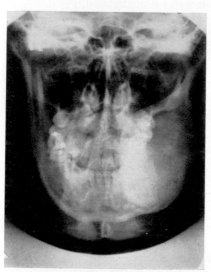 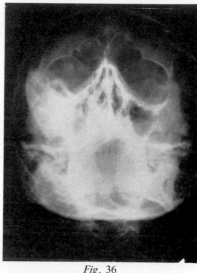

Fig. 35   *Fig.* 36

Fig. 35.—Postero-anterior radiograph showing fibrous dysplasia of the mandible. The patient is 20 years of age and the lesion has the ground-glass appearance.

Fig. 36.—Occipitomental radiograph in a patient of 40 years of age showing patchy areas of sclerosis in the region of the zygomatic bone which is affected with fibrous dysplasia.

Worth has pointed out that there is no correlation between the radiographs and the histological appearances of the bone involved. A diagnosis of fibrous dysplasia can usually be made on the radiographic appearances alone, but occasionally the lesion may assume most unusual appearances. However, whenever a long-standing bony lesion is seen, the possibility of the diagnosis of fibrous dysplasia must always be considered irrespective of its radiographic appearance.

Histopathology.—Most authorities agree that the lesions in the polyostotic and monostotic types are histologically identical. However, some workers consider that while polyostotic fibrous dysplasia is a developmental anomaly, the monostotic lesions are reparative reactions to trauma (Schlumberger, 1946).

In the area affected there is replacement of normal bone with greyish white tissue which imparts a gritty sensation to the knife due to the newly formed bony trabeculae it contains. Microscopically the cancellous spaces of the marrow are seen to be occupied by cellular fibrous tissue arranged in whorls and interlacing bundles. In this fibrous tissue newly formed woven bone is seen, the trabeculae being irregularly arranged. The original trabeculae are absent and osteoclasts are very few in number. Groups of foam cells may be seen and there is an abrupt demarcation between the affected and the adjacent normal bone, and the lesions are more vascular than normal bone. The proportion of bone in the replacement tissue is variable; in some only scattered trabeculae are seen while others contain a sponge-like arrangement of woven bone which can become quite dense.

Malignant Changes in Fibrous Dysplasia.—Although fibrous dysplasia is regarded as a relatively benign lesion, malignant changes have been recorded by numerous authorities. In 1914 Emslie reported giant-celled sarcoma in a femur with fibrous dysplasia, and further cases have been recorded by Coley and Stewart (1945), Dustin and Ley (1950), Sutro (1951), Perkinson and Higginbotham (1955), Vahkurkina (1958), Jaffe (1958a), Seth, Climie, and Tuttle (1962), and Riddell (1964).

Probably the greatest risk occurs when areas of fibrous dysplasia are irradiated and Sabanas, Dahlin, Childs, and Nins (1956) reported post-irradiation sarcoma in bone affected by fibrous dysplasia, and Van Horn, Johnson, and Dahlin (1963) reported a post-irradiation sarcoma of the maxilla which was affected by monostotic fibrous dysplasia. In a series of 50 cases of fibrous dysplasia, Harris, Dudley, and Barry (1962) reported 2 cases where sarcoma occurred in lesions that had been irradiated.

Cases in which fibrous dysplasia of the jaws have undergone malignant change have also been reported. De Marchi (1956) recorded osteogenic sarcoma occurring in the mandible which was affected by monostotic fibrous dysplasia. Tanner and others (1961) found 4 cases of sarcoma arising in lesions of fibrous dysplasia in the facial bones and in all cases the lesions had been subjected to radiation. Jäger (1962) reported osteogenic sarcoma of the maxilla in a case of Albright's syndrome. Bruckner and others (1967) reported osteogenic sarcoma arising at a site of fibrous dysplasia in the mandible, and Pilheu and Soldato (1966) reported a particularly large fibro-osteosarcoma of the jaw in a case of polyostotic fibrous dysplasia.

Treatment.—Because there is little disturbance of function in cases of craniofacial fibrous dysplasia, most patients seek treatment for cosmetic reasons. In view of the fact that areas of fibrous dysplasia continue to enlarge during the period of general skeletal growth it is advisable to defer surgery until growth has ceased. It is best to avoid operations designed to reduce the size and contour of the jaws affected by fibrous dysplasia before skeletal growth has ceased since, particularly during adolescence, extremely rapid growth of the remaining part may be induced. However, once growth has ceased contouring operations produce a pleasing and reasonably permanent result. It would appear logical, therefore, to postulate that such surgery should be deferred until the patient is about 21 years of age. However, occasionally the deformity may be so cosmetically unacceptable that earlier operation is indicated, but in such cases the patient should be warned that some relapse is to be anticipated and that a secondary operation may be necessary when general skeletal growth has ceased.

Operations on the upper and lower jaws can usually be satisfactorily effected through an intra-oral incision along the crest of the ridge in the edentulous case and round the buccal aspect of the gingival margin when teeth are present. The operation consists of exposing the affected bone and trimming the excess with chisels or Jansen-Middleton bone gouges. It is not necessary or desirable to excise all the affected bone.

In the young patient the affected bone is quite soft and feels gritty as it is cut. Surgical trimming is a simple matter in such cases, but with increasing age the bone in fibrous dysplasia becomes more sclerotic and great difficulty may be encountered in cutting it. The bone involved by fibrous dysplasia in the young is highly vascularized and haemorrhage may be brisk. It is important to achieve complete haemostasis before closing the wound or large haematoma formation may occur. Bony organization of such a haematoma may contribute to residual bony enlargement in the area. Where possible, a postoperative pressure dressing should be applied.

Elderly patients with fibrous dysplasia not only have hard sclerotic bone, but the area is relatively avascular and liable to postoperative infection. Chronic low-grade osteomyelitis may occur postoperatively in such individuals. All patients with fibrous dysplasia should be reviewed at regular intervals in view of the possible risk of malignant changes developing in the lesion.

HYPERPARATHYROIDISM

As long ago as 1877, Langedorff described a patient with cystic disease of the bones and was able to demonstrate evidence which pointed towards an upset in calcium metabolism, and in 1884 Davies-Colley described a 13-year-old girl who had generalized skeletal disease, a tumour of the jaw, and renal stones with an increased renal excretion of calcium.

When Jung reviewed Von Recklinghausen's autopsy material he felt certain that in 2 cases what had been described as a 'lymph-node' was, in fact, a parathyroid adenoma. Askanazy (1904) was the first to relate the bone disease to parathyroid disease and Mandl (1926) was the first to excise the gland for a patient.

Hyperparathyroidism may be due to the presence of one or more parathyroid adenomas, a parathyroid carcinoma, or parathyroid hyperplasia. Parathyroid hyperplasia may be primary or secondary to renal disease or occasionally steatorrhoea. Tertiary hyperparathyroidism occurs when autonomous adenomas arise in a hyperplastic gland. In children the sexes are equally affected, but in adults females are twice as common as males.

The clinical picture exhibited by these people may be presented under three headings: skeletal signs and symptoms, urinary tract signs and symptoms, and signs and symptoms of hypercalcaemia.

Skeletal Signs and Symptoms.—The patient may suffer from aches and pains in the bones which may be tender to pressure. Often such complaints are dismissed initially as muscular rheumatism. Later the bones bend, the skeleton becomes deformed, and pathological fractures occur. The ends of the terminal phalanges are resorbed so that the tips of the fingers and toes fall in, giving an appearance of clubbing. A curious, dull, wooden note may be elicited if the skull is percussed. Giant-cell tumours may develop in the bones, causing expansion of the bone. On occasions they may grow with surprising speed and may be mistaken for a sarcoma.

Finally, in advanced cases the skull may exhibit basilar inversion which carries a danger of medullary compression and death if the neck is extended during parathyroidectomy.

Urinary Tract Signs, Symptoms, and Complications.—A high serum calcium results in a high urinary calcium. This together with the increased phosphorus excretion induced by parathormone leads to calcium diabetes with polyuria and polydipsia.

Renal stones may form and migrate into the ureter, stimulating ureteric colic. Ascending infection, renal damage, and renal failure can follow. Calcification of the renal tissues or nephrocalcinosis will also disturb renal function.

Symptoms and Signs of Hypercalcaemia.—The patient may suffer from anorexia, nausea, and vomiting with abdominal cramps, weakness, wasting, and drowsiness. A parathyroid crisis can resemble an acute abdominal catastrophy. Although the reason for the relationship is unknown, duodenal ulcers and amenorrhoea are common.

Calcium salts may be deposited in the conjunctiva and, when renal impairment produces retention of phosphorus and hyperphosphataemia is added to hypercalcaemia, calcium salts are deposited in the cornea, lungs, blood-vessels, and gastric mucosa.

Curiously, even though some adenomas reach an inch or more in diameter, it is exceptional to be able to palpate them. Perhaps this is because 84 per cent develop in the inferior parathyroid gland.

Pathology.—Osteoclastic resorption of bone takes place under the stimulus of parathormone with progressive destruction of the normal bone. Much woven bone is deposited to replace the lamellar bone and zones of cellular fibrous tissue and giant-cell tissue appear.

Radiology.—Radiographically there is thinning and disappearance of the cancellous trabeculae with resultant widening of the medullary spaces. The cortex initially develops a streaky appearance as Haversian canals are widened, then it, too, is reduced in thickness. Clouds of woven bone spicules are formed and the bone takes on a 'moth-eaten' appearance. Once the cortex has been completely destroyed radiolucency may be extreme, particularly in the jaws where the bone assumes a uniform cloudy or granular pattern.

Giant-cell lesions may form before, or after, obvious generalized bone changes have occurred. They are usually similar in appearance to giant-cell granulomas and are of particular significance if multiple, or if they recur after local surgery. Sometimes giant-cell epulides are formed. In some patients a localized zone of cortex is destroyed which, when viewed from the surface, produces an oval radiolucency. This is the appearance which is loosely described as 'cystic change'.

In all such cases screening tests for hyperparathyroidism should be performed. Although investigation of this condition is now quite sophisticated, the best test for this purpose is still the serum calcium estimation. To be of value, this test should be done properly. The specimen should be taken before the first food in the morning and the vein from which the blood is to be drawn should not be occluded for sufficient time for cyanosis to occur. The tourniquet should be released before the blood is aspirated. Further, the patient must not be taking alkali even if he has a peptic ulcer.

In doubtful cases the test should be repeated at weekly or fortnightly intervals for some months.

The lamina dura will be reduced in thickness as the cancellous trabeculae are thinned, but this change is difficult to spot in the early stages. Any cause of bone atrophy will produce a similar change. A readily detectable loss of lamina dura coincides with the appearance of other obvious bony changes.

The hands are a useful part to radiograph, since detailed pictures can be made. Some even employ macroradiography, whereby an enlarged image is produced by deliberately increasing the object–film distance. The tube must, of course, have an ultra-small focal spot if resolution of detail in the image is to be maintained. Alternatively, fine grain, single emulsion film and magnification of the image can be used. The particular changes which are looked for in these films are loss of the terminal feathering of the distal phalanges and subperiosteal resorption at the junction of the base and the shaft of the phalanges. Such resorption is seen as a roughening of the surface of the bone and small hemispherical cavities.

Another site where subperiosteal resorption is seen is below the medial condyle of the tibia. A sizeable indentation in the surface results and this appearance is called 'Pugh's sign'.

For TREATMENT, *see* p. 96.

RENAL OSTEODYSTROPHY

There are basically two renal conditions which produce bone changes. The first of these is renal rickets in which as a result of a developmental error there is a renal leak of phosphorus and amino-acids. Such patients develop vitamin-D resistance, rickets in childhood, and osteomalacia in adult life. They tend to develop chronic pyelonephritis and the resulting renal damage eventually results in uraemia.

The second condition is azotaemic bone disease or renal osteodystrophy. The uraemic state appears to exert an anti-vitamin D effect and also to reduce the absorption of calcium and phosphorus from the gastro-intestinal tract. These patients have a low serum calcium and develop rickets in childhood and osteomalacia in adult life. Azotaemic bone disease can be added to the osteomalacia due to the renal leak of phosphorus of the first group as uraemia supervenes.

When renal damage becomes severe phosphorus retention tends to occur. This stimulates parathyroid hyperplasia since parathormone controls phosphorus excretion. Thus, secondary hyperparathyroidism is added to osteomalacia, though in renal rickets the rise in serum phosphorus may improve the bone disease.

In some patients certain parathyroid nodules may exhibit autonomous growth converting the secondary hyperparathyroidism into tertiary hyperparathyroidism. Management of these patients involves large doses of vitamin D and, where appropriate, parathyroidectomy.

At one time the problem of renal osteodystrophy was self-limiting since the patients ultimately died from their renal disease. Now with renal dialysis and transplantation the problem has been enhanced and, indeed, dialysis has added to the complexity of the bone disease. It is easy to wash calcium out of the dialysed patient over a period, so it is important to have the correct amount of calcium in the dialysate. Too low a calcium will result in the removal of calcium from the patient and a stimulation of parathyroid hyperplasia. In such patients a return to a normal serum calcium may be an indication of hyperparathyroidism and the need for parathyroidectomy rather than the assumption that all is well with the dialysis. On the other hand, too high a dialysate calcium can result in metastatic calcification.

In practice, because of the large volumes of solution involved, it is not easy to prevent dialysis bone disease. In many centres most patients have bone pain in the feet, knees, and shoulders by the time they have been on regular dialysis for 4–5 years.

For the reasons indicated above, patients with renal rickets and azotaemic osteodystrophy exhibit a mixed picture of bone disease; namely osteo-malacia and hyperparathyroidism. In the jaws the appearances of the latter condition dominate the picture as shown in the radiograph. Cawson (1964) described hypoplastic defects in such patients' teeth. Because the hyperparathyroidism is a response to a low serum calcium, the result of the original disease, renal stones are not a feature of secondary hyper-parathyroidism.

In dialysate bone disease the appearance more resembles osteoporosis and differs histologically in that there is the resorption of hyperparathy-roidism, but no bone deposition and hence no wide osteoid seams. Parathyroidectomy in these patients halts the bone resorption, but does not result in bone deposition and without osteoid vitamin D is useless.

Osteitis Deformans: Paget's Disease of Bone

In 1891 Von Recklinghausen published a paper on generalized osteitis fibrosa. His cases included 2 which today would be classed as polyostotic fibrous dysplasia of bone, but the remainder were either cases of hyper-parathyroidism or Paget's disease of bone. While our understanding of polyostotic fibrous dysplasia and hyperparathyroidism has increased greatly since the end of the 19th century, our understanding of Paget's disease is only a little better than that of Paget himself when he wrote his classic paper in 1877.

Aetiology.—The aetiology of osteitis deformans remains obscure and none of the many suggestions as to its cause stands careful scrutiny.

Sex Incidence.—If the skeleton as a whole is considered the sex incidence is about equal, though it is often said that males are somewhat more commonly affected than females. Schmorl (1932) found 80 cases of Paget's disease in 2279 autopsies on male patients and 58 cases among 2235 female cadavers. Barry (1969), in a series of 2630 cases of Paget's disease, found that 1420 were men and 1210 were women.

Incidence.—According to Schmorl (1932) and Collins (1956) some evi-dence of Paget's disease is present in 3–4 per cent of patients over 40 years of age. In a series of 4614 necropsies performed on unselected persons over the age of 40 years Schmorl (1932), of Dresden, found 138 cases of Paget's disease. Similarly selected post-mortem examinations on 650 persons by Collins (1956) in Leeds and Sheffield showed an incidence of 3·7 per cent cases of Paget's disease.

Figures published by Barry (1969) revealed that in Australia 2630 patients were admitted to hospital with Paget's disease out of a total of 1,769,664 admissions, an incidence of 1:673. All statistics of the disease show that Paget's disease is essentially a disease of old age.

Although the incidence of the disease increases in age-groups above 40, rare cases are known to have been affected from their late teens or early twenties. A point of importance is that usually the condition develops quite slowly. For example, it may take 20 years for the evolution of the typical thickened, cranial vault with cotton-wool radio-opacities, from the time at which osteitis circumscripta appears. Indeed, the slow progress of the disease and lack of obvious physical signs in the early stages probably lead to misunderstandings concerning the age incidence.

Racial and Geographical Distribution.—According to Barry (1969), Paget's disease is fairly common in the United Kingdom, France, and Germany, but rare in Scandinavia. The incidence also appears to be low in Spain, Italy, Central Europe, and Russia. The disease is also less common in North and South America than in England. As yet only occasional cases have been reported from Africa, the Middle East, India, Japan, and China.

Family History.—While in many cases there is no family history, this is not invariably so and periodically papers are published describing families in which several members are affected. According to Barry (1969) the evidence that the disease may have a genetic basis is by no means conclusive.

Signs and Symptoms.—Patients may complain of aching in the diseased bone, pain on weight-bearing, or headaches. When it involves the jaws the pain of the disease during periods of activity may be attributed to the teeth and demands made for their removal. As the affected bones enlarge the pressures to which the teeth are subjected by the soft tissues are altered and they tend to tilt. Their articulation changes and temporomandibular joint dysfunction can follow.

When the condition is widespread there may be stiffness of the joints, muscular weakness, and fatigue. Affected bones increase in thickness and become bent. Dilated blood-vessels are observed in the overlying soft tissues which may feel warm to the touch. Some of the thickened areas of bone are highly vascularized and on auscultation the arteriovenous shunt produces a marked bruit.

Hypercementosis makes the removal of teeth from an affected jaw difficult. (*Fig.* 37.) When they are extracted the sensation is like the pulling of a screw from rotten wood. A brisk haemorrhage follows, but usually ceases spontaneously. Following the extractions, patches of dense bone near the socket may become infected, leading to septic sockets or even to localized osteomyelitis. Other dental complications of this condition are resorption of the roots of teeth and ankylosis. Where a tooth affected by hypercementosis is adjacent to a mass of sclerosed bone, union of the two tissues tends to occur. Ankylosis then leads to submersion of the tooth as the alveolar process continues to enlarge.

Histology.—Histologically in Paget's disease there is resorption of existing bone and deposition of new. There is destruction of the cortex with widening of the Haversian canals until large, vascular, Haversian lakes are formed. The normal fatty marrow is replaced by a cellular connective tissue, the so-called 'fibrosis of the marrow', and new bone is deposited both endosteally and subperiosteally. Resorption and deposition of bone continue at an abnormal rate, leading to the formation of the classic mosaic pattern. Fluorescent marker studies suggest that the turnover of bone is ten times the normal.

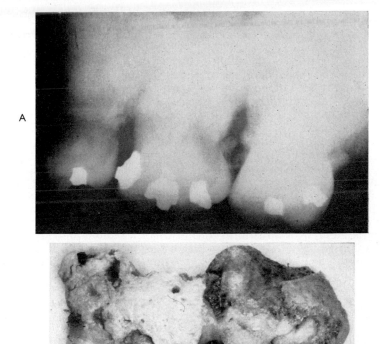

Fig. 37.—A, Intra-oral radiograph of |678 showing marked hypercementosis in a patient suffering from Paget's disease. B, The |678 removed in one block from patient shown in A.

In early cases much of the new bone which is laid down is woven bone. Later, lamellar bone is deposited and patchy sclerosis appears. In the denser bone osteones resembling Haversian systems may be formed, but true cortical bone is not produced.

Subperiosteal deposition of bone results in enlargement while minute, incomplete fractures lead to bending and bowing. Both factors produce accentuation of the natural curvatures of the bone.

At first sight Paget's disease appears to be without pattern but this is not entirely so. Some bones are affected more commonly than others; the maxilla more frequently than the mandible, and the mandible alone more often than both mandible and maxilla together.

Paget's disease of the tibia always starts near the upper end and progresses downwards. Similarly if Paget's affects the maxilla it does so before it affects the cranial vault and it enters the calvarium via the frontal bone.

What is the basic error in osteitis deformans? Is the turnover of bone increased so that there is no time for the formation of complex Haversian systems and proper cortical bone? In which case is it a result of abnormal osteoclasis? Are more osteoclasts formed or do they persist longer than the usual 48 hours? Or is the ability to lay down Haversian systems lost so that as the cortical bone is resorbed in the normal way it is not replaced and an increased surface area of bone is exposed to osteoclastic activity? Either way, the deposition of new bone both subperiosteally and endosteally can be explained as an attempt to compensate for the loss of the mechanically efficient cortex. That the bone so deposited should be woven bone in the early stages of the process is in accord with the deposition of this type of bone anywhere where rapid bone production is necessary.

The Radiology of Paget's Disease.—In long bones, the earliest lesion as seen in radiographs is a fusiform zone of cortical radiolucency. A similar appearance is to be seen in the mandible before the whole of the bone has been involved. The affected area of cortex slowly spreads round the bone, but maintains a pointed extremity in its long axis. Where it is seen tangentially the lesion again forms a fusiform radiolucent patch, outlined by a thin layer of bone on both endosteal and periosteal surfaces.

In the jaws the normal lamellar bone is at first largely replaced by woven bone and the normal cortex is destroyed. Radiographically the bone takes on a granular pattern of low radiographic density. A striated pattern may be seen in the maxillary premolar region and in the mandible. This pattern is produced by the persistence of a few of the normal trabeculae on which new bone is deposited, so increasing their thickness and radiopacity. The lamina dura is reduced in thickness and may be difficult to detect. As the disease progresses the typical cotton-wool clumps of sclerotic, mosaic patterned bone appear and they tend to form first near the apices of the teeth.

Enlargement of the affected jaw occurs. In the maxilla, the extra bone has the same texture as the rest of the jaw and is covered by a thin sheet of subperiosteal bone. In the mandible successive layers of subperiosteal bone are deposited, giving the new bone an onion-skin appearance.

As the condition spreads from the maxilla it involves the walls of the orbits and the sphenoid. It extends into the frontal bone as an advancing front of cortical bone destruction. Thus, osteoporosis circumscripta is produced which spreads backwards to involve the whole vault. Thickening occurs mainly on the outer surface since the shape of the inner surface is controlled by contact with the dura and brain. The classic cotton-wool pattern spreads in by the same route until the whole vault is involved. Finally, the heavy, structurally weak calvarium sags over the cervical spine to produce basilar inversion and a 'tam-o-shanter' skull.

In some patients enormous enlargement of the maxilla can occur. This highlights two matters of radiological interpretation. One is that where there is a considerable thickness of bone the mass is radio-opaque. But, of course, the radio opacity does not mean that the bone is sclerotic. Indeed, per unit volume the bone may still be more radiolucent than normal except for the cotton-wool patches. Furthermore, just because the outlines of the maxillary sinuses cannot be visualized it does not mean they have been obliterated. It is far more likely that they are present, even if reduced in size, and that their image is overshadowed by the masses of bone on the surface. Moreover, with the loss of cortex any linear image from the margins of the sinuses is lost.

Differentiation of Paget's disease from fibrous dysplasia of bone involves a consideration of the clinical as well as the radiographic features. Advanced cases are rarely a difficulty, but early cases in which enlargement of the jaw is localized can be a problem. Two factors are a help: the first is that radiographic involvement of the whole jaw is usually present by the time enlargement occurs in Paget's disease, whereas in fibrous dysplasia the radiographic changes remain more localized to the changes in contour. Secondly, hypercementosis of involved teeth is usual in Paget's disease and uncommon in fibrous dysplasia.

Complications.—There are many complications which may befall the patient with Paget's disease. Deformity of individual bones can lead to postural deformity and osteoarthritis of the joints. Curious transverse fractures, both complete and incomplete, may occur. If, for any reason, patients with this condition are confined to bed there is a risk that rapid resorption of bone will take place, leading to a rise in serum calcium and renal stone formation. The foramina of the skull may be narrowed, producing cranial nerve palsies and optical field defects or deafness.

The bone of osteitis deformans is unusually vascular and blood-flow may be up to 20 times the normal. Intra-bony vessels form numerous arteriovenous shunts so that the cardiac output is raised and may reach three times the normal value. Cardiac hypertrophy follows and eventually cardiac failure. In advanced cases the thoracic cage becomes deformed with an increased liability to bronchitis and bronchopneumonia. Thus, patients with Paget's disease can present an increased anaesthetic risk.

Malignant change in the form of osteogenic sarcoma or malignant osteoclastoma is an uncommon but well recognized risk. Hutter and others (1963) describe benign osteoclastomas in Paget's disease, some of which were in the jaws. Whether they were true neoplasms, or more of the nature of giant-cell granulomas, it is difficult to say. Barry (1969) describes 2 examples of benign giant-celled tumours from Australia—one seen in the tibia and one in the sacrum. Hutter and others (1963) reported 5 cases of benign giant-cell tumour at the Memorial Center for Cancer, New York. McKenna and others (1964), from the same hospital, found 12 cases of benign giant-cell tumour in patients with Paget's disease: 5 were in the calvaria and 2 each in the mandible and maxilla. In a case reported by Cones (1953) a giant-cell tumour in a patient with generalized Paget's disease was irradiated, after which the tumour rapidly recurred as a chondrosarcoma causing death in six months.

Sarcoma.—Paget's original case developed sarcoma at the elbow, and of the 23 cases reported by Paget 5 died from a malignant change in the lesion. Barry (1969) reported 116 patients with sarcoma developing in this way in Australia. Coley and Sharp (1931) reported 72 cases of sarcoma from the records of the Memorial Hospital, New York, and the American Tumour Registry. In 20 of these cases (28 per cent), the tumour had developed in patients suffering from Paget's disease.

Porretta, Dahlin, and Janes (1957) found 16 cases of bone sarcoma among 1753 patients with Paget's disease in the records of the Mayo Clinic. Coley (1960) and Lichtenstein (1959) considered the incidence of bone sarcoma in Paget's disease to be 10 per cent. Barry (1961), however, considered the incidence to be less than 1 per cent in Australia, a figure which agrees with Porretta and others' (1957) figures from the Mayo Clinic.

Aspects of Paget's Disease which affect the Oral Surgeon.—

Extractions.—Marked hypercementosis of the teeth causes considerable difficulty during their extraction with forceps and this may lead to fracture of the tooth. It is preferable to extract the teeth surgically, after which the wound should be carefully closed and sutured to prevent chronic infection in the underlying sclerotic bone which might lead to a protracted osteomyelitis of the jaw. In this respect, it is important that all fractured roots should be removed. Sometimes several upper teeth are united by masses of hypercementosis and surgical removal of the teeth and attached bone is required. Excessive force exerted on such teeth with forceps leads to fracture of the teeth concerned and also fracture of the underlying sclerotic masses which eventually sequestrate.

Bone Pain.—Pain due to Paget's disease of the jaws must be differentiated from other causes of facial pain. By and large, bone pain in the jaws is uncommon and care should be taken to exclude all other causes. In particular osteomyelitis of the Paget bone as a cause of the pain, or malignant change, should be considered. Where bone pain is severe, consideration should be given to the use of porcine serocalcitonin and the advice of a physician specializing in metabolic disease should be sought to this end. Injections of 1 unit per kg. of body-weight of serocalcitonin are given daily. Following this alkaline phosphatase levels in the blood fall, the urinary output of hydroxyproline also falls, the bone remodels and pain is relieved. Currently such treatment is expensive and hence not widely available.

Prosthetic Considerations.—When Paget's disease affects the jaws, it is usually the maxilla which is involved. Clinically the disease manifests itself by a great widening of the palate, especially in the tuberosity region, but sometimes a series of bony bumps are present in the sulcus. Such bony projections, particularly in the tuberosity region, cause difficulty in the construction of satisfactory dentures and should therefore be removed surgically. When the condition is of recent origin the bony masses can be removed fairly easily as the bone is soft, though haemorrhage may be profuse. However, in the elderly patient where the condition has been present for many years, the bone becomes exceedingly hard and resists most cutting instruments. Such bone is also very sclerotic and avascular and the introduction of infection into such an area may result in a protracted chronic osteomyelitis. Following surgery in such cases careful soft-tissue closure and suturing is necessary in order to avoid the introduction of infection. The patient should, of course, have antibiotic therapy until the area is healed. It is also a wise precaution to support the soft tissues against the bone with acrylic base plates lined with black gutta-percha. For the upper jaw circumzygomatic wires may be safely used to hold such a plate in place and circumferential wires are suitable for the lower jaw.

Osteomyelitis.—Patients with Paget's disease may also be referred with a chronic osteomyelitis, usually of the upper jaw. This has often developed following an unsuccessful extraction. At one time this condition was a cause of mortality of patients with Paget's disease who died of anaemia, septicaemia, pyaemic abscesses, or amyloid disease. However, the condition can be controlled by antibiotic therapy and the affected area of bone should be removed surgically as soon as a line of separation is established. Spontaneous sequestration may take many years and to wait for this event leaves the patient with a painful and suppurating area in the mouth (McGowan, 1974).

ACROMEGALY

Aetiology.—Acromegaly is caused by an adenoma of the eosinophil cells of the anterior lobe of the pituitary gland. When the adenoma develops after the epiphyses have closed, acromegaly occurs but prior to epiphysial closure the glandular dysfunction results in gigantism.

Clinical Features.—Acromegaly is most commonly found in males. The hands are enlarged and spade-like and the feet are similarly affected. There is an overgrowth of the nasal cartilage which results in a thick, enlarged nose. The substance of the subcutaneous tissues is also affected and this gives a coarse appearance to the skin. The lips are grossly thickened. The frontal sinuses are enlarged and this gives increased prominence to the supra-orbital ridges. Closure of the epiphyses prevents any increase in the patient's height, but periosteal appositional bone growth is not prevented and the bones increase in thickness due to surface deposition. In the mandibular condyle, however, the fibroblasts deep in the fibrous covering of the condylar head differentiate into chondroblasts and then to chondrocytes. Therefore, an anteroposterior increase in the length of the mandible is possible and an extreme mandibular protrusion occurs. The muscles attached to the angle of the mandible (masseter and medial pterygoid) cannot elongate and, therefore, resorption of bone occurs at the angle producing a more or less straight gonial angle. Because the condylar growth centre faces downwards as well as forwards, the ramus lengthens and the mandibular teeth are carried down away from the maxilla. As the freeway space is increased the prognathism is not so obvious in the resting position of the mandible as when the teeth are brought together.

The enlarging adenoma of the pituitary presses on the optic chiasma and the decussating fibres of the nasal half of the retina are affected. This results in bitemporal optic hemianopia. The patient often suffers from severe headaches and the voice becomes deep due to enlargement of the laryngeal cartilages. There may be diabetes insipidus.

Radiology.—The marked mandibular protrusion and the configuration of the lower jaw can be demonstrated by the true lateral radiograph and this film will also demonstrate the enlargement of the pituitary fossa and the destruction of the posterior clinoid process. Appositional bone growth produces an increased density of bone and osteophytic outgrowths may be seen on the vertebrae and the phalanges.

Treatment.—Successful removal of the adenoma is difficult and carries a relatively high mortality, but radiotherapy can often control the disease.

Oral Surgical Aspects of Acromegaly.—Cases of acromegaly are sometimes referred to the oral surgeon with a view to mandibular osteotomy or ostectomy. It is, of course, important to diagnose the condition, for any surgical interference would at best produce only a temporary improvement in the condition, for the mandible would continue to grow. More important, valuable time would be lost in instituting therapy for the acromegaly. The oral surgeon should always consider the possibility of acromegaly when confronted by a case of extreme mandibular protrusion and institute the appropriate investigations. Jaw surgery should not be contemplated until the mandibular growth has been arrested.

OSTEOPETROSIS, ALBERS-SCHÖNBERG, OR MARBLE BONE DISEASE

Osteopetrosis, first described by Albers-Schönberg in 1904, is a rare disease of unknown aetiology which is characterized by a generalized and extreme density of the bone. The medullary cavities tend to become obliterated due to failure of bone resorption and the continued deposition of bone. This renders the bone highly susceptible to infection since its vascular supply is decreased, and it also gives rise to a secondary anaemia.

It has been suggested (Weinmann and Sicher, 1955) that there is a delay in the appearance of osteoclasts so that remodelling resorption is out of phase with deposition and overtaken by the next wave of osteoblastic activity in the region.

Involvement of the skull leads to a reduction in the diameter of the foramina with consequent pressure on the cranial nerves. This may eventually lead to deafness and amblyopia. The disease is hereditary (McPeake, 1936) and is transmitted through both males and females as a Mendelian recessive (Hurscher and Stein, 1940). The condition is usually congenital, but occasionally the diagnosis is not made until later in life. Despite the density and thickening of the bones, they are very fragile and fractures often occur following minimal trauma. According to Thompson and others (1969) radiographic diffractions and microradiography have shown that the molecular structure is similar to that of normal bone. However, the distribution of mineral salts has an abnormal characteristic pattern and the arrangement of the collagen is irregular. This may account for the extreme fragility of the bone.

Incidence.—Gomez (1966) found 200 cases during a survey of the literature and Thompson and others (1969) reported 270.

Clinical Features.—Osteopetrosis may be characterized by either a severe or a relatively mild systemic disturbance and is usually divided into two types. The extreme or malignant form of the condition occurs early in life and may be present in utero. Such children seldom survive much beyond puberty (McPeake, 1936; Zawisch-Ossenitz, 1947) and they have marked anaemia, deafness, mental retardation, and often suffer from hydrocephalus. Their limbs are deformed as a result of multiple fractures. According to Winter (1945) they have a characteristic facies with a broad face, snub nose, hypertelorism, and frontal bossing. There is a hepato-splenomegaly due to the compensatory extramedullary haemopoiesis. According to Gomez (1966) and Thoma (1969) delayed eruption and impaction of teeth are common. The teeth are also said to be of defective quality and prone to caries.

The less extreme or benign variety is often not diagnosed until late in life, and a case reported by Dyson (1970) was first detected at the age of 74 years. Such patients tend to be asymptomatic, but they may suffer from a modified form of any of the symptoms associated with the more extreme variety of the disease.

Radiology.—Radiological examination shows extreme density of the entire skeleton with no differentiation between the cortex and marrow. In the skull views there is gross thickening at the base of the skull with increased density of the remainder of the calvarium. Long bones are club-shaped and have transverse bands at their ends, and bossing of the ribs occurs at the costo-chondral junctions. It would, of course, be incompatible with life for all the bones to have complete obliteration of their medullary cavities and, therefore, on radiological survey some bones will appear within the range of normal.

Haematological Investigations.—In the mild variety of the disease there may be a moderate iron deficiency anaemia, but in the more severe disease there may be a leuco-erythroblastic or aplastic type of anaemia. The serum calcium and phosphorus are normal (Thompson and others, 1969).

Treatment.—No effective treatment has been discovered for osteo-petrosis and the various complications are treated as they arise.

The main complications from an oral surgical point of view are fracture of the jaw and osteomyelitis, and either of these complications can arise as a result of dental extractions. The removal of teeth should therefore be effected with minimal trauma and the operation is best carried out under general anaesthesia. The raising of mucoperiosteal flaps is unwise and should be avoided whenever possible. Following extractions, accurate soft-tissue closure and suturing of the socket wounds should be carried out and an antibiotic should be used until the wounds have healed. In spite of such treatment, Radden (1949) reported a case which developed osteo-myelitis.

Fractures of the jaws tend to heal provided that they do not become infected, but in view of the risk of introducing infection to the avascular bone, the types of fixation available for treatment are of necessity limited. For example, it would be most imprudent to employ bone plating, transos-seous wiring, or extra-skeletal fixation. Osteomyelitis usually occurs in the mandible, but Wallace and Kemp (1945) reported a case from the literature of maxillary involvement. Chronic osteomyelitis of the jaws in osteopetrosis is an extremely difficult condition to eradicate, for surgical removal of the affected area only results in further areas of sound bone becoming necrotic. Surgery is, therefore, contra-indicated except to effect drainage during an acute episode. Rowe (1970) attempted to treat a case with hyperbaric oxygen in the belief that local oxygenation of the tissues would help, but the results were not especially encouraging.

The established osteomyelitis of the jaws in a case of osteopetrosis should therefore be treated conservatively, but suitable antibiotics are prescribed should an acute exacerbation occur. Probably the only effective method of curing the condition is by mandibulectomy.

CLEIDOCRANIAL DYSOSTOSIS

Cleidocranial dysostosis is a disease of unknown aetiology which is probably hereditary and when it occurs is inherited as a dominant Mendelian characteristic which can be transmitted by either sex. However, many sporadic cases occur and the sexes are equally affected.

The most striking features of the condition are the defects in ossification of the cranium and clavicles and the persistence of the primary dentition with delay or failure of eruption of the permanent dentition.

Clinical Appearances.—

1. *The head:* The head appears to be large and there is a marked median furrow in the centre of the forehead which runs vertically downwards towards the bridge of the nose. The frontal bone tends to bulge either side of the furrow. There is a depression in the region of the anterior fontanelle which may be palpable and similar depressions may be felt over the antero-lateral and posterior and posterolateral fontanelle sites. The nasal bridge may be depressed and there is a hypoplasia of the middle third of the facial skeleton with a relative mandibular protrusion.

2. The deciduous teeth erupt normally, but are retained and fail to show normal osteoclastic resorption of their roots. The permanent teeth are largely unerupted and their roots are stunted and deformed. Rushton (1937) reported on the deformity of the roots of teeth in patients with cleidocranial dysostosis. Supernumerary teeth are common. Owing to pseudo-anodontia dentures are required from an early age.

3. *The thorax:* The shoulders appear to droop and the clavicles may be completely or partially absent. The absence of clavicles imparts an extreme mobility to the shoulders and enables the patient to approximate the shoulders towards the midline until they meet. Absence of the clavicles does not appear to cause the patient any inconvenience, but occasionally they may develop the scalenus syndrome.

4. *The pelvis:* There is often a defect in the ossification of the pubic symphysis which may be detected on palpation. A coxa vara or valga deformity of the hip is present in some cases.

5. A variety of other skeletal abnormalities are reported from time to time.

Radiographic Appearances.—

1. *The skull:* Defects in ossification are seen and the anterior, antero-lateral, and posterolateral fontanelles remain patent. Small Wormian bones may be seen in their vicinity. In some cases part or all of the zygomatic bone is missing and the mastoid bone may fail to pneumatize. The middle third of the facial skeleton is hypoplastic and there is a relative mandibular protrusion. Very rarely the suture line at the mandibular symphysis may persist (Fleischer-Peters, 1967).

2. *The clavicles:* Usually the acromial end of the clavicle is absent or deficient, but the clavicle may be in two portions joined by a fibrous band. Sometimes only the sternal end is absent and occasionally the clavicle is entirely absent.

3. *The spine:* Scoliosis and kyphosis may be present as well as spina bifida occulta.

4. *The pelvis:* There may be an increase in width of the pubic symphysis and coxa vara and valga deformities of the hip may be present.

5. *The jaws:* Radiographs will demonstrate the presence of numerous unerupted and supernumerary teeth. According to Thoma (1969), if supernumerary teeth are present they are present in the incisor and premolar regions.

Oral Surgical Aspects of Cleidocranial Dysostosis.—The oral surgeon is primarily concerned with the problem of the unerupted teeth. Some success may be obtained by surgically uncovering the unerupted teeth provided the patient is operated upon during the erupting phase, and the chances of success decrease considerably with patients over 16 years of age. Thoma (1969) recommends the removal of all supernumerary teeth, but he states that good results are not obtained due to lack of erupting force. The mere presence of numerous unerupted teeth is unlikely to cause the patient any inconvenience, but due to normal alveolar atrophy with age the crowns of some of the teeth become exposed to the mouth and infection may occur, leading in some instances to osteomyelitis. At this stage extraction of the teeth presents additional difficulties. To avoid such a situation developing, it is prudent to remove the unerupted teeth earlier in life when the mandible is more substantial and infection is not present. One of the complications of removing a large number of unerupted teeth in the mandible is the possibility of jaw fracture.

REFERENCES

ALBERS-SCHÖNBERG, H. (1904), 'Röntgenbildung einer selteren knochererkrankung', *Munch. med. Wschr.*, **51**, 365.
— — (1907), 'Eine bisher nicht beschriebene allgemeinerkrankung des skelletes im röntgenbild', *Fortschr. Geb. Röntg Strahl.*, **11**, 261.
ALBRIGHT, F., BUTLER, A. M., HAMPTON, A. O., and SMITH, P. (1937), 'Syndrome Characterised by Osteitis Fibrosa Disseminata', *New Engl. med. J.*, **216**, 727.
ASKANAZY, M. (1904), 'Arbeiten auf dem gebiet der pathologischen anatomie und bakteriologie aus dem pathologisch-anatomischen', *Institut zu Tubingen*, **4**, 398.
BARRY, H. C. (1961), 'Sarcoma in Paget's Disease of Bone in Australia', *J. Bone Jt Surg.*, **43A**, 1122.
— — (1969), *Paget's Disease of Bone*. London: Churchill-Livingstone.
BRUCKNER, R., and others (1967), 'Osteogenic Sarcoma arising at a Site of Fibrous Dysplasia', *Oral Surg.*, **24**, 377.
CAFFEY, J. (1956), *Pediatric X-ray Diagnosis*, 3rd ed., p. 814. Chicago: Year Book.
CAWSON, R. (1964), 'Defects of Enamel Structure in a Case of Renal Osteodystrophy', *Br. dent. J.*, **117**, 141.
COLEY, B. L. (1960), *Neoplasms of Bone*, 2nd ed., p. 753. New York: Hoeber.
— — and SHARP, G. S. (1931), 'Paget's Disease a Predisposing Factor to Osteogenic Sarcoma', *Archs Surg., Chicago*, **23**, 918.
— — and STEWART, F. W. (1945), 'Bone Sarcoma in Polyostotic Fibrous Dysplasia', *Ann Surg*, **121**, 872.
COLLINS, D. H. (1956), 'Paget's Disease of Bone', *Lancet*, **2**, 51.
CONES, D. M. T. (1953), 'Unusual Bone Tumour complicating Paget's Disease', *J. Bone Jt Surg.*, **35B**, 101.
DAVIES-COLLEY, N. (1884), 'Bones and Kidneys in a Girl Aged 13', *Trans. Path. Soc. Lond.*, **35**, 285.
DUSTIN, P., and LEY, D. A. (1950), 'Contribution à l'étude des dysplasies osseuses', *Revue belge. Path. Méd. exp.*, **20**, 52.

DYSON, D. P. (1970), 'Osteomyelitis of the Jaws in Albers-Schönberg Disease', Br. J. oral Surg., 7, 178.
EMSLIE, R. C. (1914), 'Fibrocystic Diseases of Bones', Br. J. Surg., 2, 17.
FAIRBANK, H. (1950), 'Fibrocystic Disease of Bone', J. Bone Jt Surg., 32B, 403.
FALCONER, M. A., COPE, C. L., and SMITH, A. H. T. ROBB (1942), 'Fibrous Dysplasia of Bone with Endocrine Disorders', Q. Jl Med., 11, 121.
FLEISCHER-PETERS, A. (1967), 'Therapeutische Möglichkeiten bei der clyostosis Cleidocranialis', Dt. zahnarztl. Z., 22, 80.
GOMEZ, L. S. A. (1966), 'The Jaws in Osteopetrosis', J. oral Surg., 24, 67.
HARRIS, W. H., DUDLEY, R., and BARRY, R. J. (1962), 'The Natural History of Fibrous Dysplasia', J. Bone Jt Surg., 44A, 207.
HUNTER, D., and TURNBULL, H. M. (1931), 'Hyperparathyroidism', Br. J. Surg., 19, 203.
HURSCHER, H., and STEIN, J. J. (1940), 'Osteopetrosis associated with Hodgkin's Disease', Am. J. Roentg., 43, 74.
HUTTER, R. V. P., and others (1963), 'Giant Cell Tumours complicating Paget's Disease of Bone', Cancer, N.Y., 16, 1044.
JAFFE, H. L. (1958a), Tumerous Conditions of Bone and Joints. London: Kimpton.
— — (1958b), Desmoplastic Fibroma in Tumours and Tumerous Conditions of Bone and Joints, p. 298. Philadelphia: Lea & Febiger.
JÄGER, M. (1962), quoted by RIDDELL, D. M. (1964), 'Osteoidsarkom auf dem Boden einer fibrös-polyostotischen dysplasiel (Jaffe-Lichtenstein)', Zentbl. allg. Path. path. Anat., 103, 291.
LANGEDORFF, X. (1877), Br. med. J., 1, 667.
LICHTENSTEIN, L. (1938), 'Polyostotic Fibrous Dysplasia', Archs Surg., Chicago, 36, 874.
— — (1959), Bone Tumours, 2nd ed. St. Louis: Mosby.
— — and JAFFE, H. L. (1942), 'Fibrous Dysplasia of Bone', Archs Path., 33, 777.
LUCAS, R. B. (1962), 'Fibrous Dysplasia in the Jaws', J. R. Coll. Surg. Edinb., 7, 255.
McCUNE, D. J., and BRUCH, H. (1937), 'Osteodystrophia Fibrosa', Am. J. Dis. Child., 54, 806.
McGOWAN, D. A., (1974), 'Clinical Problems in Paget's Disease affecting the Jaws', Br. J. oral Surg., 11, 230–235.
McKENNA, R. J., and others (1964), 'Osteogenic Sarcoma arising in Paget's Disease', Cancer, N.Y., 17, 42.
McPEAKE, C. N. (1936), 'Osteopetrosis: Report of Eight Cases in Three Generations in One Family', Am. J. Roentg., 36, 816.
MANDL, F. (1926), 'Die behandlung der lokalisierten und generalisierten osteitis fibrosa', Wien. klin. Wschr., 39, 1046.
DE MARCHI, R. (1956), Sulla trasformazione sarcomatosa della displasia fibrosa monostotica', Friuli med., 11, 639.
PAGET, J. (1877), 'On a Form of Chronic Inflammation of Bones (Osteitis Deformans)', Med. chir. Trans., 60, 37.
PERKINSON, N. C., and HIGGINBOTHAM, N. L. (1955), 'Osteogenic Sarcoma arising in Polyostotic Fibrous Dysplasia', Cancer, N.Y., 8, 396.
PILHEU, F., and SOLDATO, G. (1966), 'Fibro-osteosarcoma of Jaw in a Case of Polyostotic Fibrous Dysplasia', oral Surg., 21, 778.
PORRETTA, G. A., DAHLIN, D. C., and JANES, J. M. (1957), 'Sarcoma in Paget's Disease of Bone', J. Bone Jt Surg., 39A, 1314.
PRITCHARD, J. E. (1951), 'Fibrous Dysplasia of Bone', Am. J. med. Sci., 222, 313.
RADDEN, H. G. (1949), 'Albers-Schönberg's Disease', Aust. J. Dent., 53, 353.
RAMSEY, H., STRONG, E., and FRAZELL, E. (1968), 'Fibrous Dysplasia of the Cranial Bones', Am. J. Surg., 116, 542.
ROWE, N. L. (1970), quoted by DYSON, D. P. (1970), 'Osteomyelitis of the Jaws in Albers-Schönberg Disease ', Br. J. oral Surg., 7, 178.
RIDDELL, D. M. (1964), 'Malignant Change in Fibrous Dysplasia', J. Bone Jt Surg., 46B, 251.
RUSHTON, M. A. (1937), 'Partial Gigantism of Face and Teeth', Br. dent. J., 63, 65.
SABANAS, A. O., DAHLIN, D. C., CHILDS, D. S., and NINS, J. C. (1956), 'Post-radiation Sarcoma of Bone', Cancer, N.Y., 9, 528.
SCHLUMBERGER, H. G. (1946), 'Fibrous Dysplasia of Single Bones', Milit. Surg., 99, 504.

SCHMORL, G. (1932), 'Über ostitis deformans Paget', *Virchows Arch. path. Anat. Physiol.,* **283**, 694.

SETH, R. S., CLIMIE, A. R. W., and TUTTLE, W. M. (1962), 'Fibrous Dysplasia of the Rib with Sarcomatous Change', *J. Bone Jt Surg.,* **44A**, 183.

SEWARD, G. R. (1970), personal communication.

SNAPPER, I. (1949), *Medical Clinics on Bone Diseases,* 2nd ed., p. 223. New York: Interscience.

STAFNE, E. C. (1964), *Oral Roentgenographic Diagnosis.* Philadelphia: Saunders.

STEWART, M., GILMER, S., and EDMONSON, A. (1962), 'Fibrous Dysplasia of Bone', *J. Bone Jt Surg.,* **44B**, 302.

SUTRO, C. J. (1951), 'Osteogenic Sarcoma of the Tibia in a Limb affected with Fibrous Dysplasia', *Bull. Hosp. Jt Dis.,* **12**, 217.

TANNER, H. C., DAHLIN, D. C., and CHILDS, D. S. (1961), 'Sarcoma Complicating Fibrous Dysplasia', *Oral Surg.,* **14**, 837.

TANNHAUSER, S. J. (1944), 'Neurofibromatosis and Osteitis Fibrosa Cystica Localisata et Disseminata', *Medicine, Baltimore,* **23**, 105.

THOMA, K. H. (1969), *Oral Surgery,* 5th ed., Vol. 1. St. Louis: Mosby.

THOMPSON, R. D., HALE, M. L., MONTGOMERY, J. C., and MONTANA-VILLAMIZAR, E. (1969), 'Manifestations of Osteopetrosis', *J. Oral Surg.,* **27**, 63.

TRUBNIKOV, V. F., and SKOBLIN, A. P. (1956), 'Transformation of the Local Fibrous Osteodystrophy into a Sarcoma', *Ortop. Traumat. Protez.,* **17**, 53.

VAHKURKINA, A. M. (1958), 'Malignant Osteoblastoclastoma developing on the Background of Fibrous Osteodysplasia', *Arkh. Patol.,* **20**, 18.

VAN HORN, P. E., JOHNSON, E. W., and DAHLIN, D. C. (1963), 'Fibrous Dysplasia of the Femur with Sarcomatous Change', *Am. J. Orthop.,* **5**, 6.

VON RECKLINGHAUSEN, F. (1891), *Die fibrose oder deformirende ostitis die osteomalacie carcinose in ihren gegenseitigen beziehungen.* Berlin: Reimer.

WALLACE, E. S., and KEMP, H. R. (1945), 'Marble Bone Disease', *Dent. J. Aust.,* **17**, 81.

WEIL, P. (1922), 'Jähriges Mädchen mit pubertas praecox und Knochenbrüchigkeit', *Klin. Wschr.,* **1**, 2114.

WEINMANN, J. P., and SICHER, H. (1955), *Bone and Bones: Fundamentals of Bone Biology,* 2nd ed., p. 151. London: Kimpton.

WINTER, G. R. (1945), 'Albers-Schönberg Disease', *Am. J. Orthod.,* **31**, 637.

WORTH, H. M. (1963), *Principles and Practice of Oral Radiologic Interpretation.* Chicago: Year Book.

ZAWISCH-OSSENITZ, C. (1947), 'Marble Bone Disease: Study of Osteogenesis', *Archs Path.,* **43**, 55.

ZIMMERMAN, D. C., STAFNE, E. C., and DAHLIN, D. C. (1958), 'Fibrous Dysplasia of the Maxilla and Mandible', *Oral Surg.,* **11**, 55.

Chapter XVIII

THE MAJOR SALIVARY GLANDS

ACUTE sialo-adenitis, recurrent swelling, and a persistent swelling are the three most common conditions of the major salivary glands with which patients present to the dental surgeon.

A. ACUTE SIALO-ADENITIS

The most frequent cause of an acute sialo-adenitis is infection of secretions retained behind an obstruction to the main duct. Indeed, such an episode may be the first intimation of the presence of such an obstruction.

Far less common in these days is an ascending infection, usually of a parotid gland, occurring in a dehydrated and debilitated patient. The affected gland becomes swollen, tender, and very painful. There is considerable oedema of the surrounding soft tissues or even a frank cellulitis. There may be some difficulty in distinguishing between an acute infection of the parotid gland and a submasseteric abscess and between an acute infection of the submandibular gland and a sublingual or submandibular cellulitis due to other causes. In the case of salivary gland infections the duct is also inflamed and, if the clinician is gentle, pus can be expressed from it. Furthermore, the maximum swelling in acute parotitis is rather more posterior than that produced by a submasseteric infection and it involves the tissues beneath the lobe of the ear.

Fortunately, in these days most infections can be controlled by vigorous antibiotic treatment with drainage occurring via the duct. In a few instances, a considerable abscess may form either in the gland or within the associated lymph-nodes. There is no problem with the submandibular gland since drainage by Hilton's method can be effected in the usual manner. With the parotid, however, the site of the abscess can be difficult to detect on clinical grounds and, indeed, one occurring in the deep part of the gland may burst into the external auditory canal before its presence is suspected.

Most sizeable parotid abscesses form in the lower pole. An incision is made in the crease in front of the pinna and curved downwards behind the angle of the mandible. The anterior flap is reflected a short distance over the deep fascia and the gland explored with a pair of fine sinus forceps or straight mosquito artery forceps. If the fascia is tough it may be incised parallel to the branches of the facial nerve. A corrugated rubber drain is placed in situ and the skin closed above and below its point of exit.

B. RECURRENT SWELLING

Recurrent swellings occur with two types of periodicity. The first type appears only when a flow of saliva is stimulated. This is usually due to the thought, sight, or taste of food, but the smoking of tobacco can produce a profuse salivary flow. The second type comes up at intervals of weeks, months, or even years and lasts for periods of days or weeks. These swellings are due to attacks of ascending infection.

The Causes of Recurrent Salivary Gland Swellings
1. *Sialo-angiectasis* or punctate sialectasis.
2. *Papillary Obstruction:*—
   a. Acute (ulcerative) papillary obstruction.
   b. Chronic (fibrotic) papillary stenosis.
   c. Relative papillary obstruction.
3. *Duct Obstruction* due to:—
   a. Causes in the lumen.
   b. Causes in the wall.
   c. Causes outside the wall.
4. *Gland Distension* due to:—
   a. The effect of drugs.
   b. An allergic reaction.

Sialo-angiectasis:—The characteristic sialographic appearance in this condition is of multiple small cavities occurring proximally in the duct tree. Patey and Thackray (1955) attribute these cavities to rupture of the diseased intralobular ducts under the pressure of the sialographic injection. However, the cavities start to fill quite early on during the injection, before any quantity of fluid has been introduced. Moreover, from time to time cases are seen in which multiple calculi have formed in the periphery of the gland, each one in a sialographic cavity, suggesting that the cavities existed before the injection and are not the result of duct rupture.

The aetiology is obscure. Rose (1954) suggests a developmental cause. Maynard (1965) considers that a reduction in salivary flow is the first change, with sialectasis, large duct dilatation and stricture formation, ascending infection, the production of abnormal mucous saliva, and calculi all playing a part in different cases. Patey (1965) appears to view the condition as an aspect of Sjögren's syndrome. Infection by an unknown virus or an auto-immune condition separate from Sjögren's syndrome have also been suggested as possible causes. In fact, there seem to be two varieties of sialo-angiectasis: primary sialo-angiectasis, which is the condition seen in childhood, and secondary sialo-angiectasis.

Primary sialo-angiectasis manifests itself in childhood as recurrent subacute infections of a parotid gland. Both sides may be affected, but rarely at the same time. Attacks of pain and swelling last for 3 to 14 days at intervals of 3 or more months. During these episodes the spontaneously discharged saliva is clear, but massage of the gland produces streaks and flakes of pus. Children as young as 3 months or as old as 12 years may suffer the first attack, but the commonest age of onset is 4–6 years. Occasionally brothers and sisters and even aunts and uncles have been similarly affected. Katzen (1969), in a longitudinal study of 45 patients, found that most cases spontaneously remitted by 15 years of age.

Patey and Thackray (1955) and Katzen (1969) examined histological material and found duct epithelial hypoplasia, periductal lymphocytic infiltration, acinar atrophy, and fibrosis. Katzen (1969) records that the basement membrane of the acini was absent or fragmentary.

Acute attacks should be treated with systemic penicillin since the causal organisms are usually *Streptococcus viridans*, staphylococci or pneumococci sensitive to this drug. Treatment is important as a few cases progress to a chronically infected state with severe gland destruction.

Sialography frequently produces a remission, perhaps because some of the contrast medium remains in the cavities and is antiseptic. The use of sugar-free chewing gum between meals can be tried to maintain a flow of saliva, so discouraging ascending infection.

Secondary sialo-angiectasis is the occurrence of similar cavities in a gland affected by a number of conditions: chronic infection, Sjögren's disease, and the effects of irradiation. These changes do not occur in all such cases nor do they appear early in the disease, but when present they are accompanied by changes in the diameter of the large ducts. If anything, the cavities are rather larger and more irregular in shape than those seen in primary sialo-angiectasis.

Papillary Obstruction.—Papillary obstruction may be acute and due to an ulcer affecting the papilla, or chronic when fibrosis follows repeated trauma to the papilla.

Swelling is of the obstructive type, although attacks of ascending infection may occur once the stage of papillary stenosis is reached. If the obstruction is due to the oedematous swelling caused by an acute ulcer, then the symptoms last only for the time that the ulcer is present and are of comparatively sudden onset. If, on the other hand, obstruction is caused by steadily increasing fibrosis, then the onset of mealtime swelling will be insidious and only when it becomes severe, or when an ascending infection occurs, will the patient complain.

The commonest cause of both types of papillary obstruction is trauma, from such things as a sharp tooth, a cross-bite on a denture, a denture with a high occlusal plane, a projecting clasp, or the large lingual flange of a lower denture.

If the condition is chronic the opening to the duct will be difficult to find and will feel rigid when a probe is inserted into it. Milking the gland may fill the dilated duct behind the papilla with saliva, thereby producing a bluish swelling.

Sialography will demonstrate the narrowed papillary segment and the dilated duct behind. Treatment involves removal of the source of the irritation and, if there is stenosis, a papillotomy with careful suture of the duct lining to the mucosa of the mouth.

Relative papillary stenosis occurs when the saliva is unusually viscous. In some patients it resembles a clear jelly and will only pass the duct orifice if the gland is massaged. Chronic obstruction, chronic infection, and auto-immune disease can produce this change and mucous gland metaplasia of the duct epithelium is said to account for it. Papillotomy may permit the material to pass with symptomatic relief.

Duct Obstruction.—

Duct Obstruction due to Causes in the Lumen.—Calculi are the commonest intraluminal cause of recurrent salivary gland swelling. Submandibular calculi are the most common, but parotid stones occur more often than is frequently believed. Sublingual calculi may occasionally be seen. If the calculus becomes impacted at the papilla or enlarges to fill the lumen of the duct, then obstructive symptoms follow. Alternatively, an acute infection behind the calculus may make the patient seek aid. Should the inflamed duct wall clamp down upon the stone, then distension of the gland at mealtimes will add to the discomforts of the acute infection. In such cases temporary relief can be obtained by treatment with antibiotics. As the oedema subsides duct obstruction will be reduced.

Calculi in the submandibular duct are often visible or palpable through the floor of the mouth. Those in the parotid papilla may likewise be seen or felt.

Inspection of the face when the gland is swollen may give an indication of the situation of a parotid calculus, since, if it is well within the gland, only the lower pole will become enlarged. Palpation of calculi in the upper pole of the submandibular gland is performed bimanually with the intra-oral finger facing downwards and outwards in the lingual sulcus and with the other hand displacing the lower pole of the gland upwards. A small, hard, submandibular gland is probably chronically infected and should be considered for excision.

Radio-opaque calculi can be demonstrated by plain radiographs. A central true occlusal view of the floor of the mouth, together with a posterior oblique occlusal and an oblique lateral jaw film, will be required for the detection of submandibular stones. A periapical film inside the cheek, a maxillary posterior oblique occlusal, a tangential film with the cheek blown out (Stafne, 1958), or an off-centred P.A. projection can be used to demonstrate parotid calculi.

A sialogram is required when a radiolucent calculus is suspected, where the calculus is close to or within the gland, or where considerable damage to the gland may have occurred.

The removal of anterior submandibular calculi is performed under local anaesthesia. A suture is passed around the duct behind the calculus and tied once, not too tightly. An incision in the floor of the mouth is deepened with scissors until the duct is identified. The duct is mobilized and a silk thread passed around it and clamped with artery forceps. This steadies the duct while a longitudinal incision is made over the calculus. Should the calculus be adherent to the duct a stitch is passed through one edge of the incision in the duct wall before it is levered out. The lumen is irrigated and sucked out, the posterior stitch removed and the gland squeezed to express any tiny calculi which might have formed behind the major one, and then the stay sutures removed. Only the mucosal wound should be closed. Indeed, attempts to suture the incision in the duct can lead to formation of a stricture.

Posterior submandibular calculi are surgically approached under endo-tracheal anaesthesia. The floor of the mouth is infiltrated with 1 : 100,000 adrenaline solution and the submandibular duct isolated towards its anterior end. By following the duct backwards the lingual nerve is identi-fied and a tape passed around it to draw it laterally. Once the lingual nerve is safe the duct is traced back to the upper pole of the gland. A calculus in the posterior duct can be released at this point. One just inside the upper pole may be attempted by raising the duct upwards and incising into the anterior part of the gland just beneath the duct. On no account should the posterior part of the upper pole be incised lest the facial artery be divided. Control of bleeding from the vessel in this situation could be most difficult.

Where the length of history, number of inflammatory episodes, con-sistency of the gland, and appearance in the sialogram suggest gross gland damage the whole gland should be excised. Calculi which lie below the junction with Wharton's duct of the most distal intralobular duct should not be tackled from the mouth and again the gland should be excised. A gland with dilatation of the intra- and interlobular ducts seems able to recover. Irregular cavitation represents frank intraglandular abscess formation, and once this stage is reached permanent freedom from infection is unlikely.

Excision of the submandibular gland is accomplished through a 5-cm. long submandibular incision. The incision should be placed in, or parallel to, a skin crease at the junction of the upper two-thirds and lower one-third of the palpable part of the gland. The wound is deepened through platysma

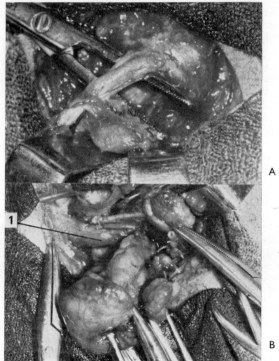

Fig. 38.—A, The gland has been separated from the lower border of the mandible and the facial artery is exposed where it emerges from the outside of the mandible. It is divided again at this point.

B, The anterior border of the gland has been freed from the mylohyoid muscle which is shown at 1. The groove between the superficial and deep parts of the gland is clearly seen now that it has been separated from the muscle. The submandibular branch of the facial artery runs forward just above the muscle.

and deep fascia and the local branches of the facial nerve identified. With care they can be mobilized and retracted. After the anterior facial vein has been taken, the lower pole of the gland is separated, grasped with Allis' forceps and turned upwards and forwards. The posterior belly of the digastric and the stylohyoid muscles are retracted downwards and backwards to expose the facial artery deep to the gland. It is doubly ligated and divided at this point.

Separation of the gland from the lower border of the mandible reveals
the facial artery lateral to the gland where it is divided and ligated again.
(*Fig.* 38.) The Allis' forceps are transferred to the front of the lower pole
and the gland turned backwards so that the attachment to the posterior

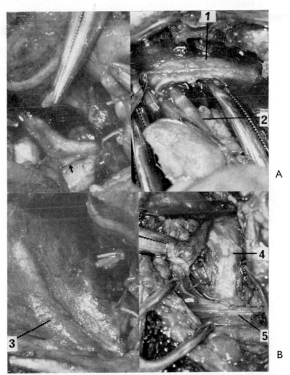

Fig. 39.—A, The gland has been mobilized sufficiently to draw it downward,
bringing the lingual nerve into view. The arrow points to the sublingual ganglion.
Right, the lingual nerve (1) has been separated from the upper pole of the gland
and has been displaced upward so as to expose the duct of the submandibular
gland (2). The duct contains two calculi which can be seen shining through its wall.
The posterior root of the sublingual ganglion is seen leaving the nerve where it
crosses the duct, but the ganglion itself is now hidden by the deep part of the gland
which is passing anterolateral to, and parallel with, the duct.

B, The gland bed as it is normally seen, with the muscles covered by a thin layer
of connective tissue. 3, The tendon of the digastric muscle. Right, the connective
tissue has been removed from part of the gland bed so that a small vein which
passed from the deep surface of the gland through the hyoglossus could be controlled. It is seen clamped by the artery forceps. The hypoglossal nerve (4) has been
uncovered where it passes upwards and forwards over the hyoglossus. The
stylohyoid tendon (5) divides at this point to embrace the digastric.

border of the mylohyoid can be uncovered. Once this has been separated
the gland can be mobilized and drawn down to display the lingual nerve.
(*Fig.* 39.) The latter is attached to the upper pole of the gland lateral to the
point from which the duct emerges. Careful scissor dissection is usually

necessary. Sometimes the nerve is most adherent, due to scarring induced by inflammation around an adjacent calculus.

Once the lingual nerve has been freed, the deep part of the gland can be enucleated and the duct ligated and divided. The wound is closed in layers with vacuum drainage.

Parotid calculi anterior to the accessory parotid may be removed through the mouth. A Y-shaped incision encloses the parotid papilla and the submucosal part of the duct is raised on the underside of a V-shaped flap. The duct is traced through the buccinator and a loop from lateral to

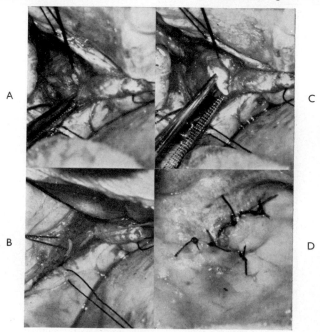

Fig. 40.—Removal of an extraglandular parotid calculus. A triangular flap has been raised from the inner surface of the buccinator which contains the parotid duct and a loop of duct from external to the buccinator is mobilized.

A, Shows an incision in the loop of duct over the calculus and a stay suture inserted.

B, The calculus is withdrawn.

C, The opening in the buccinator is approximated with a continuous 5/0 plain catgut suture.

D, The flap is sutured with black waxed silk.

this muscle drawn into the mouth. A longitudinal slit is made over the calculus and a silk suture passed through one edge to steady the duct while the stone is removed. Closure of the buccinator with plain catgut is necessary to prevent herniation of the buccal pad of fat. The mucosa is closed with silk in the usual manner. (Fig. 40.)

Calculi more posterior than this in the parotid duct should be tackled through a parotidectomy incision. A flap is raised from the surface of the gland and the duct identified at the anterior border. From this point it can be followed backwards through the substance of the gland until the calculus is uncovered. Due attention is given to the preservation of branches of the facial nerve, particularly the lower zygomatic branch which lies on the surface of the duct just below the accessory parotid.

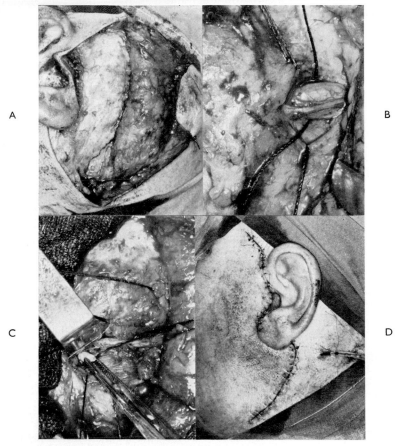

Fig. 41.—The removal of an intraglandular parotid calculus.

A, A flap is raised from over the parotid gland and sutured forward.

B, The deep fascia is incised in line with the duct and the duct isolated. A branch of the facial nerve lies on the surface of the duct.

C, By tracing the duct backwards through the gland, the calculus is uncovered.

D, The wound is closed in layers and vacuum drainage instituted. A pressure dressing is applied to keep the flap firmly in contact with the underlying tissues.

The fascial sheath of the gland is closed with care to prevent a leak of saliva into the tissues and the wound closed in layers with vacuum drainage. (*Fig.* 41.) Further details of these procedures can be found in papers by Seward (1968).

Obstruction due to Causes in the Wall.—Strictures are the most important cause of duct obstruction in this group and ulceration around a calculus the most common cause of stricture of the submandibular duct. Parotid calculi may present at the duct orifice and may be discharged spontaneously if small. The orifice of the submandibular duct, however, is small compared with the lumen of the duct and it is exceptional for calculi to pass through it. Instead, even quite small ones will ulcerate through into the mouth. A characteristic short stricture can be a sequel to such a happening, particularly if the resulting fistula closes. Traumatic injury to the ducts is another cause of strictures. Where the stricture is reasonably well forwards, the dilated duct behind the narrowing can be anastomosed to the mucosa of the mouth. This should be by an 'end to side' procedure for a 'side to side' procedure will narrow down and become ineffective.

Certain parotid duct strictures are less easy to explain. Some occur bilaterally either opposite the anterior border of the coronoid or opposite the posterior border of the mandible. Perhaps friction from the movement of the ramus is a factor in these cases. Perhaps auto-immune processes play a part, for in a few instances duct dilatation precedes the appearance of the stricture. The retromandibular strictures are of special interest since the patient's complaint may closely mimic temporomandibular joint arthrosis. Diagnosis may be difficult as there is no visible swelling because only the deep part of the parotid is involved.

Dilatation of these strictures with graduated sizes of gum-elastic urethral bougies is the safest form of treatment. The bougies are lubricated with lignocaine urethral gel and this will often give symptomatic relief for up to three years.

In order to avoid the formation of strictures or external salivary fistulae, the correct management of traumatic injuries to ducts needs to be mentioned. If a duct is transected by a facial laceration or during the course of an operation anastomosis of the two ends should be attempted. To prevent narrowing of the healed suture line each duct end is slit longitudinally for a short distance. Where it is difficult to repair the duct the proximal end may be implanted in the mucosa of the mouth. A tube pedicle of oral mucosa as advised by Anderson and Byers (1965) may help repair of a damaged parotid duct.

Duct Obstruction due to Causes Outside the Wall.—Both benign and malignant neoplasms can compress one of the salivary gland ducts. Benign neoplasms simply compress the duct, inducing dilatation proximal to the point of compression. Removal of the neoplasm cures the obstruction.

Malignant neoplasms may also produce simple compression but, alternatively, they may invade the duct wall. If the latter event occurs, a stricture may be produced with dilatation proximally, or the neoplasm may ulcerate into the lumen of the duct. Sialographically, such ulceration produces an irregular enlargement of the lumen of the duct.

Sjögren's syndrome may be discussed under this heading. Patients with this condition suffer from a dry mouth, dry eyes, difficulty in swallowing, and rheumatoid arthritis, or varying combinations of these complaints. The damage to the lacrimal and salivary glands is thought to be auto-immune in nature. In well-established cases there is a positive latex test for rheumatoid factor, a positive antinuclear factor test and salivary duct antibody test. There may be an increase in serum globulin, and where the eyes are affected by kerato-conjunctivitis sicca this can be demonstrated by Rose-Bengal staining. Labial salivary gland biopsy can provide a specimen of salivary gland for study which is relatively unaffected by ascending infection.

Histologically, destruction of gland acini and their replacement by a lymphocytic and plasma-cell infiltration is seen; features which account for the decreased salivary secretion. Epithelial hyperplasia leads to obstruction of the smaller ducts, the formation of 'casts' in the larger ducts, and possibly predisposes to calculus formation. The jelly-like saliva mentioned previously may be formed in some cases.

In the early stages there are no sialographic changes. Then, by comparison with normal glands, the intralobular ducts are seen to be more sparse than usual. Finally many changes occur: the ducts may be grossly dilated, strictures may be found or re-duplication of the lumen suggestive of the presence of epithelial casts. The periphery of the gland becomes difficult to demonstrate and gross, irregular cavitation of the gland occurs. A coarse sialectasis may appear in some patients.

Apart from a progressive dryness of the mouth the patient may suffer from attacks of infection of the salivary glands or distension of the gland with jelly-like material. In some patients a nodular enlargement of a gland occurs resembling neoplastic disease. Where a more uniform, symmetrical enlargement of the salivary and lacrimal glands is found the condition is described as 'Mikulicz's disease'.

Treatment is difficult. Nothing can be done to restore the glandular tissue which has been destroyed, so that the dryness of the mouth cannot be cured. Demulcent mouthwashes and tablets, sips of water with the food, and cream on the lips are all that can be tried. Because the progress of the condition is so variable the effect of steroid therapy is difficult to assess. The well-known hazards of long-term systemic steroid therapy need to be balanced against the possibilities of slowing the progress of the disease. The risk that the exhibition of steroids will increase the susceptibility to secondary infection has also to be considered. Chronic or subacute attacks of infection of the parotids add to the patient's discomfort and further damage the glandular substance. Such infections must, of course, be treated with systemic antibiotics.

Single glands which are enlarged or show nodular enlargement may require exploration and biopsy to exclude the presence of a neoplasm. Where the enlargement of Mikulicz's disease is embarrassing, surgical reduction may be considered. However, it is obvious that superficial parotidectomy with conservation of the facial nerve may be far from easy as the gland may well be adherent, inflamed, and fibrosed. Furthermore, the operation may increase the dryness of the mouth. These are factors which must be weighed carefully in individual cases.

Swelling due to Gland Distension and Infiltration.—Certain drugs can cause enlargement of the salivary glands. Iodine, thiouracil, and thiocyanates used in the treatment of thyrotoxicosis may occasionally have this effect. The minor as well as the major glands may enlarge and interfere with mastication.

Phenyl and oxyphenbutazone can cause water and salt retention with parotid enlargement and certain curious dietary habits, like the eating of clay, which can produce the same effect.

In some people fat is deposited in the gland causing it to enlarge, although such enlargement is progressive rather than recurrent. Allergic parotitis is a further cause of gland enlargement. An association of the swelling with a particular time of year or part of the week's routine may suggest this as a cause. Other allergic phenomena such as hay fever or asthma may coexist, and it may be possible to establish a cause-effect relationship with a particular antigen.

A normal sialogram, a sterile saliva, plugs of mucus containing eosinophils in the saliva, or a high eosinophil count in the peripheral blood may support the diagnosis. Antihistamine preparations frequently reduce the swelling and discomfort.

Differential Diagnosis.—A number of calcified objects must be distinguished from salivary calculi. These are calcified tuberculous lymph-nodes, phleboliths in a haemangioma, tonsilloliths, calcified parasites in cysticercosis in the masticatory muscles, developmental bone islands in the hyoid and the stylohyoid ligament, and calcification in an atheromatous facial artery. Many of these calcified structures differ in detail in their appearance compared with salivary calculi. Two-plane radiography and sialography will show that they are in a position outside the salivary glands.

Recurrent subacute infection of pre-auricular lymph-nodes or those in the lower pole of the parotid can simulate lobular parotid infection. The difference is that lobular parotid infection is usually secondary to duct obstruction, the cause of which can be demonstrated by sialography.

Finally, it must be remembered that mumps and a number of other virus infections cause salivary gland swelling, though not recurrent enlargement. In particular, not all such patients are obviously ill and, in some, one or both submandibular glands may be affected rather than the parotids. Determination of S and V antibody titres in the patient's serum on two occasions two to three weeks apart will confirm or refute a diagnosis of mumps in difficult cases.

C. Persistent Swellings of the Salivary Glands

Where a patient has a persistent, localized swelling of a salivary gland the likelihood of its being a neoplasm springs to mind. Other possibilities are chronic enlargement of the associated lymph-nodes, for example as a result of chronic infection, sarcoid, Hodgkin's disease, or (rarely these days) tuberculosis. Occasionally auto-immune disease may produce a nodular rather than a diffuse enlargement. Neoplasms of associated tissues such as neurofibromas, haemangiomas, lipomas, or even simple cysts may be encountered. Sialography can help to distinguish the salivary from the non-salivary masses, although difficulties exist. A peripheral neoplastic mass cannot be distinguished from an extra-salivary mass indenting the gland. Furthermore, lymph-nodes adjacent to the parotid can contain salivary tissue, and neoplasms have been known to arise in these enclaves. Such neoplasms may then be outside the parotid capsule but do *not* represent metastases.

Neoplasms of the Major Salivary Glands.—Both the histopathology and the surgery of these neoplasms have their difficulties. As a result, the responsibility for the care and treatment of these cases tends to gravitate into the hands of those with special knowledge and experience in the field.

The parotid gland is more commonly the site of neoplastic change, the submandibular gland next, and the sublingual last.

The Pleomorphic Adenoma (*Fig.* 42).—Pleomorphic adenomas are the most common salivary gland neoplasms and usually they are benign.

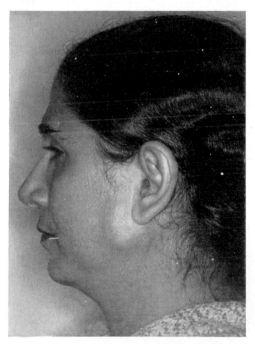

Fig. 42.—Pleomorphic adenoma of the left parotid region.

That is, they neither invade the facial nerve nor do they metastasize. Indeed, because they are slow-growing and cause the patient little trouble, they may be permitted to remain for many years and to attain a considerable size. Their benign behaviour, however, is deceptive and their periphery is lobulated and complex and any capsule is thin and histologically penetrated in places by growth. What is more, they 'seed' readily if penetrated at operation, so that the wound is contaminated with tumour cells. Hence they require to be removed with a narrow margin of apparently normal tissue. Fortunately, the narrow sheath of connective tissue which surrounds the facial nerve branches is an adequate margin at these points. Once the position of the related branches has been established, it is not too difficult to include an adequate layer of adjacent tissue at intermediate places and separate the mass.

The pleomorphic adenoma usually presents as a firm, lobulated mass, although soft or even fluctuant areas may be demonstrated if part of the tumour contains large amounts of mucus.

As the neoplasm enlarges it displaces the normal gland and its duct system to the periphery producing the so-called 'grasping fingers' appearance in a sialogram. Many are in the part of the gland superficial to the facial nerve, but others start in the deep part of the gland. The latter may not manifest themselves until they have reached a large size. The styloid process and posterior border of the ramus of the mandible constitute a bony tunnel for these neoplasms: the deeper part bulging into the lateral wall of the pharynx and soft palate, the more superficial part ultimately pushing up to the surface between the branches of the facial nerve. Because of their shape they are described as 'dumb-bell' tumours. Adequate access to them is most difficult to achieve and an approach may be required from both a preauricular incision and one across the soft palate and pterygomandibular fold. It may be necessary to perform a vertical subsigmoid osteotomy of the mandibular ramus to permit delivery of the mass. Obviously both the internal carotid and jugular vein are in close posterior relationship to the tumour and constitute an additional surgical hazard.

Because excision of the submandibular salivary gland is a far easier surgical problem, the results of the excision of pleomorphic adenomas of this gland should be better than those of the parotid. This, however, is by no means always so. One reason is the temptation to grasp the gland with instruments during the removal, particularly during display of the lingual nerve. Unfortunately, such instrumentation can rupture the tumour, disseminating cells into the wound.

A few pleomorphic adenomas both clinically and histologically are malignant. They should be excised radically like other malignant tumours.

Papillary Cystadenoma Lymphomatosum (Warthin's Tumour).—This is a benign tumour which affects men more often than women, and the middle-aged and elderly rather than young subjects. The tumour is smooth, soft and rounded, and may well be fluctuant. There may be more than one papillary cystadenoma present so that a recurrence after the excision of one neoplasm may really represent the appearance of a new one. The cut surface has a reddish-brown appearance in contrast to the pale yellowish grey of the pleomorphic adenoma. Treatment is by excision.

Adenocystic Carcinoma (Cylindroma).—Some adenocystic carcinomas grow comparatively slowly, but this does not necessarily improve the prognosis for the patient since they are likely to be looked upon as a pleomorphic adenoma and excised in too conservative a fashion. Indeed, these neoplasms can penetrate surprising distances away from the main mass; particularly along the perineural lymphatics. This means, unfortunately, that cells may have penetrated far beyond the reach of surgery with little to show for it macroscopically.

Over-generous surgical excision combined with postoperative radiotherapy offer the best chance of control. Some advocate the use of frozen sections of related nerves at the time of operation to try to ensure that perineural extensions are removed. Although there can be a depressingly high recurrence rate with this tumour, patients may be free of symptoms of the disease for many years after such treatment. An otherwise inexplicable pain or paralysis can be the first sign of recurrence.

Muco-epidermoid Carcinoma.—This is another malignant neoplasm exhibiting a very variable degree of aggressiveness. Some examples grow very slowly indeed, and again may be mistaken for a pleomorphic adenoma on clinical grounds so that once more there is a risk of inadequate excision. Fortunately, once the correct diagnosis is understood, adequate excision presents less of a problem than with the adenocystic carcinoma.

Squamous-cell Carcinoma.—There is little clinical difference between the more rapidly progressive and invasive salivary tumours. Fixation of the tumour mass, pain, involvement of related motor nerves, radiographic evidence of invasion of the adjacent bones all point to their malignant nature. However, as elsewhere, squamous-cell carcinoma tends to feel very hard and to metastasize early to the regional lymph-nodes.

Treatment.—Radical neck dissection may be required as part of the treatment of the more aggressive malignant neoplasms.

Biopsy of Neoplasms of the Major Salivary Glands.—It is an obvious advantage for the clinician to have histological evidence of the nature of any neoplasm about which he has to advise a patient. The problem with other than superficial lesions is that biopsy carries a risk of spillage of viable cells into the tissue planes opened up by the surgery. The risk of such contamination is particularly great if fluid in cystic parts of the tumour is released and flows into the wound. Widespread dissemination of the lesion can result. Because of this risk some surgeons prefer not to biopsy salivary neoplasms, but to rely upon the clinical findings plus the general feel of the mass at operation.

Others consider that a drill biopsy carries little risk of contamination of the drill track. This is probably true if the drill penetrates only as far as the neoplasm, but there would appear to be a risk if the neoplasm were transfixed and the drill went on into sound tissue beyond. Furthermore, the sample obtained by a drill biopsy may be very small.

In some centres frozen sections made during the operation are advocated, but special experience in interpreting these is required if the report is to be relied upon.

Where the pathologist prefers to use paraffin sections for this, often difficult, corner of pathology, an incisional biopsy may be preferred. An accessible part of the mass should be approached through a short incision, the wound should not be opened laterally and should be closed carefully after the specimen has been taken. The biopsy incision should be so sited that the entire wound, with a margin, can be conveniently excised when the definitive surgery is undertaken.

Dissection of the Facial Nerve.—The main trunk of the facial nerve is found by reflecting the lower pole of the parotid gland forwards, detaching it from the mastoid process and external auditory canal. It curves round below the external auditory canal just deep to the junction of the cartilagenous and bony part. It can be found anterior to the mastoid process and above the posterior belly of the digastric, curving forwards over the origin of the stylohyoid muscle. It is quite deeply placed, but a pointed process of the cartilaginous part of the canal points to its path.

The branches of the nerve are readily picked up as they leave the gland; the lower zygomatic branch lies on Stenson's duct and the mandibular branch lies near to the posterior facial vein (retromandibular vein).

If a neoplasm is to be excised, a flap is reflected from the surface of the gland, care being taken neither to thin out the flap too much, nor to pass too close to the surface of the mass. The tumour is outlined to delineate an adequate margin. Both the main nerve-trunk and the peripheral branches should be identified as convenient and separation of the lesion started by working first along the most accessible parts of the nerve. As in all cancer surgery, the aim when removing the neoplasm is to think in three dimensions and never approach nearer to the tumour than the width of apparently normal tissue considered necessary to include all outgrowths from the periphery (*Fig.* 43).

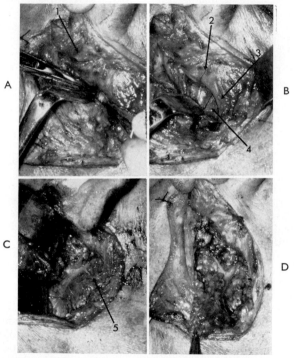

Fig. 43.—The exposure of the facial nerve during conservative parotidectomy.

A, The view of the main trunk immediately the overlying temporoparotid fascia has been divided. The pointed end of the tragal cartilage is outlined in black (1).

B, The parotid gland has been retracted anteriorly to show: the relationship of the main trunk to the temporo-mastoid fissure (2), to which the temporoparotid fascia was previously attached; the sterno-mastoid muscle (3); and the posterior belly of the digastric muscle (4).

C, The cervico-mandibular division of the nerve has been identified and branches to the stylohyoid and posterior belly of the digastric are seen arising from the main trunk of the facial nerve (5).

D, The zygomatico-facial division has now been identified and a small pleomorphic adenoma of the lower pole of the gland removed.

Stimulation with an electrical stimulator or by pinching with forceps is a wise precaution to avoid section of an unsuspected branch of the nerve, but the ability to recognize the peripheral branches on sight is perhaps the most valuable safeguard.

Where branches of the nerve must be sacrificed they can be replaced by grafts taken from the great auricular nerve.

Frey's Syndrome.—Frey's syndrome is sweating and sometimes flushing of the skin over the distribution of the auriculo-temporal nerve which is occasioned by a stimulus to salivary secretion. It is thought that as a result of damage to the auriculo-temporal nerve post-ganglionic parasympathetic fibres from the otic ganglion become united to sympathetic nerves from the superior cervical ganglion going to supply the sweat-glands of the skin.

The syndrome can follow parotid surgery, temporomandibular joint surgery, and injuries and injections in this region. Congenital cases probably follow birth injuries. The condition is rarely sufficiently severe to warrant any treatment. If this is necessary, a neurosurgeon may be asked to consider interrupting the intracranial course of the secreto-motor fibres.

REFERENCES

ANDERSON, R., and BYERS, L. T. (1965), *Surgery of the Parotid Gland.* St. Louis: Mosby.
KATZEN, M. (1969), 'Recurrent Parotitis in Children', *S. Afr. med. J.,* **7,** 37.
MAYNARD, J. D. (1965), 'Recurrent Parotid Enlargement', *Br. J. Surg.,* **52,** 784.
PATEY, D. H. (1965), 'Inflammation of the Salivary Glands with particular reference to Chronic and Recurrent Parotitis', *Ann. R. Coll. Surg.,* **36,** 26.
— — and THACKRAY, A. C. (1955), 'Chronic "Sialectatic" Parotitis in the Light of Pathological Studies on Parotidectomy Material', *Br. J. Surg.,* **43,** 43.
ROSE, S. S. (1954), 'A Clinical and Radiological Survey of 192 Cases of Recurrent Swellings of the Salivary Glands', *Ann. R. Coll. Surg.,* **15,** 374.
SEWARD, G. R. (1968), 'Anatomic Surgery for Salivary Calculi', *Oral Surg.,* **25,** 150, 287, 525, 670, 810; **26,** 1, 137.
STAFNE, E. C. (1958), *Oral Roentgenographic Diagnosis,* p.132. London: Saunders.

CHAPTER XIX

DISEASES OF THE TEMPOROMANDIBULAR JOINT

DEVELOPMENTAL DISTURBANCES

Hypoplasia of the Joint.—Hypoplasia of the condyle head can occur as part of unilateral or bilateral hypoplasia of the mandible. In such cases the joint is small, although the zygomatic arch is normal. In other instances, as, for example, in the case of the so-called 'first arch' syndrome, not only is the condyle head diminutive but the zygomatic process of the temporal bone also is small. This state of affairs, together with deficient zygomatic bones, is seen too as a symmetrical deformity in the genetically determined Treacher-Collins syndrome.

Hemifacial microsomia, first and second arch syndrome or otomandibular dysostosis occurs about once in 300–500 live-births and with no sex preference. The abnormalities are usually unilateral and of varying degrees of severity, with reduction in size or abnormality of the shape of the pinna and tragus, irregularities of the auditory ossicles, hypoplasia of the ramus and condyle of the mandible, deficiency of the muscles attached to the ramus and paresis of the muscles of facial expression. The external ear is also set lower on the head. In severe cases the external ear and auditory canal may be absent and the condyle and posterior part of the mandible fail to develop. Eruption of the teeth is frequently incomplete so that multiple impactions in the ramus are seen and teeth fail to reach the occlusal plane. Teeth may also be absent. Poswillo (1973a, b; 1974a) has shown that a haemorrhage occurs from the anastomosis of developing vessels which initiate the stapedial arterial stem at about the 6th week of embryonic life. The resultant haematoma produces a varying degree of tissue damage dependant on its size. Depending on the amount of destruction and the time required to resorb the debris and effect repair, so will the potential for 'catch up' differentiation be affected before the end of that phase of morphogenesis. Since the functional matrix of the face is affected in that region, so will secondary growth disturbances become manifest as growth proceeds.

In the Treacher-Collins' syndrome or mandibulofacial dysostosis the symmetrical defect is inherited as an autosomal dominant trait with equal sex incidence. There are an antimongoloid slope to the palpebral fissures, colobomas of the outer third of the lower lid, absence of cilia medial to the coloboma, deformed pinna, not uncommonly an absent external auditory canal, anomalies of the middle ear, extra ear tags, deficient malar bones, a receding chin and hypoplastic condyles and ramus. Poswillo (1973b; 1974b) suggests that there is a destruction of neural crest cells destined for the face and affecting those moving later in development rather than earlier. The severity depends on the degree of destruction. As a result of the destruction the developing otic pit moves up into first arch territory and the ear becomes located closer to the angle of the mandible. Since the genetic programme is now carried out, but with smaller amounts of material, the tissues affected are hypoplastic and to this extent a caricature of the normal part is found, rather than an absent part. Unlike the first and second arch syndrome cases, the degree of deformity is not increased as somatic growth proceeds, so that the appearance does not deteriorate as the child grows older.

Hyperplasia of the Joint.—Bony hyperplasia of all components of the joint probably only occurs with facial hemi-hypertrophy. Thus, although the cavity is increased in size to accommodate the enlarged head of unilateral condylar hyperplasia, there is no comparable enlargement of the zygomatic process of the temporal bone. This usually applies even though there may be some enlargement of other elements of the patient's face on the same side.

Basically, there are two types of unilateral condylar hyperplasia and a variety of terms are used to indicate this. One type has a not very greatly enlarged condyle head. The condyle neck, which is moderately elongated, is inclined downwards and forwards along the usual axis. Thus, the rest of the mandible on that side is pushed forwards. The angle is also farther forwards, the patient has mandibular prognathism, and the midline of the mandible is pushed to the opposite side. The point to note is that the joint functions normally, i.e., the condyle translates as well as rotates. Therefore, excision of the condyle should *never* be considered as a means of surgical correction. If this is done a normal jaw relationship may be restored together with a symmetrical face at rest, but deviation of the chin towards the side of surgery will occur as the patient opens the mouth. Instead, the Obwegeser sagittal splitting operation or the vertical sub-sigmoid procedure should be used. In a few patients it may be sufficient to shorten the elongated side of the mandible, rotating the jaw round the normal joint. The twisting of the condyle in its fossa produces no ill-effects. Usually, however, it is necessary to operate on both sides to produce a satisfactory occlusion. This is a further reason why simple condylectomy is unsatisfactory.

In the other form of condylar hyperplasia the condyle head is greatly enlarged, the neck elongated and directed downwards. A lateral open bite is established on that side, but the mandible is neither displaced forwards nor is the midline shifted to the other side. Many other associated changes may occur, some of them compensatory in nature. Hovell (1970) has shown that condylectomy practised at the correct time can produce a near-normal face for some of these patients. Therefore, in such cases, this method of management is acceptable since the greatly enlarged condyle only rotates in its fossa and there is no translatory movement to be lost.

TRAUMATIC INJURY TO THE TEMPOROMANDIBULAR JOINT

Traumatic Arthritis.—An injury which is insufficient to produce a fracture of the condyle or condyle neck, or a dislocation, may yet be sufficient to produce a traumatic arthritis.

Following the injury the patient complains of pain and limitation of movement of the joint. There is slight puffiness over the affected regions, the joint is markedly tender and the condyle head may appear more prominent than usual. This is usually due to a slight deviation of the mandible towards the opposite side, but there may be a unilateral posterior open bite without deviation. Whichever posture is adopted the patient is unwilling to close the teeth in centric occlusion because of pain. A joint radiograph will demonstrate widening of the radiographic jiont space.

Immobilization of the jaw with a pair of eyelet wires on each side for a few days can give comfort, but the patient may require an occlusal wafer of acrylic resin which is inserted between the occlusal surfaces of the teeth before the intermaxillary wires are tightened. Often reassurance and analgesics are all that is required.

Acute Subluxation.—In this condition there is a sudden onset of limitation of opening, pain with movement of the affected joint, and reluctance to close in centric occlusion. Equally suddenly, and usually after some days, the patient will be aware of a jolt in the joint and normal movement is restored. Exactly what happens within the joint is not known. It is usually postulated that the condyle head manages to slip backwards over the posterior thickening of the disk. Muscle spasm leads to the other phenomena observed, including the slight deviation of the chin towards the *opposite* side seen when the patient is at rest.

Chronic Subluxation.—Some people can open their jaws to the point where the joints 'stick', then they free the joints, one at a time. The habit is a dangerous one since it can progress to recurrent subluxation of the joint. Should the latter develop, the patient should still be persuaded to try to control the situation voluntarily, for although there are many ingenious operations for this condition little is written about their long-term effectiveness.

Dislocation.—Dislocation of the condyle head upwards and forwards into the temporal fossa occurs when the masticatory muscles contract at a time when the mouth is open to its greatest extent, or when a blow is delivered to the point of the chin, again when the jaw is wide open. Cineradiography of the joint demonstrates that the condyle moves normally to a point beyond and above the lowest point on the eminentia. The jaw is controlled at this point by the balanced pull of the muscles and can be brought back smoothly under the eminentia and up into the fossa. Thus, there need only be a temporary lack of balance in the muscular pull for dislocation to occur.

Reduction is accomplished by downward pressure with the padded thumbs on the lower molars, together with an upwards and backwards force applied to the underside of the chin with the fingers. Once the patient's confidence has been gained most acute dislocations may be reduced in this manner. Rarely will it be necessary to resort to anaesthesia to produce the muscular relaxation necessary for success.

Chronic dislocation is seen almost always in edentulous patients, for where teeth are present the matter is drawn to everyone's attention by the gagged occlusion. Once the muscles are relaxed in a patient under a general anaesthetic, the condyles can be dislocated and replaced in their fossae with the greatest of ease for it is the muscles which normally prevent this occurrence. Both the operator and the anaesthetist maintain a forward displacement of the jaw to ensure a free airway. With a prop or gag between the molar teeth acting as a fulcrum, this pressure easily pushes the condyles over the eminentia. If, during the anaesthetic, the patient's teeth are extracted, all reference points between the upper and lower jaw are removed. Postoperatively the patient expects both some discomfort in the jaw and a change in appearance, so a dislocation is easily overlooked. Muscle spasm and then fibrosis and muscle-shortening prevent reduction of the dislocation.

Once such a state of affairs has persisted for some months treatment is difficult. There are several alternatives. First, the situation can be accepted, but, alternatively, condylectomy can be performed with replacement of the mandible. Open reduction has been tried, but this can prove very difficult. Hayward (1965) has had success with manipulation and muscle relaxation, and Popesca (1960) uses a roll of gauze placed between the molars to act as a fulcrum and an upward force applied to the chin.

An unusual injury to the joint is fracture of the roof of the articular fossa with dislocation of the condyle head into the middle cranial fossa. The injury is of importance because the patient may have some degree of opening of the mouth (Pirok and Merrill, 1970) and derangement of the occlusion may be the only clue to the nature of the occurrence.

Tearing of the Disk.—Campbell (1965) has shown by some beautiful arthrography and radiography that the meniscus may be torn free at one margin and crumpled up within the cavity. Movement of the condyle head is then restricted. If the disk lies behind the condyle the latter cannot return to its proper position in the fossa. Badly torn and crumpled disks should be removed. This constitutes one of the few indications for menisectomy.

A damaged meniscus used to be blamed as the cause of the painful and locking joint. It is now realized that such damage is uncommon. Further, removal of the disk gives only temporary relief in this particular type of case.

Damage to the Condyle.—Injury or disease affecting the condyle during childhood can affect the condylar growth centre and produce changes in mandibular growth. (*Fig.* 44.) Trauma to the condyle, infection, and Still's disease are the main offenders. Infection may reach the condyle by direct spread from osteomyelitis, or as a result of a suppurative arthritis, in some cases secondary to otitis media.

The mandible can be considered as composed of three elements, a bar of bone which stretches from the condyle to the mental eminence, the alveolar process, and the muscular processes of the coronoid and angle. The condylar growth centre is responsible for the growth in length of the basic bar or arch of bone. If growth ceases the distance between the condyle and the point of the chin remains the same. As the maxilla grows downwards in relation to the joint the chin end of the bar is tilted down into the neck. In an attempt to compensate, the alveolar process, particularly that in the incisor region, grows upwards and forwards towards the maxilla. Both the muscular processes achieve a near normal size, so by comparison with the condyle the coronoid is elongated and the sizeable angle accentuates the facial notch.

Ankylosis of the Temporomandibular Joint.—Ankylosis can be a sequel to an intracapsular fracture of the condyle (particularly in members of

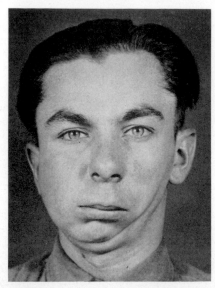

Fig. 44.—Osteomyelitis of the right ramus in childhood has resulted in damage to the condylar growth centre and deviation of the mandible to the right.

the coloured races), severe infection of the joint (particularly suppurative infections), and long-standing active rheumatoid arthritis, Still's disease, and, of course, to ankylosing spondylitis. Ankylosis may be either bony or fibrous. When the union is fibrous it may be possible to demonstrate a joint space by radiography, particularly short-distance radiography of the condyle head, or tomography. Also with fibrous ankylosis there is frequently a considerable rotational movement of the joint. (*Fig.* 45.)

Curiously, a unilateral bony ankylosis seems to be compatible with some degree of jaw movement, even when the bony union seems to be quite extensive at operation. When bony ankylosis follows a fracture the area of bony union may be considerable in extent, involving the condyle, sigmoid notch, coronoid, and lingula, on the one hand, and the joint, zygomatic arch, pterygoid plates, and the base of the skull on the other.

Operations to free an ankylosis seek to produce a pseudarthrosis. The bony or fibrous attachment is divided and the abnormal tissue removed. Three manœuvres are employed to try to prevent reattachment: the part of the mandible adjacent to the joint may be widely excised; a soft tissue, such as muscle or dermis, may be interposed between the bone-ends; alternatively, an allograft material can be inserted in the gap or over one of the bone-ends. The disadvantage of creating a wide gap is that, subsequently, muscle pull shortens the jaw towards the joint producing a micrognathic appearance and an anterior open bite.

Ward (1961) pointed out that a direct attack on the joint region can involve the operator in a difficult dissection. He devised a curved, low ramus section which avoids these problems. His operative technique consists essentially of fitting a plate of chrome-cobalt over the bone-end to discourage bony union. A new joint made in this fashion tends to become stiff as the area of contact is too great for the length of false capsule which develops. Reducing the end of the upper fragment to a point can cure this difficulty.

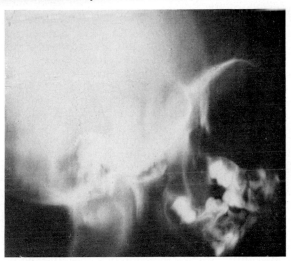

Fig. 45.—A radiograph of a congenitally ankylosed mandible. A band of radio-lucent cartilage separates the condylar bone from that of the temporal like an irregular epiphysial plate.

Both muscle and dermis have been used to discourage osteogenesis. The dermal graft is cut by raising a Thiersch graft. The epidermal graft is left attached by one edge while the dermal graft is dissected off the underlying fat. The epidermis can then be replaced to cover the wound. The bone-end is rounded and holes drilled just behind the end. The dermal sheet is stretched over the bone-end and fixed by sutures which are passed through the holes.

Silastic has been used freely in recent years as a barrier between the bone-ends, but the long-term results with this material are not yet known.

OTHER CAUSES OF LIMITED OPENING

Mechanical Causes.—In some patients the tissue which prevents proper mandibular movement is outside the capsule of the joint (extracapsular ankylosis) or even at a distance from the joint. A fractured zygomatic arch, for example, can interfere with movement of the coronoid process.

Conversely, the coronoid process may be enlarged as in the condition called 'coronoid hyperplasia'. Cartilage, and as a result bone, proliferate so as to elongate the coronoid and produce a knob-like expansion. An adventitious bursa develops between the coronoid and the inside of the zygomatic arch, which may be resorbed on its inner aspect so as to accommodate the mass. Compensatory deposition of bone on the outer aspect of the zygomatic bone produces an enlargement of the cheek.

Quite often the hyperplasia affects both coronoid processes. Because an accessory cartilaginous growth centre is formed for a while in the coronoid process during development, it has been suggested that persistence of this cartilage is the cause of the hyperplasia. As the coronoid enlarges, first lateral movements of the jaw and then opening of the mouth become restricted. Excision of the coronoid process gives good results.

The operation is carried out in the following manner. Anaesthesia is induced and blind endotracheal intubation is performed. A vasoconstrictor is infiltrated into the operation site and an incision is made vertically through the mucous membrane and buccinator over the anterior border of the ramus. The deep facial vein and buccal artery have to be divided and must be ligated. At first sight, access is very limited since the patient's jaw cannot be separated very far. However, the cheek wound is distensible and only the buccal pad of fat is likely to reduce visibility. If the latter cannot be satisfactorily retracted, it should be drawn out of the wound, ligated, and excised. The masseter and temporalis insertion are elevated to clear the mandible in a line from the wound to the sigmoid notch and a hole is drilled in the base of the coronoid. A wire must be passed through this to prevent the temporalis from pulling the coronoid upwards out of sight once it has been separated. The coronoid is sectioned with a bur. Once the cut has been completed, with an osteotome if necessary, the jaws can be separated unless the other side is affected. Traction is applied to the wire and the mass separated from the temporalis and removed. A vacuum drain is threaded through the submandibular skin and the wound closed. A new coronoid forms from the periosteum, but it is of normal size.

Dense fibrous bands can develop in the muscles of mastication which limit mandibular movement. This reaction may be seen on occasions in the temporalis after the injection of alcohol into the ganglion in cases of trigeminal neuralgia. A similar response can follow the injection of dental local anaesthetic solutions suggesting that a haematoma, or possibly a low-grade infection, has been caused by the injection.

Cleft palate operations can produce fibrosis of the pterygomandibular raphe and, consequently, limitation of opening. Moderate degrees of fibrosis can be released or a coronoidectomy performed if the temporalis is involved. The jaw should be propped wide open, and although it may be removed at mealtimes the prop must be replaced afterwards for at least a fortnight.

Submucous fibrosis (see also p. 126) results in dense fibrous bands in the cheeks and pillars of the fauces which stretch from mandible to maxilla. While almost all the cases have been recorded in Indians and a few other Asians and Europeans living in India, a few similar cases in white people have, however, been reported outside India: one by Lemmer and Shear (1967), in South Africa, and one by Simpson (1969), in Manchester. The latter had been married to a Pakistani for 12 years and had been eating Indian food. Sirsat and Khanolkar (1962) have produced a similar response in rats' palates by painting them with capsaicin, a constituent of chillies, and it is thought that this may be the aetiological factor. Affected individuals are usually between 20 and 40 years of age, but cases from 10 to 70 years of age are seen. Dense acellular masses of collagen and strands of an elastic-like material form in the submucosa limiting movement of the mandible, tongue, and soft palate and occluding the Eustachian tube. The overlying epithelium is thin and lacks rete pegs. There is no effective treatment.

In some subjects myositis ossificans develops as a response to injury. Many cases of myositis ossificans of the masseter have now been recorded. The probable mechanism is a tear of the muscle origin or insertion such that the periosteum is also damaged. As a result, bone develops in the healing haematoma. Usually the new bone is resorbed, which is fortunate. The excision of myositis ossificans, as in the case of scar bands, can be followed in some patients by a recurrence to a greater degree than before.

Rarely the progressive, generalized myositis ossificans affects the tissues of the face, uniting mandible to maxilla. There is also a rare congenital deformity in which the upper and lower alveolar processes are conjoined on one or both sides.

Functional Causes.—The most frequent cause of limited opening is an inflammation affecting the tissues about the jaws. Usually this is described as trismus, but is not strictly so as it is not due to muscle spasm. Indeed, Moore and Greenfield (1967) have shown that inhibition of muscular activity is a reason for limited mandibular movement after 3rd molar surgery, and this seems to be a logical way for the part to be rested. Oedema of the elevators of the mandible such that they cannot lengthen to permit depression of the mandible is another cause.

Two cases of tetanus have been seen by the authors which presented as cases of limitation of opening. In both cases the patient had been referred as a suspected case of temporomandibular joint disorder. One was due to a penetration wound in the foot, the other to a similar small wound in the hand.

In an unusual neurological case true muscular spasm resulted in inability to open the mouth, or part the cords in the larynx. The patient required a permanent tracheostomy. So severe was the spasm of the masticatory muscles that a considerable dose of curare was required to abolish electromyographic evidence of activity and to permit the jaws to be separated. The remaining few teeth were sheathed in deep pits in the opposing alveolar ridge.

Occasionally there is no physical cause for the inability to open and the patient is a hysteric. Such cases can be baffling until it is realized that the patient is mentally disturbed.

ARTHRITIS AND ARTHROSIS

Infective Arthritis of the Temporomandibular Joint.—Infective arthritis of the temporomandibular joint is by no means a common complaint. Suppurative arthritis from staphylococcal infection may arise as a result of a penetrating injury of the joint or by the spread of infection from adjacent structures. Involvement of the condyle head following an osteo-myelitis of the ramus is one mechanism and extension of infection from otitis media is another. The latter may develop as a complication of measles in children, but can also occur in adults where the mastoid air cells extend into the zygomatic process of the temporal bone. Rarely, a boil or an infected pre-auricular sinus is the source of the infection. Many of the older clinicians can recall cases of gonococcal arthritis of the temporomandibular joint.

Suppurative arthritis should be treated by aspiration of the joint, the instillation of an antibiotic solution, and the administration of a systemic antibiotic. A smear should be made from the aspirate and a sample sent for culture and sensitivity tests.

Even less common are non-suppurative infections such as tuberculosis, but an acutely swollen joint from Reiter's disease may be seen from time to time.

Rheumatoid Diseases.—Rheumatoid arthritis, psoriatic arthritis, and, in children, Still's disease can affect the temporomandibular joint. However, this joint is only one of many which may be affected and, in general, the patient's management will be in the hands of a rheumatologist. The manifestations of the disorder in the temporomandibular joint differ little from those in joints elsewhere. There will be pain particularly on movement, some swelling of the overlying tissues, and limitation of opening. Radiographically the condyle head and articular fossa will be less radio-opaque than usual and erosion of the articular surface of the condyle may be seen.

In Still's disease there may be damage to the growth centre of the condyle and the development of both extra- and intracapsular adhesions which limit joint movement.

In addition to the general measures recommended for the patient, all local causes of joint strain should be eliminated. Courses of short-wave diathermy may give comfort, and the cautious use of intra-articular hydrocortisone can be of benefit.

One factor of importance is the effect of systemic steroids on condyles affected by rheumatoid arthritis. The bone is progressively resorbed, sometimes over quite a short period of time, until no condyle remains. The first intimation of this effect may be the development of an anterior open bite.

Gout.—Gout of the temporomandibular joint is most uncommon. One of the authors has seen a case in a child with leukaemia. The importance of the condition lies in the presentation of acute inflammation of the joint in such a way that the condition can be mistaken for a suppurative arthritis.

Osteoarthritis.—Osteoarthritis is detected mostly in the older age-groups, but can be found affecting joints which have previously suffered a fracture. The joint is painful, often has a palpable and audible grate when the mouth is opened, and is tender to palpation. Careful radiography can demonstrate localized resorption cavities in the condyle head, sclerosis of the underlying bone, osteophytic masses particularly anteriorly, and occasionally small cystic cavities.

As with other joints, there are probably many osteoarthritic ones which are symptomless, and not a few which return to a painless state after months or years of causing trouble.

The full range of conservative measures should be tried: analgesics, attention to the occlusion, the use of shortwave diathermy. Altering the mechanics of the joint with a bite-raising appliance or the provision of new dentures which restore the proper vertical dimension may both help.

The mechanism, presumably, is similar to that seen in the femur where an osteotomy which permits a slight displacement of the femoral head can improve an osteoarthritic hip. In some patients the occasional intra-articular injection of hydrocortisone will give quite long periods of relief.

Henny (1957, 1968) employs a high condylectomy for those cases in which bony changes can be demonstrated and where the patient has considerable trouble with the joint. In a large series of middle-aged women he obtained good results with this operation. Through a pre-auricular incision he uncovers the joint, incises the capsule over the condyle, and removes a thin layer of articular surface with a drill. There should be minimal occlusal changes as a result of this procedure.

Functional Derangement of the Temporomandibular Joint.—That so many young people suffer pain and disordered function of the temporo-mandibular joint makes it a quite unusual condition, for often it affects fit subjects in whom it is impossible to demonstrate either disease of the surfaces of that particular joint or of any other joints. In what ways then are the temporomandibular joints unusual anatomically? First, they are the only joints at each end of a bone which have to function in concert with one another, a situation which arises because of the horseshoe shape of the mandible. Secondly, the path of movement of all other joints is dictated solely by the articular surfaces of the joint and the muscles. With the temporomandibular joints the path of movement is in part imposed upon the joints from without, by the articulation of the teeth and by the movement of the opposite joint. Finally, each joint has two compartments separated by a disk, and both the condyle head and the disk are to be found balanced on the posterior sloping surface of the eminentia when the maximum masticatory force is exerted. It is in order to control the final movement of condyle head and disk from the eminentia into the fossa under this heavy load, that the lateral pterygoid has such a complex insertion into both condyle and disk. A malfunction of this muscular control by the lateral pterygoid could permit the condyle head to move separately in relation to the disk, starting the chain of events that gives rise to clinical clicking.

Much has been written about the derangements of the temporo-mandibular joint, but much is, of necessity, pure speculation. The condition appears to be more common in women than men. The complaint may be of pain in the joint, limitation of opening, locking of the joint, or a click. Not infrequently the pain is less clearly related to the joint and may be described as passing across the face or down the ramus and either into the neck or along the mandible. Other patients may complain of pain in the ear.

On examination the joint is usually tender to pressure. Limitation of opening may vary from the barely perceptible to the extreme. There may be deviation of the mandible as the mouth is opened: the chin coming back into the midline after the condyle has moved laterally apparently around an obstruction, or after a click or palpable thud.

Many aetiological factors have been suggested for this condition. Frequently when a patient is examined not one, but several, possible precipitants are uncovered. What causes the joint to give symptoms in one patient, but not in others with similar anomalies, remains an enigma. The main factors include abnormalities of the occlusion, particularly Angle's Class II, division 1, which require the patient to protrude in order to incise, and deep overbites which deny affected persons the facility of lateral chewing movements. Alterations and adaptations in the chewing mechanism, which a patient may have to effect because of the ravages of dental disease, can throw a considerable strain on the joints. Habitual chewing on one side of the arch and chewing on the incisors are examples of this type of disturbance. The avoidance of gaps, a sore pericoronal gum flap, or elongated unopposed teeth are other provocants. Even the insertion of a restoration with a high spot or the wrong angle of a cusp plane can precipitate symptoms.

Certain habits seem to strain the joint. Sleeping with the side of the face pressed against the pillow will displace the jaw laterally and the patient may wake with a stiff, aching joint. Nocturnal bruxism, pencil-chewing, and other habits which cause pressure on the mouth and lips can play their part.

Just as there are many aetiological factors so there are many treatments. If possible, the factor which precipitated symptoms should be identified and reversed. If this is not feasible, another factor which is amenable to alteration should be tackled. For example, if as a result of the extraction of the posterior teeth the patient is overclosing, dentures should be provided. Where there are gaps in the dental arch, these can be filled to provide more uniform use of both sides for chewing.

Advice can be given about posture during sleep, recommending that the back of the head should rest on the pillow. If a patient cannot follow this advice, a bite-locking plate can be tried. This is similar to a lower acrylic bite-raising plate, but made to fill the freeway space and with deep indentations in the upper surface for the upper teeth. Such a plate prevents lateral displacement of the jaw during sleep.

The bite-raising appliance is a standby of much temporomandibular joint treatment. In many cases the effect is probably just to alter the mechanics of joint function, at the same time providing free lateral articulation. If the patient's major complaint is of an early click, a bite-raising appliance may prevent the condyle from going back into the pre-click position.

Occlusal grinding, drugs which reduce muscle spasm, exercises, and short-wave diathermy are other forms of treatment which may prove beneficial.

Condylectomy and meniscectomy have no place in the treatment of this condition and, in general, operations of any kind should be avoided. In a few carefully selected patients the Ward condylotomy may be performed (Ward, 1961). In this procedure the condyle neck is sectioned with a Gigli saw, passed round the back of the ramus with the mouth open so that it emerges in front of the condyle neck through the sigmoid notch. When the saw is almost through, section is completed by pressure with the thumbs. Following the operation the jaw is immobilized for two weeks. Slight displacement of the condyle head occurs. As with the bite-raising appliance, it is probably the slight alteration in joint mechanics which produces the benefit.

RADIOGRAPHY AND RADIOLOGY OF THE TEMPOROMANDIBULAR JOINT

Many of the techniques and interpretations of temporomandibular joint radiography in the past were based on a narrow concept of normal function and an incomplete understanding of the applied anatomy. For the most part, disturbances of joint movement are as easily observed clinically as radiographically. Thus, the place of radiography is to confirm, or refute, the presence of overt joint disease. For this purpose the orthopantomograph emerges as the best diagnostic weapon so far (Tammisalo, 1964). Where the bony structure of the condyle and condyle neck are to be recorded, Toller's variant of the short distance, transpharyngeal technique is advocated (Toller, 1969). For an A.P. view of the condyle head and neck the transorbital A.P. is advised.

While some excellent arthrograms have been produced by a number of experts in the field, this technique has its hazards. The yield in diagnostic information is probably not enough to warrant its routine use.

SURGICAL EXPLORATION OF THE TEMPOROMANDIBULAR JOINT

Of the many surgical approaches to the temporomandibular joint that of Henny (1968) seems to have many advantages. The pre-auricular tissues are infiltrated with a vasoconstrictor and the skin incision begins in front of the pinna, runs downwards to join the crease above the tragus, and then follows the free edge of the tragus. It ends in the crease in front of the lobe of the ear. The wound is deepened by keeping the edge of a number 15 blade against the outer surface of the cartilage of the auditory canal. This separates the auriculo-temporal nerve, the superficial temporal vessels, and the upper pole of the parotid from the auditory canal. The facial nerve is safe provided that the dissection is not carried below the canal. Once the zygomatic arch is reached the temporalis fascia is divided and the tissues are swept forwards with the rounded blade of the Howarth's rugine. The middle temporal vein passes horizontally just above the zygomatic arch and this is picked up, divided, and ligated.

If the correct plane of dissection is used the tissues strip readily off the surface of the joint capsule. An L-shaped incision with one limb parallel with the floor of the articular fossa and the other vertically behind the condyle head will open the capsule.

Careful haemostasis is secured after the operative procedure has been completed and the wound closed in layers without drainage. A pressure dressing is applied for 48 hours.

REFERENCES

CAMPBELL, W. (1965), 'Clinical Radiological Investigations of the Mandibular Joint,' Br. J. Radiol., 38, 401.

HAYWARD, J. R. (1965), 'Prolonged Dislocation of the Mandible', J. oral Surg., 23, 585.

HENNY, F. A. (1957), 'Treatment of the Painful Temporomandibular Joint', Ibid. 15,. 214.

—— (1968), in Textbook of Oral Surgery 3rd ed. (ed. KRUGER, G. O.), p. 379. St. Louis: Mosby.

HOVELL, J. H. (1970), 'Surgical Correction of Facial Deformity', Ann. R. Coll. Surg., 46, 92.

LEMMER, J., and SHEAR, M. (1967), 'Oral Submucous Fibrosis', Br. dent. J., 122, 343.

MOORE, J. R., and GREENFIELD, B. E. (1967), 'Electromyographic Investigation into Postoperative Trismus'. Lecture, Meeting of the British Association of Oral Surgeons, Edinburgh, July, 1967.

PIROK, D. J., and MERRILL, R. G. (1970), 'Dislocation of the Mandibular Condyle into the Middle Cranial Fossa', *Oral Surg.*, **29**, 13.

POPESCA, V. (1960), 'A Practical Method for the Reduction of Temporomandibular Dislocation', *Stomatologia*, **4**, 87.

POSWILLO, D. E. (1973a), 'The Pathogenesis of the First and Second Branchial Arch Syndrome', *Oral Surg.*, **35**, 302–328.

— — (1973b), 'The Pathogenesis of the Treacher-Collins Syndrome', Paper presented at British Association of Oral Surgeons meeting, October 1973.

— — (1974a), 'Orofacial Malformations', *Proc. R. Soc. Med.*, **67**, 343–349.

— — (1974b), 'Otomandibular Deformity: Pathogenesis as a Guide to Reconstruction', *J. Max. fac. Surg.*, **2**, 64–72.

SIMPSON W. (1969), 'Submucous Fibrosis', *Br. J. oral Surg.*, **6**, 196.

SIRSAT, S. M. and KHANOLKAR, V. K. (1962), 'Submucous Fibrosis of the Palate and Pillars of the Fauces', *Indian J. med. Sci.*, **16**, 189.

TAMMISALO, E. H. (1964), 'Orthopantomographic Roentgenography of the Temporo-mandibular Joint', *Suom. Hammaslääk. Seur. Toim.*, **60**, 139.

TOLLER, P. A. (1969), 'The Transpharyngeal Radiography for Arthritis of the Mandibular Condyle', *Br. J. oral Surg.*, **7**, 47.

WARD, T. G. (1961), 'Surgery of the Mandibular Joint', *Ann. R. Coll. Surg.*, **28**, 139.

Chapter XX

NERVE INJURIES OF INTEREST TO THE ORAL SURGEON

THE nerves most likely to sustain damage as a result of an oral surgical procedure or a facial fracture are the facial, auriculo-temporal, mandibular, lingual, and infra-orbital.

THE FACIAL NERVE

Injury to the facial nerve results in facial paralysis.

Differential Diagnosis of Causes of Facial Paralysis.—Dealt with in detail, the differential diagnosis of causes of facial paralysis is a complex subject. Those interested in this degree of detail are referred to neurological texts. Briefly, facial paralysis may be supranuclear, nuclear, and infranuclear in origin or due to primary degeneration of the muscles of facial expression.

Supranuclear Paralysis.—The commonest cause of supranuclear facial nerve paralysis is a stroke. Movements of the lower part of the face are more severely affected than those of the upper. There is no reaction of degeneration when the nerve is electrically stimulated and emotional facial movements are unimpaired. Rarely the reverse state is seen and there is loss of emotional facial expression.

Nuclear and Infranuclear Paralysis.—Lesions within the pons may affect the VI nucleus because of the curvature of the facial nerve-fibres around the nucleus. More extensive lesions will involve the spinal tract of V, the motor fibres of V, and spinothalamic and pyramidal tracts destined for the upper and lower limb of the other side.

Within the posterior cranial fossa facial paralysis is associated with deafness and vestibular disturbances, due to damage to the VIII nerve. There is an associated loss of taste in the anterior two-thirds of the tongue.

Damage to the nerve within the facial canal is usually associated with damage to the taste fibres of the anterior two-thirds of the tongue, either while they are with the nerve or in the chorda tympani. Should the branch to the stapedius be involved there will be hyperacusis, but loss of salivary secretion due to damage to secreto-motor fibres is not easily appreciated. Lesions in the last part of the facial canal do not affect taste and the commonest cause here is Bell's palsy. Occasionally the lesion in Bell's palsy migrates sufficiently far proximally to affect the chorda tympani and then taste is affected.

Outside the stylomastoid foramen the nerve branches almost immediately, but loss of function in the stylohyoid muscle, the posterior belly of the digastric, and occipital belly of the occipito-frontalis, which are supplied by the first branches, is difficult to spot clinically. Damage to individual branches within, or distal to, the parotid gland is more easily distinguished.

Primary Muscular Weakness and Degeneration.—Myasthenia gravis, muscular dystrophy, and dystrophia myotonica are possible causes of facial weakness in this group. Other muscular groups elsewhere in the body will be involved.

Electrical Stimulation Tests.—Following inadvertent trauma to the facial nerve, tests with electrical stimulation are of some value in ascertaining the extent of the nerve damage.

The Reaction of Degeneration.—Normal muscles respond to stimulation by faradic and galvanic current (interrupted and constant). Faradism causes a muscular contraction which persists as long as the current is passing, but galvanism causes a muscular contraction only when the current is made or broken. In normal muscle, if the kathode is used (a kathodal closing current, KCC) a more vigorous response is obtained than when the anode (anodal closing current, ACC) is used. Following a lower motor neuron lesion a muscle ceases to respond to faradic stimulation of its motor point in 4–7 days and after 10 days a normal response to galvanism ceases, though the muscle may respond with a sluggish contraction. At this time the ACC is more effective than the KCC, a condition known as 'polar reversal'. Taken collectively these phenomena constitute the reaction of degeneration.

According to Brain (1962) electrical records obtained directly from muscles by electromyography give much more detailed and accurate information of muscular function than the test for reaction of degeneration which will be superseded by electromyography.

Oral surgical procedures may occasionally produce a temporary or a permanent facial paralysis if one or more branches of the seventh nerve are inadvertently severed (neurotmesis) or bruised (neurapraxia). The possibility of cutting the facial nerve or one or more of its branches must always be considered when incisions are made on the face, especially when carrying out surgery in the temporomandibular joint area. Nerve damage may also occur through misplaced incisions when opening facial abscesses, but the most commonly damaged branch of the facial nerve is the mandibular branch which can be inadvertently severed during a submandibular surgical approach to the mandible. This injury leaves the patient with an ugly weakness of the angle of the lower lip. All submandibular incisions must therefore be made at least 1 cm. beneath the lower border of the mandible in order to avoid this mishap. Branches of the facial nerve may also be bruised as a result of rough retraction, excessive postoperative swelling of the cheek, or by blunt dissection in the vicinity of the facial nerve. Temporary facial paralysis may also be caused through a misdirected mandibular injection in which the analgesic solution is deposited too far posteriorly and diffuses within the parotid gland. The resultant unilateral facial paralysis is complete and, though it is alarming to both patient and operator, it is a purely temporary phenomenon and normal muscle movement is gradually restored as the effect of the local analgesic wears off.

Treatment.—Facial paralysis is an ugly deformity and the management of the case depends upon whether the condition is likely to be permanent or if there is hope of recovery. Most cases of Bell's palsy tend to recover though progress is slow in the older patient. When recovery is anticipated the musculature of the cheek should be lifted by fitting an intra-oral prosthetic appliance attached to the patient's teeth or denture which is designed to lift the cheek and side of the lip. This helps to mask the facial deformity and removes tension on the cheek. The rheumatologist may suggest electrical stimulation of the muscles to improve their tone until re-innervation begins. When the nerve begins to recover, feeble muscular movement is seen and at this stage the patient should be instructed to exercise the affected side while facing a mirror. In order to prevent the overaction of the unaffected side of the face interfering with the exercise, the patient should hold one hand firmly over the normal side of the face to prevent its muscle pull interfering with muscular movements on the affected side. In most instances recovery is a slow process.

The treatment of facial paralysis where there is no hope of recovery is not particularly rewarding and none of the suggested treatments is uniformly effective. The possibilities are:—

1. *A Nerve Graft.*

2. *An Anastomosis* of the proximal section of the facial nerve to the spinal accessory.

3. *Sling Operations* where the angle of the mouth and cheek are connected by a sling within the tissues to some stable point such as a hole drilled in the zygomatic bone. The slings are made of fascia lata, kangaroo tendon, floss silk, polythene tape, stainless-steel wire, etc., which are threaded through the tissues with a straight needle. The results are not particularly impressive and many of the materials such as fascia lata stretch, so leading to a relapse of the deformity. On the other hand, materials such as stainless-steel or tantalum wire do not stretch, but they tend to become unduly prominent beneath the skin and constitute an unacceptable deformity.

4. *Re-animation Procedures.*—Various re-animation procedures have been suggested where strips of active muscle, such as the temporalis or masseter muscle, are connected to the angle of the mouth and cheek. If the operation is successful considerable training of the patient is necessary to enable the best use to be made of the new muscle connexion.

5. *Disguising Procedures.*—This treatment consists of a series of cosmetic operations to restore an appearance of normality to the affected side. The main procedures are a unilateral face-lifting procedure and a partial tarsorrhaphy to correct the droop of the lower lid. An incision is made in the nasolabial fold on the affected side and incisions are made to correspond with the creases in the normal side of the forehead. These incisions are sutured so that an inverted scar is formed and the two sides of the face are then relatively similar. If these procedures are skilfully performed the results are quite good.

6. *Selective Neurectomy.*—It has been suggested that by cutting the corresponding branches of the facial nerve on the unaffected side of the face, a harmonious muscular balance can be achieved. In practice this procedure produces a most lugubrious expression.

THE AURICULO-TEMPORAL NERVE

Gustatory Sweating and Flushing.—Frey-Baillarger syndrome. Dupuy's syndrome, auriculo-temporal and chorda tympani syndromes.

The auriculo-temporal nerve, in addition to supplying sensory fibres to the pre-auricular and temporal areas, carries parasympathetic fibres to the parotid gland and sympathetic vasomotor and pseudomotor fibres to the skin of the same area. Injury to the auriculo-temporal nerve denervates the sweat-glands and vessels of the skin over its distribution in addition to producing sensory disturbances. Both the parasympathetic and sympathetic nerves of the face are cholinergic and in the process of regeneration parasympathetic fibres become misdirected and grow along sympathetic pathways. Thus, a gustatory stimulus produces sweating and flushing. This syndrome develops about five or more weeks after injury to the auriculo-temporal nerve. The syndrome is usually permanent, but regression and even disappearance of the symptoms may occur in a very small proportion of cases. There is no effective treatment.

THE MANDIBULAR NERVE

The mandibular nerve may be inadvertently severed as a result of fracture of the mandible or it may be bruised or sectioned during surgery. The most common sites of injury are in the lower 3rd molar area and where the nerve emerges from the mental foramen. The mandibular nerve supplies a small area to one side of the lower lip and cutting or bruising the nerve results in anaesthesia of this section of the lower lip. Fortunately, this area of the lower lip has an accessory nerve-supply from C2 and C3 and some recovery of sensation can be confidently anticipated in all instances, though the patient may complain of a variation in quality of the sensation compared with the normal side. Recovery following neurapraxia may take from 6 weeks to 3 months and following neurotmesis recovery takes 18 months to 2 years. Some patients experience protracted hyperaesthesia during the recovery period, but in the course of time recovery is more or less complete. In all the long-term follow-up surveys of mandibular fractures complete recovery of sensation in the lower lip is found in almost all cases.

Since anaesthesia of the lower lip is not particularly uncommon after the removal of impacted 3rd molars, this situation can be considered further to illustrate the ways in which this nerve may be damaged. Anaesthesia may be present immediately following recovery from the effects of the anaesthetic. Such anaesthesia may be due to pressure on the nerve during elevation of the tooth or a transmitted shock wave during tooth division with an osteotome. A neurapraxia results and early and complete recovery of normal sensation will occur. Alternatively, the nerve may have been crushed, but continuity of the bundle remains. Degeneration occurs and the condition is known as 'axonotmesis'. Recovery will be delayed and will be accompanied by paraesthesia (unpleasant, abnormal sensation), but this will be short-lived and ultimate recovery will be complete.

If the nerve has been completely severed (neurotmesis) recovery will again be delayed until regeneration occurs and the paraesthesiae will persist until cortical reorientation has taken place. Ultimate recovery may not be perfect.

It may be possible with an intelligent patient to distinguish between neurapraxia and neurotmesis, even within 48 hours of the operation, since the loss of sensation is usually more profound with the latter.

In some cases lip sensation is normal immediately after recovery from the anaesthetic, but sensory impairment develops over the next 24 hours.

This is often due to a rise in pressure within the inferior dental canal as a result of postoperative oedema. The defect is a neurapraxia and resolves quite rapidly. A similar sequence may follow the handling of the nerve in circumstances which make it unlikely that there is a postoperative increase in pressure.

THE LINGUAL NERVE

If the lingual nerve is severed loss of sensation in the anterior two-thirds of the tongue occurs. This area of the tongue has no accessory nerve supply and neurotmesis results in loss of sensation. The lingual nerve may be inadvertently severed during lower 3rd molar surgery, for the nerve runs very superficially on the lingual aspect of the mandible in this area. The nerve must be retracted and protected by an instrument such as a Howarth's periosteal elevator when operating on lower 3rd molars. Retraction should be gentle or neurapraxia may occur. The nerve may also be kinked at the pterygo-mandibular raphe or under-run with a suture, particularly if much bone has to be removed to uncover the 3rd molar. Such an injury usually recovers comparatively rapidly, but occasionally unilateral anaesthesia of the anterior two-thirds of the tongue may be protracted. Surgical exploration of the lingual nerve in patients where the nerve has been severed has shown a neuroma on the proximal end of the nerve. Muscular movements of the tongue probably preclude the possibility of regeneration of the lingual nerve following neurotmesis.

THE NERVE TO THE MYLOHYOID

Recently (Roberts and Harris, 1973) attention has been drawn to the occurrence of small patches of anaesthesia in the lower part of the chin and close to the midline as a sequel to lower 3rd molar surgery. It has been shown by these authors that selective infiltration of the nerve to the mylohyoid will produce an identical area of anaesthesia. They postulate that neurapraxia of the nerve may be caused by the retraction of the soft tissues in an attempt to protect the lingual nerve.

THE INFRA-ORBITAL NERVE

Neurapraxia or neurotmesis of the infra-orbital nerve occurs as a result of fracture of the zygomatic bone and in Le Fort 2- and 3-type fractures. It results in anaesthesia of one side of the upper lip, the side of the nose, and an area of the cheek. Recovery of sensation in the affected area can be confidently expected in almost all cases, though if the nerve is severed it may take 8–12 months.

REFERENCES

BRAIN, R. (1962), *Diseases of the Nervous System*, 6th ed. London: Oxford University Press.
ROBERTS, E. D. D., and HARRIS, M. (1973), 'Neurapraxia of the Mylohyoid Nerve and Sub-mental Analgesia', *Br. J. oral Surg.*, **11**, 110.

CHAPTER XXI

SOME NON-PYOGENIC INFECTIONS OF THE SOFT TISSUES

ALL non-pyogenic infections are of interest and importance to the oral surgeon, but it is obviously impractical in a work of this nature to discuss such infections as leprosy and yaws, etc. Even the non-pyogenic infections such as syphilis and tuberculosis are becoming rarer at the present time in countries where effective therapy is available. In any case, only limited features of these diseases are of particular concern to the oral surgeon, and discussion will be confined to the relevant aspects of these infections.

SYPHILIS

It is of primary importance that syphilitic lesions are recognized early in view of the risk to both operator and patient. It is therefore imperative that the possibility of a syphilitic infection should always be considered whenever an unusual ulcerative lesion is encountered and when operation sites fail to heal in the usual manner. Soft tissue manifestations of syphilis can occur anywhere in the oral cavity, but lesions are most commonly encountered on the lip and tongue and occur during the primary, second-ary, or tertiary stage. Meyer and Shklar (1967) published 81 cases of oral lesions in acquired syphilis, and they concluded that oral manifestations were rare in the primary and secondary stages since 84 per cent of their cases occurred in the tertiary stage.

The Lip.—The lip is said to be the most common extragenital site for chancre. The lesion presents as a smooth elevated, painless, coppery-coloured ulcer which is about 0·5–1 cm. in diameter and is surrounded by an area of induration. The upper lip is usually affected and within a few weeks the regional lymph-nodes undergo a shotty enlargement. The condition must be distinguished from a neoplasm. However, carcinoma usually affects the lower lip and a chancre develops much more rapidly than a malignant ulcer. The diagnosis is, of course, confirmed by identifica-tion of the spirochaete on dark ground illumination from a direct smear of the ulcer or after scarification of the lesion. It should be remembered that few patients will admit to contact which would have resulted in a venereal infection and, therefore, a history of exposure is seldom obtained. It is also important to remember that the Wassermann and Kahn reactions and V.D.R.L. slide test do not become positive until infection has been present for 6 weeks to 3 months.

Mucous Patches.—Mucous patches in the mouth are sometimes seen by the oral surgeon when examining a patient suffering from the secondary stage of syphilis, and a speedy diagnosis is essential in view of the increased risk of infection to both patient and operator at this period.

The Tongue.—Primary syphilis can affect the tongue and the chancre usually occurs on or near the tip. There is a lymphadenopathy of the cervical nodes within 10 days. The secondary rash can also involve the tongue and in tertiary syphilis the tongue may be affected by a midline gumma which, on breaking down, forms a characteristic punched-out type of ulcer with a washleather slough.

Leucoplakia.—Leucoplakia of syphilitic origin has already been discussed. (*See* p. 122.)

Primary Syphilis of the Gingiva.—In 1921 Klauder reviewed the literature and found 113 reported cases of primary syphilis of the gingiva. Straith (1937) added a further 42 cases. In 1966 Steiner and Alexander reported 2 more cases. The typical primary manifestation is an erosive ulcerative lesion with a smooth red surface which may be as much as 2–3 cm. in diameter. There is a regional lymphadenopathy.

TUBERCULOSIS

It is generally agreed that oral manifestations of tuberculosis are usually secondary to lesions elsewhere in the body, especially the lungs. However, primary tubercular lesions have been reported by Boyes (1956), Brand and Ballard (1951), Miller (1953), Galloway and Horne (1953). Darlington and Salman (1937) reported 27 cases of tubercular lesions in the mouth. Tuberculous lesions may appear anywhere in the oral cavity, and according to Carmody, Appleton, and Ivy (1923) the most common site is the tongue, especially the tip. Brodsky (1942) lists the following sites for his 72 patients: pharynx, 22; tonsils, 19; tongue, 16; cheeks, gingiva, and floor of mouth, 9; lips, 6.

Tuberculosis of the Tongue.—Tuberculosis may reach the tongue from the exterior, by auto-inoculation from affected sputum, by haematogenous or lymphatic spread, and by direct spread from neighbouring structures. The infection may take the form of tubercles, tuberculoma, cold abscess, tuberculous fissures, or papillomas and ulcers.

The Tuberculoma.—The tuberculoma usually ulcerates early, but occasionally it may reach a considerable size before ulcerating and when this occurs it must be distinguished from a gumma on the tongue.

Tuberculous Fissures.—Tuberculous fissures occur at the sides or tip of the tongue and are often stellate or branched.

Tuberculous Papillomas.—Tuberculous papillomas occur as an overgrowth of epithelium at the edges of tuberculous fissures.

The Tuberculous Ulcer.—The tuberculous ulcer is the most common tuberculous lesion and usually develops as a tiny tubercle which ulcerates. The ulcers are always at the tip of the tongue and may extend backwards along its sides. They are shallow, yellowish, and are usually very painful, but not always, while their edges are sloping rather than undermined and the ulcer is deeper than it appears. Unlike tuberculous ulcers in other situations, they are usually painful and extremely tender. The tubercle bacillus may be found, but bacteriological identification is often difficult if the ulcer is secondarily infected. The patient is usually suffering from pulmonary tuberculosis and the ulcers in the mouth tend to reflect the progress of the lesion in the lungs and improve with the pulmonary disease.

However, the tongue is seldom affected until the pulmonary disease is well advanced. The oral surgeon may also encounter tuberculous ulceration on the neck and if it is associated with severe oral sepsis the patient may have been referred in the erroneous belief that the oral sepsis is responsible for the breakdown of the lymph-nodes. Tuberculous ulceration in the neck is due to breakdown of an affected lymph-node which has formed a cold abscess. Characteristically the base of the ulcer is soft and pale and it is covered with granulations. The edges of the ulcer tend to be bluish and undermined. The outline is serpigenous and there may be a watery discharge. Bacteriological examination of the ulcer reveals the characteristic acid-fast tubercle bacillus. More than one broken-down lymph-node may be present. Bailey (1933) recorded tuberculosis infection in a branchial cyst. Occasionally the oral surgeon is confronted with a cold abscess which has resulted from the breakdown of a submandibular lymph-node. It is important to diagnose the lesion by aspiration before incising the abscess for tuberculous lesions are notoriously slow to heal and the incisions tend to produce ugly keloid scarring.

LUPUS VULGARIS

The dusky red, slightly elevated lesions with pale pink scarred areas interspersed have sharp margins and pale apple-jelly nodules which can be demonstrated with a glass slide. They occasionally may become ulcerative lesions of lupus vulgaris (tuberculous infection of the skin), but are virtually never seen these days, and with them has gone one cause of carcinoma of the face. Patients with destruction of the nose from old, healed lesions are still seen from time to time.

ANTHRAX

Anthrax is a disease caused by the *Bacillus anthracis* which occurs in both man and animals. The oral surgeon may occasionally encounter the cutaneous variety of the disease in patients who work with animal skins such as tanners, butchers, veterinary surgeons, etc. This condition is called the 'malignant pustule' which occurs as a result of the entrance of the anthrax bacillus through a cutaneous abrasion on some exposed body surface such as the face. The lesion is usually solitary and commonly on the face. The incubation period is 2 hours to 7 days, but is usually 24–48 hours. Itching is followed by pain and the appearance of a red papule. This develops a central vesicle surrounded by an area of hyperaemia and by the third day the vesicle bursts and the centre of the papule becomes a black necrotic area which is surrounded by secondary vesicles which also slough. The area is surrounded by marked oedema. Even a tiny pustule may be followed by septicaemia when it occurs on the face. The oedema may spread to the glottis. Onset of septicaemia usually leads to a fatal termination. This dangerous condition must always be considered in patients who may have been at risk due to their occupation. The condition must be distinguished from a virulent furuncle and accidental vaccinia.

Treatment: The *B. anthracis* is susceptible to penicillin which should be used in large doses.

ECTHYMA CONTAGIOSUM (ORF)

This is the infection in man caused by the virus of ovine pustular dermatitis and is transmitted to man by direct contact with live or dead affected lambs and sheep or indirectly through fomites. Three to seven days after inoculation there is a macule at the portal of entry and then a papule. The papule enlarges rapidly up to 1–4 cm. in diameter and is covered with small vesicles containing clear fluid. The vesicles coalesce into a flaccid, white, umbilicated bulla which breaks down and then the lesion crusts over. Healing can take 4–8 weeks and the regional nodes are enlarged.

These rather florid lesions may be mistaken for a variety of infective and inflammatory processes about the jaws such as tuberculosis, and even for malignant neoplasms. Diagnosis depends in part on obtaining a suggestive history of contact with sheep. The topical application of Dermevan Iodophor speeds resolution of the lesions (Parnell, 1965).

REFERENCES

BAILEY, H. (1933), 'The Clinical Aspects of Branchial Fistulae', *Br. J. Surg.*, **21**, 173.
BOYES, J. (1956), 'Oral Pathology in Children', *Proc. R. Soc. Med.*, **43**, 503.
BRAND, T. A., and BALLARD, C. F. (1951), 'Oral Tuberculosis', *Archs Dis. Childh.*, **26**, 261.
BRODSKY, R. H. (1942), 'Oral Tuberculous Lesions', *Am. J. Orthod.*, **28**, 132.
CARMODY, T. E., APPLETON, J. L., and IVY, R. H. (1923), 'Diagnostic Importance of Tuberculous Lesions of Oral Cavity', *Dent. Summary*, **44**, 233.
DARLINGTON, C. G., and SALMAN, I. (1937), 'Oral Tuberculous Lesions', *Am. Revue Tuberc.*, **35**, 147.
GALLOWAY, W. J., and HORNE, N. W. (1953), 'Primary Tuberculosis Infection of the Gum', *Br. dent. J.*, **15**, 9.
KLAUDER, J. (1921), 'Wassermann Test with Secretions, Transudates and Exudates in Syphilis', *Dent. Cosmos*, **53**, 1067.
MEYER, I., and SHKLAR, G. (1967), 'The Oral Manifestations of Acquired Syphilis', *Oral Surg.*, **23**, 45.
MILLER, F. J. W. (1953), 'Recognition of Primary Tuberculous Infection of Skin and Mucosae', *Lancet*, **1**, 5.
PARNELL, A. G. (1965), 'Ecthyma contagiosum (Orf)', *Br. J. oral Surg.*, **3**, 128.
STEINER, M., and ALEXANDER, W. N. (1966), 'Primary Syphilis of the Gingiva', *Oral Surg.*, **21**, 530.
STRAITH, F. (1937), 'Chancre of the Gingiva', *Am. dent. Ass. J.*, **24**, 196.

CHAPTER XXII

THE FUNGAL DISEASES

ACTINOMYCOSIS

HUMAN cervicofacial actinomycosis is a comparatively rare disease, but even so it is one of the most common of the systemic mycoses. It is caused by an anaerobic, Gram-positive, branched filamentous organism, the *Actinomyces israeli*, which was first isolated by Wolff and Israel in 1891, though many authorities consider that it is a variant of the *Actinomyces bovis* which causes 'lumpy jaw' in cattle. However, Ajello (1968) states that *A. israeli* is an exclusively human parasite while *A. bovis* causes actinomycosis in animals and that, on biochemical and antigenic properties, they have been proved to be distinct and separate entities. At one time some confusion occurred between the human pathogen and some saprophytic varieties of the organism that were found outside the body, and this gave rise to the myth that the disease could be introduced into the mouth by sucking a straw. Even so, actinomycosis is more common in country populations (Aird, 1957).

The usual pattern of the condition is one of a chronic granulomatous infection which eventually results in abscess formation and drainage via multiple fistulae. Macroscopic examination of pus from the abscess may show small bright yellow or grey lumps known as 'sulphur granules'. Microscopic examination of these granules shows colonies of the actinomyces. Sulphur granules are not found in all cases and in a series of 32 patients with actinomycosis, sulphur granules were only seen in 5 instances (Thoma, 1969). The actinomycete has long been known to be a commensal in the oral cavity of man where it lives in competitive existence with other micro-organisms and the actinomycete israeli can be demonstrated in and cultured from carious teeth, crypts of the tonsils, and dental calculus. There are no authenticated records of the isolation of *A. israeli* from soil or any other inanimate source (Ajello, 1968).

The pathogenesis of actinomycosis is imperfectly understood, but it may occur following trauma such as the extraction of a tooth or a jaw fracture which provides a portal of entry for the organism into underlying tissues. Goldin (1945) and Rowe and Killey (1970) reported actinomycosis following a jaw fracture. Zachary Cope (1920) considered that actinomycosis would not occur in the absence of a carious cavity in a tooth, and Aird (1958) says that the disease is of low incidence in the edentulous. It has been suggested that organisms can enter the tissues via a carious cavity or a periodontal pocket, but this is not proved.

Actinomycosis is classified anatomically as: (1) Cervicofacial, (2) Pulmonary, (3) Abdominal. The cervicofacial form is the most common variety of the disease and comprises two-thirds of all cases (New and Figi, 1923). It is of prime interest to the oral surgeon, though Zachary Cope (1962) reported a case of a dental surgeon who attempted an extraction for a colleague, a general surgeon, and inadvertently displaced the fractured crown of the tooth into the surgeon's lung, a mishap which resulted in the unfortunate patient developing pulmonary actinomycosis.

Clinical Features.—Organisms which enter the underlying tissues through the oral mucosa may remain localized in the soft tissues or spread to involve the salivary glands, bone, or skin of the face and neck. The fungus has a preference for growth in the fascia and subcutaneous tissues.

Actinomycosis in the upper jaw may extend to involve the meninges and Zitka (1952) reported a case in which a fatal meningitis occurred. He also reported cases from the German literature with metastatic involvement of the lungs, liver, kidney, and brain. Once the organism gains admittance to the tissues it gives rise to an infection which results in a low-grade swelling and induration of the tissues. Eventually, abscess formation occurs and the pus is discharged extra-orally through multiple skin sinuses. (*Fig.* 46.)

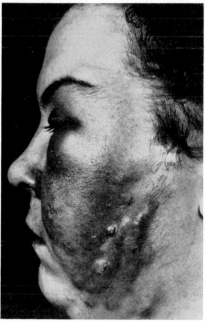

Fig. 46.—Actinomycosis of the cheek. After the cervical region this is the most common site for this infection about the jaws. The skin is a purplish-red colour and there are multiple subcutaneous hemispherical abscesses and multiple sinuses.

This results in scarring and cosmetic deformity due to puckering of the skin. The soft tissue infections may extend to involve the bone. Usually the mandible is affected, but the condition can also occur in the maxillae and it results in fungal osteomyelitis which causes extensive bone destruction. The radiological appearance of such a lesion resembles an osteitis.

On rare occasions the salivary glands are involved. In a case seen by the authors the patient presented with a hard, painless swelling of the right submandibular gland. There was no history of dental extractions on that side and the patient did not have a rise in temperature. The white-cell count and the sedimentation rate were normal. A sialogram showed an irregular space-occupying lesion and the pathological process continued to increase in size in spite of two courses of antibiotic therapy. A neoplasm was suspected and a very experienced general surgeon confirmed the diagnosis. At operation he encountered extreme difficulty in removing the gland owing to the marked induration of the tissues. The submandibular gland appeared to be the seat of a squamous-cell carcinoma when it was examined macroscopically after removal, but pathological examination proved the condition to be actinomycosis.

When the soft tissues are affected there is usually a history of extraction or fracture in the area some five weeks previously. The swelling is hard, indurated, and painless and resistant to antibiotic therapy administered empirically. Later, it may or may not break down to discharge pus through multiple sinuses and at this stage the sulphur granules may be seen. In the absence of a discharge the swelling should be aspirated to obtain pus for bacteriological examination. Actinomycosis should be suspected whenever an abscess-like swelling in the region of the jaws fails to respond to anti-biotic therapy of the customary duration, 7–10 days, and which shows no signs of improvement or worsening. Routine investigations such as the white cell-count and sedimentation rate are often normal.

Treatment.—Treatment is by protracted antibiotic therapy and penicillin remains the drug of choice. Of the various preparations available, fortified procaine penicillin B.P. in 2–3 ml. doses daily or phenoxymethylpenicillin 250 mg. 6-hourly for a period of six to eight weeks are suitable. It has been demonstrated by Holm (1948) that some strains of actinomyces develop a resistance to penicillin. However, Blake (1964) demonstrated that the resistance of the colonies to antibiotics has been shown to be solely a resistance to bactericidal effect, and he found no evidence of strain variation to the bacteriostatic effect of antibiotics. Oxytetracycline 250 mg. 6-hourly is an alternative to penicillin when patients are hypersensitive to that drug, and recent work by Blake (1970) shows that lincomycin is efficacious in the treatment of actinomycosis. Occasionally a low-grade abscess-like swelling is found to contain actinomycete on bacteriological examination of the pus following aspiration or incision and drainage, and yet the lesion will resolve on minimal antibiotic therapy and in some instances incision and drainage of the area alone is sufficient to eradicate the disease. This raises the possibility that there are two varieties of the disease with organisms which appear bacteriologically similar, or that there is a variation in the pathogenicity of the organism. Hertz (1960) employed the term 'pseudoactinomycosis' for cases in which the smear shows only a few mycelia and where a tender swelling contains foul-smelling pus. Anomalies in the clinical behaviour and response to treat-ment of some abscesses which appear to be due to actinomycosis may result from an inability in the present state of knowledge to distinguish organisms which resemble the actinomycete israeli.

CANDIDIASIS

Candidiasis, or monilial infection, is an acute or chronic fungal disease involving the superficial tissues of skin or mucous membrane and more rarely it may disseminate haematogenously to produce systemic disease. Septicaemic candidiasis is often not diagnosed until the post mortem and according to Wright and Symmers (1966) the incidence has risen with the introduction of the corticosteroids. Chronic candidiasis can affect the skin, nails, and hair follicles, while in the lungs it may present as a pneumonia or a lung abscess.

Man can be infected with a variety of candida organisms which are commonly present in the mouth, vagina, sputum, and stools of otherwise normal persons. Monilial infection in the form of oral thrush, skin lesions, or disseminated disease can arise in patients with other diseases or under special circumstances, i.e., in infancy, old age, diabetes, debilitation, antibacterial treatment, pregnancy, etc. Barlow and Chattaway (1969) found a 45 per cent incidence of candida in 125 patients. There tends to be an exacerbation of monilial infection of the vagina before menstruation and in pregnancy. Oral thrush in infants may be the result of infection from the vagina during childbirth (Winner and Hurley, 1964). It is not uncommon to find oral thrush in one or more young children in a family when the mother is known to have severe monilial infection of the vagina. The source of the children's infection probably results from poor hygiene on the part of the mother.

Clinical Features.—The oral lesions may occur on any mucosal surface and are white or greyish-white, discrete or confluent patches which resemble curdled milk. If the patch is removed a raw bleeding area is left in the underlying membrane. Various clinical types have been described in the oral cavity. In infants the condition is referred to as thrush, but in adults the plaque-like lesions are less friable and are thicker. Atrophic candidiasis has been recognized in various conditions such as denture-sore mouth, angular cheilitis, and glossitis. Chronic lesions may become hyperkeratinized and develop pseudoepitheliomatous hyperplasia. *Candida leucoplakia* or chronic hyperplastic or hypertrophic candidiasis may show a strong tendency to undergo neoplastic change and such cases cannot be clinically differentiated from leucoplakia due to other causes. Oral candidiasis is sometimes seen during protracted antibiotic therapy especially when tetracycline is used. Angular cheilitis in edentulous patients with a markedly overclosed bite often has the commissural fissures infected with *Candida albicans*.

Systemic candidiasis with a fatal outcome has been reported in 4 patients following dental extractions and these cases have been reviewed by Lehner (1964), though in an experimental study of the blood of 50 post-extraction cases candida was not cultured. According to Zegarelli and Kutschner (1964), 4 of their cases under treatment with topically applied corticosteroid developed monilial infection. Denture-sore mouth may be due to monilial infection in some instances and Cawson (1963) isolated *C. albicans* in 23 patients out of a series of 35 cases suffering from denture-sore mouth.

Treatment.—Thrush in infants is best treated with a 1 per cent aqueous solution of one of the aniline dyes such as gentian violet, brilliant green, neutral red, etc., while adults and children over 5 years of age can be treated with nystatin or amphotericin B—4 tablets or lozenges respectively should be taken daily and sucked slowly. Severe monilial infection arising as a result of protracted antibiotic therapy should be treated by stopping the antibiotic and prescribing nystatin, or by painting the area with one of the aniline dyes in a 1 per cent aqueous solution. Candidal leucoplakia is best treated by excision of the leucoplakic patch, but if this is impractical a protracted course of nystatin is often efficacious. Angular cheilitis due to monilial infection may be associated with an overclosed bite or iron deficiency, and this should be corrected. Nystatin should be used if the condition fails to improve after the correction of the bite and if this is not effective, the area should be excised and a Z-plasty performed.

Often secondary to the antifungal treatment of denture sore-mouth, one or more of the following measures may be necessary:—

1. Correct denture hygiene by using a detergent to clean it, e.g. cetrimide.

2. Correct the height of bite of the denture.

3. Correct the fit and eliminate roughness on the underside of the denture which abrades the palate as a result of:—

a. Alginate impressions—mucus on the palate.

b. Bubbles in models.

c. Too much detail in the model.

4. Process new dentures against burnished foil.

5. Use vacuumed or vibrated stone model.

6. Free lateral articulation of teeth to reduce movement over the ridge.

7. Treat papillary palatal hyperplasia.

8. Correct posture of lip by placing canines in proper buccopalatal position and use of 'plumpers'.

9. Use nystatin cream under the denture, but better still leave the denture out while taking nystatin tablets, on a dosage basis of 4 daily.

It is also advisable to investigate the haemoglobin level, the serum iron concentrate, and iron absorption and utilization to exclude iron deficiency. If the condition is recurrent in a young person, the possibility of *Candida vaginitis* must be considered in women, and proctitis must also be excluded, for either of these conditions may re-infect the mouth.

HISTOPLASMOSIS

Histoplasmosis is a systemic fungal disease which is respiratory in origin and spreads via the pulmonary lymphatics and blood to mediastinal lymph-nodes, spleen, liver, kidneys, and skin. The central nervous system, heart, and other organs may also be affected. The disease may be asymptomatic, acute, or progressive and eventually fatal.

Aetiology.—The causative organism is the *Histoplasma capsulatum*. The disease usually occurs in infancy or old age and it affects the sexes equally. Man is infected by inhalation of dust contaminated with the organisms, and soil from chicken houses or bat and bird droppings are rich in the organisms. The disease can also affect animals such as dogs and cats.

Clinical Manifestations.—Primary infection is usually asymptomatic, but there is often a febrile respiratory disease, cough, shortness of breath, chest pain, and even haemoptysis. The pulmonary symptoms may resolve completely, but occasionally the disease may progress to the severe disseminated form in which there is pyrexia, weight-loss, lymphadenopathy, and anaemia. There may be local lesions in the mouth which are nodular, ulcerative or vegetative, and these are associated with a marked lymphadenopathy. The tongue, lips, and cheeks are most commonly affected and biopsy of the lesions may be suggestive of neoplastic change.

Diagnosis.—The isolation, culture, and identification of the fungus microscopically are required in order to diagnose the disease. There are also skin and complement-fixation tests available. Biopsies of mucosal lesions may be suggestive of carcinoma and the material must be cultured to confirm the disease.

Treatment.—Amphotericin B is the most effective antifungal drug available at present, but X-5079, a polypeptide drug, has been shown to have strong antifungal activity.

NORTH AMERICAN BLASTOMYCOSIS

This disease, commonly known as 'North American Blastomycosis', is caused by the fungus *Blastomyces dermatitidis*. It used to be thought that the condition was confined to North America, but there have been recent reports of the condition from several African countries such as the Republics of Zaïre (formerly Congo), and of South Africa, Tanzania, Tunisia, and Uganda (Destombes and Drouhet, 1964; Emmons and others, 1964). Cases have also been reported from Latin America (Arias Luzardo, 1962). The source of the infection in human beings is unknown, but it is a chronic systemic fungal disease which is respiratory in origin that clinically disseminates to skin, subcutaneous tissue, bone, and other organs. The disease is found more commonly in men than in women.

Clinical Features.—The disease starts as an acute respiratory infection and, although the cutaneous lesions are respiratory in origin, they are often the presenting symptom. The cutaneous lesions start as small, red papules which increase in size and form tiny pustules which ulcerate and discharge pus through tiny fistulae. These coalesce and crateriform lesions with elevated borders are formed, but sometimes the lesion becomes warty. Systemic spread can occur as a result of the infection becoming disseminated through the subcutaneous tissues into the blood-stream. This results in pyrexia, weight-loss, and, if the lungs are infected, a productive cough.

When the condition occurs in the mouth a chronic granulomatous lesion arises with multiple sinuses which resembles actinomycosis.

Diagnosis.—The diagnosis is made by culture of the *B. dermatitidis* from pus or lesions.

Treatment.—Amphotericin B has been used extensively for all forms of the disease.

SOUTH AMERICAN BLASTOMYCOSIS

This type of blastomycosis is caused by *Paracoccidioides brasiliensis*, which affects workers in the coffee-growing regions of Brazil. The fungus is related to the North American form of the disease, the South American fungus being considerably larger, varying in size between 10 and 60 microns.

Clinical Findings.—The disease starts as a small papular lesion often on the cutaneous surface of the lip and resembles a squamous-cell carcinoma. The condition may also involve the gingiva and may begin following a dental extraction. The regional lymph-nodes are enlarged and hard and may resemble either tubercular adenitis or those of Hodgkin's disease. The lungs may become secondarily infected.

Diagnosis.—Diagnosis is by culture of the organism.

Treatment.—Treatment is with amphotericin B.

REFERENCES

AIRD, I. (1957), *A Companion in Surgical Studies*, 2nd ed., p. 91. Edinburgh: Livingstone.

AJELLO, L. (1968), *Systemic Mycoses*, p. 130. Ciba Foundation Symposium. London: Churchill.

ARIAS LUZARDO, J. J. (1962), Doctoral Thesis, Universidad Nacional Autonoma de Mexico, Escuela National de Medicina.

BARLOW, A. J. E., and CHATTAWAY, F. W. (1969), 'Observations on the Carriage of *Candida Albicans* in Man', *Br. J. Dermat.*, **81**, 103.

BLAKE, G. C. (1964), 'Sensitivities of Colonies and Suspensions of *Actinomyces Israeli* to Penicillins, Tetracyclines and Erythromycin', *Br. med. J.*, **1**, 145.

— — (1970), personal communication.

CAWSON, R. A. (1963), 'Denture Sore Mouth and Angular Cheilitis. Oral Candidiasis in Adults', *Br. dent. J.*, **115**, 441.

COPE, V. Z. (1920), 'Actinomycosis considered specially in its Relationship to the Jaws', *Ibid.*, **41**, 649.

— — (1962), Lecture at Rooksdown House, Basingstoke.

DESTOMBES, P., and DROUHET, E. (1964), 'Mycoses d'importation', *Bull. Soc. Path. exot.*, **57**, 848.

EMMONS, C. W., and others (1964), *Sabouraudia*, **3**, 306.

GOLDIN, H. (1945), 'Case of Cervicofacial Actinomycosis following Fractured Mandible', *S. Afr. dent. J.*, **19**, 392.

HERTZ, J. (1960), 'Actinomycosis Borderline Cases', *J. int. Coll. Surg.*, **34**, 148.

HOLM, P. (1948), 'Some Investigations into Penicillin Sensitivity of Human Pathogenic Actinomycetes and some Comments on Penicillin Treatment of Actinomycosis', *Acta path. microbiol. scand.*, **25**, 376.

LEHNER, T. (1964), 'Oral Candidiasis', *Dent. Abstr.*, Chicago, **9**, 104.

NEW, G. E., and FIGI, F. A. (1923), 'Actinomycosis of the Head and Neck: A Report of 107 Cases ', *Surgery Gynec. Obstet.*, **37**, 617.

ROWE, N. L., and KILLEY, H. C. (1970), *Fractures of the Facial Skeleton*. Edinburgh: Livingstone.

THOMA, K. H. (1969), *Oral Surgery*, 5th ed. St. Louis: Mosby.

WINNER, H. L., and HURLEY, R. (1964), *Candida albicans*. London: Churchill.

WOLFF, M., and ISRAEL, J. (1891), 'Ueber reinkultur des actinomyces und seine ueber-tragbarkeit auf tiere', *Virchows Arch. Path. Anat. Physiol.*, **126**, 11.

WRIGHT, P., and SYMMERS, W. (1966), *Systemic Pathology*, p. 828. London: Longmans.

ZEGARELLI, E. V., and KUTSCHNER, A. H., (1964), 'Oral Moniliasis following Intra-oral Topical Corticosteroid Therapy', *J. oral. Ther.*, **1**, 304.

ZITKA, E. (1952), 'Toplich verlaufene falle von cervicofacialer aktinomykose', *Wien. med. Wschr.*, **102**, 939.

CHAPTER XXIII

THE MANAGEMENT OF SOME OF THE FOREIGN BODIES SEEN IN AND AROUND THE JAWS

SOME of the more common foreign bodies which may be lodged in the soft tissues, the paranasal sinuses, or the bony structure of the upper or lower jaw can be considered under the following headings:—

1. BROKEN HYPODERMIC NEEDLES

The main causes of hypodermic needles being broken during an injection in the mouth are a violent movement on the part of the patient, a structural fault in the needle, or faulty technique on the part of the operator. The breaking of a hypodermic needle in the tissues, is, fortunately, an uncommon accident, but the injections most likely to result in an accident of this nature are the inferior dental nerve block and the posterior superior dental nerve block. (*Fig.* 47.) Infiltration injections round the

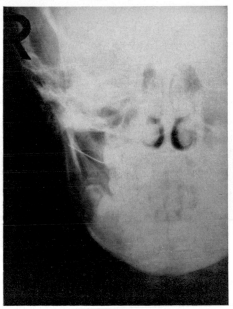

Fig. 47.—Postero-anterior radiograph showing a broken hypodermic needle lying in the soft tissue on the lingual aspect of the ramus.

teeth are so superficial that if the needle breaks the fragment can usually be recovered with little difficulty. In the case of the mandibular and posterior superior dental injections, it is easy to retrieve the broken fragment of needle if it is projecting from the tissues, and whenever an injection is being carried out an instrument such as an artery forceps should be at hand in order to grasp the needle fragment should this accident occur.

Removal of a Fragment of Needle.—The decision to remove a fragment of needle must depend upon the size of the fragment and its situation in the tissues, for there is little point in operating to remove a minute portion of needle buried under the periosteum and. therefore, unlikely to move in the tissues. Hypodermic needles broken elsewhere in the body in muscle, or even worse in veins, are liable to travel considerable distances and may come to rest in vital organs such as the heart, but most hypodermic needles broken in the mouth are firmly sited under the periosteum. Occasionally a needle broken in the oral cavity may be in thick muscle such as the medial pterygoid and the fragment may be propelled deep into the tissues by muscular action. Therefore, if a needle is considered to be lying free in the tissues, there is some urgency in arranging for its removal.

Small portions of needle in the tissues which show no tendency to move do not give rise to symptoms but, unfortunately, once a patient knows there is a needle broken in the tissues he tends to become extremely anxious about its presence. For this reason, it may be advisable to remove fractured portions of hypodermic needle provided that the operation is considered feasible.

The Surgical Removal of a Needle Medial to the Ramus.—Many techniques have been described for localizing a needle lying medial to the ramus. Most of them depend on the insertion of one or more additional needles and then taking radiographs in order to localize the broken fragment in relation to the needles inserted. Ingenious methods have also been devised to enable the guide marker needles to be held in place during radiography. A simple device can be constructed by jamming a sterile cork between the teeth and passing the guide needles through the cork and into the tissues. However, personal experience has shown that such marker needles are of little practical help in searching for a needle, and not only interfere with the operator's access but cause additional oedema in the tissues. A true lateral and a postero-anterior radiograph taken with the mouth open, since this is how the patient will be during the operation, are quite adequate to establish the presence of the needle and its approximate location.

Provided that the operator is familiar with the anatomy of the region, it is a simple matter to search the area systematically to locate the fragment. The mouth is gagged open wide and an incision is made down the anterior aspect of the ramus from almost the tip of the coronoid process to the retromolar fossa and then down into the buccal sulcus. The soft tissue is raised from the bone, exposing the subperiosteal area. Often the needle is seen sticking through the periosteum and can be grasped with mosquito forceps. If there is no sign of the needle, the medial tail of the temporalis tendon and the inferior dental neurovascular bundle should be separated so that the pterygomandibular space can be searched. If the needle is neither beneath the periosteum nor in the pterygomandibular space, it must be within the medial pterygoid muscle. In the line of the muscle-fibres a Howarth's periosteal elevator can be used to separate the fibres so as to systematically search the muscle.

As soon as the needle is seen, a pair of mosquito forceps is clamped on it and then the needle is worked anteriorly in its direction of insertion. As soon as the needle end is visible, it is grasped with another pair of mosquito forceps and withdrawn. No attempt should be made to pull the needle laterally through the tissues with the first mosquito forceps or the needle will bend, so making it more difficult to remove, or it may even break and it is then necessary to remove two broken fragments. The search for a needle should be carried out largely by blunt dissection in a good light, and the operative field should be as avascular as possible to facilitate the search.

Ingenious electrical devices have been advocated whereby one electrode of an electrical circuit is made with the patient and the other is connected to a probe which is passed through the tissues. When the probe touches the broken portion of needle a bell or buzzer sounds. The use of such devices poses further problems. For example, plastic retractors must be used, as metal ones are bound to be touched by the probe in such confined quarters. Also, some locators are so sensitive that they buzz when 0·5 cm. from the needle. This is a help in a limb, but in this particular instance it can be easy to predict where the needle will be within 0·5 cm., but still difficult to find it.

The only postoperative complication is limitation of opening, but if the operation is carried out carefully and the medial pterygoid muscle is not damaged, this symptom is trivial and temporary.

Needles broken during the Posterior Superior Dental Injection.—Needles broken during a posterior superior dental injection usually penetrate the periosteum and their broken end projects downwards towards the mouth in the line of the injection. To obtain adequate access an incision is made anterior to the upper 2nd molar and a soft tissue flap is raised superficial to the periosteum. The flap is retracted and the area overlying the tuberosity is inspected. If the needle is not seen, the tip of a finger is gently inserted into the wound and the fragment, which feels like a stiff bristle, is usually palpated quite easily. It is useful to remember that a needle in the tissues feels less stiff than one would expect. Care must be taken not to dislodge the needle further up into the soft tissues by milking movements with the finger, but usually the tip of the needle has penetrated the periosteum and jammed into the bone and so this is unlikely. However, every care must be taken to avoid dislodging the needle with the finger tip. Once the needle is palpated a pair of curved mosquito forceps is guided into the area with the other hand and the needle is grasped and withdrawn along its line of insertion.

2. TOOTH OR ROOT IN THE SOFT TISSUES

Teeth or roots can be inadvertently displaced into the soft tissues during exodontia or as a result of trauma such as road traffic accidents and fights. Common situations from which teeth or roots have to be extricated are as follows.

The Lingual Space.—Lower 3rd molars or their roots can be inadvertently displaced into the so-called 'lingual space' or 'pouch' during lower 3rd molar surgery. This potential space is bounded by the periosteum and the lingual aspect of the mandible, and it extends vertically down the neck.

An entire tooth may be dislodged into this area and the usual reason for the accident is that force is applied to an impacted lower 3rd molar when a gingival flap is still covering the posterior part of its crown. During delivery the crown of the tooth is impeded by the resistant gum flap and is levered over the upper border of the lingual plate and slips down the lingual side of the mandible. The apices of many lower 3rd molars actually penetrate the lingual plate of the mandible and attempts to elevate out such roots may result in their deflexion through the lingual plate into the lingual space.

When this accident occurs the operator should place a finger on the lingual side of the mandible beneath the tooth or root which can be easily palpated beneath the mucosa. The tooth is then gently pressed upwards towards the operation site. Sometimes the incision must be lengthened to enable the dislodged tooth or root to be properly visualized. When the fragment can be seen, it is grasped with a small pair of Allis forceps and lifted out of the wound. A finger must be positioned on the lingual mucosa beneath the tooth or root until the fragment is retrieved, for attempts to grasp the tooth or root without taking this precaution will only result in further displacement of the object. The passage of a conically rooted tooth through the tissues is facilitated by rotating the tooth with the fingers over the mucosa covering the lingual plate so that the conical apex is directed towards the original socket.

Tooth or Root in the Lateral Pharyngeal Space.—Occasionally during surgery in the area a lower 3rd molar or its root is inadvertently displaced backwards into the lateral pharyngeal space. This unfortunate accident causes the patient considerable pain especially on deglutition and the tooth should be removed as soon as possible, for infection in this region could have serious consequences. Following such an accident the patient has marked limitation of opening and the tooth can travel backwards and become positioned beneath the mucosa on the posterior pharyngeal wall. Usually, however, the displaced tooth can be palpated beneath the overlying mucosa reasonably near to the operation site and can then be gently pushed towards the original incision by pressure with the operator's finger through the mucosa behind the tooth or root. As soon as the fragment can be seen through the original operation incision, it should be grasped with Allis forceps. Again, no attempt should be made to grasp the tooth or root with an instrument without anchoring the fragment by finger pressure behind it or the foreign body will be pushed backwards. If the original operation wound is small, it should be enlarged by extending the incision up the ramus. Suitable antibiotic therapy should be maintained until there is no risk of a residual infection in the lateral pharyngeal space.

Tooth or Root in the Pterygoid Plexus Region.—Occasionally an upper 3rd molar or its root is displaced into the soft tissues between the coronoid process and the maxillary tuberosity. It can then pass upwards towards the pterygoid plexus. This is not only a surgically inaccessible region, but it is a very haemorrhagic area and due to the vascular anastomosis with the cavernous sinus any infection in the area must be regarded as extremely serious. The incision in the area should be widened by bringing it forwards from the tuberosity to the upper 1st molar area. The incision should be on the crest of the ridge in the edentulous case and round the gingival margins when teeth are standing. It should be deepened down to, but not through, the periosteum. Careful retraction usually allows the tooth or root to be visualized deep in the wound. Occasionally a Howarth's periosteal elevator can be inserted on either side of the tooth or root and the fragment can be gently levered down into the wound. On other occasions it can be grasped with a narrow-bladed pair of Allis forceps. Blind manipulation within the wound using a finger or an instrument usually results in the tooth or root being displaced further into the soft tissues.

Tooth Fragments in the Soft Tissues following Facial Trauma.—Teeth or tooth fragments can be displaced into any of the facial soft tissues as a result of trauma. Retrieval is usually a simple matter of palpating the object beneath the tissues and then immobilizing it by finger pressure beneath and to one side before approaching it surgically by a direct incision. The cut is made over the fragment from either an extra-oral or intra-oral approach depending whether it is nearer the outer or inner surface of the face. As soon as the tooth or tooth fragment is exposed it can be carefully dissected out of the wound. The most common area for such displaced teeth or fragments is the upper or lower lip. As a result of an accident either the maxillary or mandibular teeth may be driven into the inside of the lip and broken off. Such fragments are readily palpated and radiographs held behind the lip confirm the diagnosis. They are most easily removed before the original wound has been sutured. Mosquito artery forceps are inserted closed into the wound until the fragment is touched. When they are opened the piece will enter the gap between the blades. Once the wound has healed no attempt should be made until the scar has softened. Infected fragments can be reached by inserting a probe along the resulting sinus. Small, uninfected, impalpable fragments are best left alone.

Tooth or Root in the Maxillary Sinus.—The problem of the tooth or root in the maxillary sinus has already been discussed. (*See* AN OUTLINE OF ORAL SURGERY, PART I, revised reprint, p. 157).

Other Foreign Bodies in the Maxillary Sinus.—If a patient has a patent oro-antral fistula almost any foreign body can enter the sinus from the mouth. When these objects have been in the maxillary sinus for any considerable time they tend to become encrusted with calcific concretions. The authors have removed mummified peas, nuts, cotton-wool, and other articles from the maxillary sinus including from one patient sufficient chewing gum to fill the entire cavity. The broken blade of an upper extraction forceps has also been reported in the maxillary sinus. Probably the most common foreign body in the maxillary sinus is impression material such as an alginate impression compound or plaster-of-Paris, and these substances should not be used in the presence of an oro-antral fistula. Root canal instruments and filling materials are also easily introduced through the apices of the molar and premolar teeth.

Tooth or Root in the Floor of the Nose.—Occasionally a tooth or root is displaced either into the floor of the nose or between the undersurface of the palatal shelf and the overlying soft tissue of the floor of the nose. The deflected tooth is usually the maxillary canine, but supernumeraries and incisors can also be involved. The tooth may have developed in this position or been displaced there as a result of attempted exodontia. Most teeth which have grown in such a situation can be approached and removed through the routine intra-oral surgical approach, but as an additional precaution, to prevent the entire tooth being inadvertently displaced into the nasal passage during operation, it is helpful to have the anaesthetist position the endotracheal tube in the nostril overlying the operation site. If a tooth or root is displaced into the nasal cavity during an operation under general anaesthesia, the patient's head should be extended so that it will pass into the nasopharynx and fall on to the throat pack where it can be retrieved. If it remains stuck in the nose, it can be gently pushed back with a nasopharyngeal airway, unless it can be seen and grasped with Allis forceps pushed up the nostril.

The more usual problem is a tooth or root displaced beneath the nasal mucosa and against the upper surface of the palatal shelf. A horizontal incision is made in the upper buccal sulcus and deepened to bone. It should be of sufficient length to expose the anterior bony aperture of the nose. The nasal mucosa forming the floor of the nose is then gently retracted from the bone and the tooth or root is pulled forwards on the tip of the sucker. If the fragment is stuck and cannot be removed in this fashion, the end of a silver probe is bent to form a large hook which is gently passed round the tooth or root after which it can be pulled forwards towards the incision.

3. RHINOLITHS

Rhinoliths are calcareous bodies which are occasionally found in the nose and very rarely in the maxillary sinus. Polson (1943), in a review of the literature, found 384 cases and he reported 6 personal cases. These objects are usually single and unilateral and consist chiefly of calcium carbonate and phosphate which originate mainly from inflammatory exudates. If sectioned, it is seen that they have been deposited round a nucleus which may be endogenous or exogenous in origin. The exogenous nucleus can be any small foreign body such as a fruit stone, bead, etc., while the endogenous nucleus can be nasal crusts, mucus, sequestra, etc. They are often spherical and their surface is a rough greyish-white, grey, or dark brown in colour. Symptoms of a nasal rhinolith are usually a unilateral purulent nasal discharge and/or obstruction. Cases have been reported of nasal rhinoliths which have ulcerated through the palate and presented in the mouth (Gilbert, 1952; Allen, 1967).

Treatment.—Rhinoliths are removed through either the anterior or posterior nasal aperture. Large ones are fragmented and removed in pieces.

Antroliths.—Those rhinoliths which occur in the maxillary sinus are also known as 'antral stones', 'antral calculi', 'antroliths', 'antral rhinoliths', and 'maxillary rhinoliths'. Bowerman (1969) defined them as a complete or partial encrustation of an antral foreign body usually of endogenous or occasionally of exogenous origin. They are hard calcareous bodies found within the maxillary sinus consisting of a central nucleus upon which are deposited mineral salts, especially calcium phosphate and carbonate, forming a rough surface, blackish-grey in colour. The salts are probably derived from antral secretions or inflammatory exudates and the foreign body with complete or partial encrustation may have been in situ for several years and associated with long-term chronic infection.

Clinical Features.—Usually the lesion is asymptomatic and is discovered on routine radiography as a radio-opaque mass, but it may give rise to a maxillary sinusitis, produce a foul smell, nasal discharge, an oro-antral fistula, and destroy alveolar or palatal bone.

Treatment.—Treatment is removal through a routine Caldwell-Luc incision.

4. FOREIGN BODIES IN THE TISSUES AS A RESULT OF GUNSHOT WOUNDS

Shell fragments and bullets may be lodged in the hard or soft tissues for many years without causing symptoms. Much depends on the size and the site of the fragment. The presence of a small metallic foreign body in the lip, for example, can be felt by the patient and should be removed, but a larger fragment can be deeply buried in the tissues and remain asymptomatic. Fragments of metal which project into the maxillary sinus or nose may become infected and should be removed, though this may in some instances be technically difficult. It is important to remember when searching for such foreign bodies that those which are palpable through the intact skin are *less* easily rather than more easily felt through the open wound at operation. Further, a readily palpable object can be quite impalpable once a solution of local anaesthetic or vasoconstrictor has been injected. Multiple lead shots from a shot gun injury are extremely hard to find at operation and as they are usually asymptomatic they should be left in situ.

OTHER FOREIGN BODIES IN THE TISSUES

Following severe trauma such as a road traffic accident, almost any type of object can be implanted into the tissues. Some of the more common foreign bodies of interest to the oral surgeon are:

Tar and Road Dirt.—If a patient's face has been scraped along the road the soft tissue lacerations may be ingrained with road dirt, including tar. If this is not cleaned away before the wound is sutured, it produces an ugly tattoo when it heals which is difficult to eradicate surgically even by excising all the scars. This road dirt must be cleaned out before suturing and a satisfactory method of cleaning such wounds is to use a toothbrush with 1 per cent cetrimide. Only when all tar and other road debris has been removed should the wound be closed.

Pieces of Glass.—Glass fragments may enter the soft tissues at the time of an accident. Sometimes the patient or operator can feel these fragments in the soft tissues and they should then be removed. Almost all glass in common use is sufficiently radio-opaque to produce a shadow when displaced into the soft tissues. The degree of opacity varies, of course, with the composition. The few which may not produce a shadow on radiological examination include some of the high soda translucent tubular lights of American pattern, some of the textile glass fibres (borates) and a few special glasses not likely to be met in everyday life (Cameron, 1970).

Wood.—Wood is radiolucent and if splinters enter the tissues it may be difficult to locate them on the radiographs. However, if the wood is painted, the paint usually shows up quite well (Gerry and Kopp, 1966).

Dentures.—The patient's dentures may be shattered as a result of an accident and portions of the dentures may enter the soft tissues or be impacted into the maxillary sinus or throat. Unfortunately, acrylic denture material is radiolucent and if the objects are not palpable it may be difficult to demonstrate their presence and locate them surgically. The older denture materials such as vulcanite are, however, radio-opaque. A radiolucent denture impacted in the throat can be demonstrated as a space-occupying lesion following a barium swallow. Patients engaged in bad risk occupations or sports should be fitted with special dentures made of a radio-opaque acrylic.

Rubber Base Impression Material.—This substance may be closely confined in a special impression tray in order to obtain a detailed and defect-free impression of inlay crown or bridge preparations.

Where one of the preparations includes the canal of a root-filled tooth, the situation can be hazardous because there may be an unsuspected lateral canal or other perforation in the wall of the root canal. Unrecognized, localized, deep, periodontal pockets present a similar hazard. One of us has seen a case in which rubber base material gained access to the medullary cavity of the jaw during the taking of an impression of mandibular teeth. The material infiltrated the bone from 1st premolar to 2nd molar region and provoked a severe inflammatory reaction with much oedema of the face. Fortunately, removal was easy once the mandible had been decorticated on that side as the impression material pulled out in long irregular strands.

Other Plastic Objects.—Many items such as internal trim in cars and instrument knobs are made of plastic. These again are often radiolucent or only slightly radio-opaque. Surprisingly large objects can be accommodated in the swollen tissues, in the paranasal sinuses, and in regions of thick muscle.

Grease-gun Grease.—An injury from a grease gun is similar to the wound produced by a jet injection device. Hence, if the nozzle is at right angles to the skin surface a puncture wound is formed, or if it is at an angle a cut results. The grease is forced widely into the tissue planes and is highly irritant. Enormous oedema results, and when the injury is to the face or neck a tracheostomy may be required. Vascular impairment in the part due to the pressure produced by the swelling and gross infection are other hazards. Early and thorough wound débridement and drainage are essential in treatment.

Indelible Pencil.—Laceration of the palate occurs when a child falls with a toy, stick, or pencil in the mouth. Usually such injuries are easily dealt with. However, if fragments of lead from an indelible pencil remain in the wound, a troublesome and persistent granulomatous reaction results.

REFERENCES

ALLEN, S. G. (1967), 'A Rhinolith presenting in the Palate', *Br. J. oral Surg.*, **4**, 240.
BOWERMAN, J. E. (1969), 'The Maxillary Antrolith', *J. Lar. Otol.*, **83**, 873.
CAMERON, J. D. (1970), 'The Treatment of Glass Injuries to the Hand at Work', *Hand*, **2**, 52.
GERRY, R. G., and KOPP, W. K. (1966), 'Wooden Foreign Body in the Parapharyngeal Space', *J. oral Surg.*, **24**, 545.
GILBERT, R. K. (1952), 'Case of a Rhinolith', *Br. dent. J.*, **93**, 75.
POLSON, C. J. (1943), 'Rhinolith in Palate', *J. Lar. Otol.*, **58**, 79.

INDEX